KUMAR & CLARK'S

Cases
in **Clinical**
Medicine

T0200385

KUMAR & CLARK'S

Cases
in Clinical
Medicine

4th edition

PROFESSOR DAME PARVEEN J KUMAR
DBE, MD, FRCP

Professor of Medicine and Education
Barts and The London School of Medicine and Dentistry, QMUL,
and Honorary Consultant Physician and Gastroenterologist
Barts Health NHS Trust and Princess Grace Hospital
London, UK

MICHAEL L CLARK
MD, FRCP

Honorary Senior Lecturer
Barts and The London School of Medicine and Dentistry, QMUL,
and Princess Grace Hospital
London, UK

For additional online content visit StudentConsult.com

ELSEVIER

London   New York   Oxford
Philadelphia   St Louis   Sydney   2021

First edition 2000
Second edition 2006
Third edition 2013
Fourth edition 2021

Notices

Practitioners and researchers must always rely on their own experience and knowledge in evaluating and using any information, methods, compounds or experiments described herein. Because of rapid advances in the medical sciences, in particular, independent verification of diagnoses and drug dosages should be made. To the fullest extent of the law, no responsibility is assumed by Elsevier, authors, editors or contributors for any injury and/or damage to persons or property as a matter of products liability, negligence or otherwise, or from any use or operation of any methods, products, instructions, or ideas contained in the material herein.

ISBN: 978-0-7020-7732-6

Printed in Poland
Last digit is the print number: 9 8 7 6 5 4 3

Content Strategist: Alexandra Mortimer
Senior Content Development Specialist: Helen Leng/Louise Cook
Project Manager: Anne Collett
Design: Amy Buxton
Illustration Manager: Paula Catalano
Marketing Manager: Deborah Watkins

Working together
to grow libraries in
developing countries

www.elsevier.com • www.bookaid.org

Contents

Contents

Preface

There are many ways of teaching and learning medicine, and education is forever evolving. This is shown by the fact that medical curricula change with great frequency, as each generation of teachers finds a better way to transmit the complex medical facts. Over the years the curriculum has altered from one that consisted of didactic lectures and learned facts, to one where the student takes the initiative in the learning process. Problem- and case-based learning, along with self-directed learning, has taken over. Nevertheless, the main factor in learning must be the individual enthusiasm of the student to study medicine.

When we started designing *Kumar and Clark's Clinical Medicine* many years ago, we wanted to make it fun to read and easy to understand. We added colour, algorithms and bulleted facts that were clearly displayed for easy learning: a design that has now been followed by many other textbooks. This smaller book of case reports is also designed in an easy-to-read format. We have extracted various clinical scenarios to follow the journey of a patient with symptoms in a logical manner. These cases have been written to reflect the way that real patients present to their local doctors or to the emergency and outpatient departments in hospitals. We have provided the questions and given you the answers stage by stage, so that a large differential diagnosis is gradually whittled down to one or two of the most likely diagnoses. We take you through the process of logical thought using the medical knowledge you have already acquired.

Cases in Clinical Medicine has been read by many students around the world, who have been kind enough to say that they have found the book and its approach most useful. We hope you enjoy it as much as they did!

Despite the hard work, medicine is always enjoyable. It is a privilege to care for our patients and to see them return to good health and happiness.

We both wish you the very best in your careers.

Good luck!

Parveen Kumar and Michael Clark
2020

Acknowledgements

This edition is based on the original contributions of skilled clinicians who were regularly on take for acute general medicine: their expertise is warmly acknowledged.

We would like to thank the original contributors:

Jane Anderson PhD FRCP
Simon Aylwin MA MB BChir PhD MRCP
Mark Caulfield MB MD FRCP FAHA
Charles R A Clarke MA FRCP MB BCh
David P D'Cruz MD FRCP
Ramesh C Joshi MD FRCP
Karim Meeran MD FRCP
David G Paige MA MB BS FRCP
Drew Provan MD FRCP FRCPath
M J Raftery MD FRCP
G S Rai MD MSc FRCP
A Sefton MB BS MSc MD FRCP(Edin) FRCPath
David Watson BSc (Hons) MB BS FRCA
Mark Weaver MBBS MRCPsych
James R Wilkinson MRCP(UK) MB BS BSc (Hons)
Mahummad M Yaqoob MD FRCP

PYREXIA OF UNKNOWN ORIGIN (PUO)

Pyrexia of unknown origin (sometimes called fever of unknown origin, FUO) is best defined as a fever persisting for more than 2 weeks with no clear diagnosis despite intelligent and intensive investigation.

Not all cases of PUO are due to infection. Approximately two-thirds of cases with recent-onset PUO are due to infection, compared with only about one-third of cases with long-standing PUO. Other causes include malignancy and autoimmune rheumatic disorders (Box 1.1).

Case history

A 25-year-old male is seen in the A&E department, at the request of his doctor, with a history of fever, anorexia and malaise. He had returned the previous week from a month's backpacking trip around India, where he had lost 5 kg in weight. The A&E doctor asks you to see this patient with PUO. The preliminary blood investigations by the GP were normal.

On examination, the patient was found to be febrile with a temperature of 39.5°C. He had no lymphadenopathy or pallor of mucous membranes.

BP 110/70; pulse 90; heart sounds normal.

Chest: clinically clear.

Examination of abdomen: slight generalised tenderness. Liver, kidneys and spleen not palpable. Examination of CNS unremarkable.

Where would you manage this patient?

Admit to a MAU side room until an infectious aetiology has been ruled out.

What questions should you specifically ask when you see a patient with PUO (in addition to routine questions)?

- Full travel history, including exactly where the patient has been and the type of accommodation stayed in.
- Vaccination/prophylaxis history.
- Contact with animals/sick people.
- Occupation: exactly what does the patient do?
- Water exposure: occupational/recreational.
- Food history: eating shellfish or reheated/raw foods, drinking dirty water.
- Risk behaviour: IV drug usage, unprotected sexual contact.
- Factors that might predispose to infection.

What initial investigations should you perform in a patient presenting with PUO?

Perform minimally invasive tests before highly invasive and expensive ones. It is always worth repeating previously performed tests (see Investigations box).

Box 1.1 Causes of PUO

- Infections (see later)
- Neoplasms, especially lymphomas, renal cell carcinoma
- Autoimmune rheumatic disease
- Vasculitides, e.g. giant cell arteritis
- Others, e.g. granulomatous disease, drug reactions, factitious

Infective causes

General

- Abscesses, e.g. liver, abdomen, pelvis, ear, sinus or dental infection
- Infective endocarditis
- Urinary tract infection

Specific

- Bacterial:
  - *Mycobacterium tuberculosis*
  - *Salmonella typhi* or *S. paratyphi*
  - *Brucella* spp.
  - Leptospirosis
  - Lyme disease
- Viral:
  - Epstein−Barr
  - Hepatitis
  - Cytomegalovirus
  - HIV
  - Dengue fever
- Protozoal:
  - Malaria
  - Amoebiasis
  - Leishmaniasis
  - Toxoplasmosis
  - Trypanosomiasis
- Rickettsial:
  - Typhus
  - Q fever
- Chlamydophila:
  - Psittacosis

Investigations

PUO

- FBC
- CRP/ESR
- U&Es
- Liver biochemistry
- Blood cultures — repeated
- Urine analysis and microscopy, culture and sensitivity
- CXR
- Sputum (if producing any) for microscopy, culture and sensitivity, and for acid-fast bacilli

- Stools for ova, cysts and parasites, and culture and sensitivity
- Store serum for future serological tests if required
- Wounds: take swabs for culture
- Screen for autoimmune rheumatic disorders
- Additional investigations in this man because of travel abroad: thick and thin blood films for malaria

Results in this patient

- WCC: slightly raised at $12\,000 \times 10^9/L$.
- ALT: 92 IU/L (normal range 5–40 IU/L).
- Alkaline phosphatase: 190 IU/L (normal range 25–115 IU/L).
- All other initial investigations normal.

What should you do now?

- Recheck his travel history.
- Recheck his risk factors for hepatitis and HIV.
- Send blood for viral markers for hepatitis.
- Arrange a liver ultrasound.

  The ultrasound shows a **liver abscess** in the right lobe and, in view of his travel history, an amoebic abscess is a strong possibility. Fortunately, you had sent off an amoebic complement fixation text (CFT) sample and you ring the reference laboratory urgently. The test is positive (usually positive with an amoebic liver abscess).

Treatment

Treat with metronidazole 800 mg × 3 daily for 10 days followed by diloxanide furoate 500 mg × 3 daily for 10 days to clear the luminal infection, even if a stool microscopy is negative. Aspiration of the abscess under ultrasound or CT guidance is required only if the cyst is at risk of rupture or medical therapy fails.

Remember

- Take a careful history: *always repeat*.
- Examine the patient thoroughly: *always repeat*.
- Initial investigations often give a clue to the diagnosis: often need repeating.
- Be patient and don't give antibiotics until diagnosis is made, unless the patient is very sick.
- Perform invasive and/or expensive investigations only when appropriate, e.g. echo, CT scan/MRI, bone marrow and culture, lymph node/liver biopsy.

Progress. This man responded quickly to therapy, with loss of pain and improvement in appetite, becoming apyrexial after 4 days. A repeat ultrasound 3 weeks later still showed a small residual cavity.

SEPSIS AND SEPTIC SHOCK

Sepsis is defined as life-threatening organ dysfunction caused by a dysregulated host response to infection.

  Septic shock is defined as sepsis that has circulatory, cellular and metabolic abnormalities profound enough to increase mortality substantially.

  Criteria for septic shock: see page 365.

Case history

A 70-year-old woman was admitted to hospital with fever, confusion and hypotension. She lived on her own and was unable to give a history.

On examination, she was clinically dehydrated and confused, and had cold, clammy peripheries. Pulse rate 108/min, respiratory rate 22/min.

She was also hypotensive with a BP 90/50 mmHg and had a temperature of 39°C.

Diagnosis: Sepsis.

What are the most common causes of sepsis in patients presenting from the community?

The most common organisms isolated are *Escherichia coli*, *Staphylococcus aureus*, *Streptococcus pneumoniae* and pyogenic streptococci — especially group A streptococci. *Neisseria meningitidis* should not be forgotten as a possible cause of community-acquired sepsis.

In hospital, coagulase-negative staphylococci can also cause sepsis in immunosuppressed patients with IV lines in situ. Wounds, the respiratory tract (especially in ventilated patients) and the urinary tract (in catheterised patients) are other sources of sepsis in hospitalised patients.

What factors predispose to sepsis?

In both Gram-positive and Gram-negative septicaemia, impaired host defences, surgery or instrumentation (including intravenous cannulae, urinary catheters and mechanical ventilation) predispose to septicaemia (Box 1.2).

What is the differential diagnosis of septic shock?

Non-infective disorders, such as acute myocardial infarction, pulmonary embolism or drug reactions, must be excluded. Toxic shock (e.g. toxic shock syndrome) can also present in a similar manner.

Box 1.2 Predisposing factors for sepsis

Gram-negative sepsis

- Urinary tract infections
- Hospital-acquired pneumonia, especially ventilator-associated
- Pre-existing abdominal sepsis, biliary tract infections
- Severe burns
- Obstetric or neonatal infections
- Meningococcal septicaemia

Gram-positive sepsis

- IV catheters
- Skin/wound infections
- Bone and joint infections
- IV drug usage
- Respiratory tract infections/pneumonia
- Obstetric or neonatal infections
- Meningitis, endocarditis

What would be your initial management of this woman and what investigations would you do?

Quick SOFA (qSOFA) (see p. 367)

- Respiratory rate ≥ 22/min.
- Altered mentation (GCS ↓).
- Systolic BP ≤ 100 mmHg.
  If >2, to outreach ICU and then transfer to HDU/ITU.

SOFA (Sequential Organ Failure Assessment Score)

This patient required supportive therapy (e.g. fluid replacement) because she was dehydrated; oxygen was given and inotropes. Broad-spectrum antibiotics were started after blood and urine cultures had been taken. The antibiotic therapy varies according to local hospital policy and the likely focus of infection.

The National Early Warning Score (NEWS) system and the NEWS thresholds and triggers are shown in Figs. 1.1 and 1.2.

Investigations

- FBC and differential
- U&Es, blood sugar, liver biochemistry, serum lactate
- ESR/CRP
- Blood cultures
- Blood gases
- Urine for microscopy, culture and sensitivity
- Sputum (if any produced) for microscopy, culture and sensitivity
- Swabs of any infected-looking lesions (including throat swab if throat appears inflamed)
- Pus (if present) for microscopy, culture and sensitivity
- High vaginal swab in women
- NAAT (nuclear acid amplification test)
- CXR
- ECG

  If a **urinary tract infection** is thought to be the likely source, a broad-spectrum cephalosporin is often appropriate (e.g. cefuroxime) or a quinolone (e.g. ciprofloxacin).

  If there is no obvious focus of infection, blind therapy must be broad-spectrum and cover streptococci, staphylococci and coliforms.

  Suitable choices are:

- A broad-spectrum cephalosporin, e.g. IV cefuroxime or IV cefotaxime or IV ceftriaxone
- Metronidazole in addition if an anaerobic infection is considered likely
- A broad-spectrum penicillin with β-lactamase inhibitor (e.g. piperacillin/tazobactam); gentamicin in addition if the patient is very ill
- A carbapenem (e.g. imipenem, although this is a restricted antibiotic in many hospitals).

Antibiotic usage

'Start smart'

- Don't start antibiotics in absence of clinical evidence of bacterial infection.
- Take a thorough allergy history.
- Note local guidelines.

Kumar & Clark's Cases in Clinical Medicine

Physiological parameter	3	2	1	Score 0	1	2	3
Respiration rate (per minute)	≤8		9–11	12–20		21–24	≥25
SpO₂ Scale 1(%)	≤91	92–93	94–95	≥96			
SpO₂ Scale 2(%)	≤83	84–85	86–87	88–92 ≥93 on air	93–94 on oxygen	95–96 on oxygen	≥97 on oxygen
Air or oxygen?		Oxygen		Air			
Systolic blood pressure (mmHg)	≤90	91–100	101–110	111–219			≥220
Pulse (per minute)	≤40		41–50	51–90	91–110	111–130	≥131
Consciousness				Alert			CVPU
Temperature (°C)	≤35.0		35.1–36.0	36.1–38.0	38.1–39.0	≥39.1	

Figure 1.1 The National Early Warning Score (NEWS) system. CVPU: Confused, Responds to voice, Responds to pain, Unresponsive. (Reproduced from Royal College of Physicians. *National Early Warning Score (NEWS) 2: Standardising the Assessment of Acute-illness Severity in the NHS. Updated Report of a Working*

NEW score	Clinical risk	Response
Aggregate score 0–4	Low	Ward-based response
Red score Score of 3 in any individual parameter	Low–medium	Urgent ward-based response*
Aggregate score 5–6	Medium	Key threshold for urgent response*
Aggregate score 7 or more	High	Urgent or emergency response**

*Response by a clinician or team with competence in the assessment and treatment of acutely ill patients and in recognising when the escalation of care to a critical care team is appropriate.

**The response team must also include staff with critical care skills, including airway management.

Figure 1.2 NEWS thresholds and triggers. (Reproduced from Royal College of Physicians. *National Early Warning Score (NEWS) 2: Standardising the Assessment of Acute-illness Severity in the NHS. Updated Report of a Working Party.* London: RCP, 2017.)

- Take a blood culture before therapy.
- Document on drug chart and notes: clinical indication, duration or review/stop dates, route and dose.

'Focus'

Review clinical diagnosis and continuing need for antibiotics by 48 h.
   Options are:

- Stop
- Switch IV to oral antibiotics
- Change to more appropriate antibiotic
- Continue
- Change to outpatient antibiotic therapy.

Remember

- If you give gentamicin, you will need to monitor serum levels. Combining it with a cephalosporin can potentiate its nephrotoxicity.
- Cefuroxime, ceftriaxone and cefotaxime have fairly good activity against staphylococci and streptococci, as well as against many Gram-negative rods; they have poor activity against *Pseudomonas* spp. Ceftazidime has poor activity against streptococci and staphylococci but excellent activity against *Pseudomonas* spp. and other Gram-negative organisms. No cephalosporins are active against *Enterococcus* spp.
- Cephalosporins are associated with *Clostridium difficile* diarrhoea and should be avoided if possible.
- If a patient develops sepsis while in hospital, it is possibly due to resistant organisms, e.g. meticillin-resistant *S. aureus* (MRSA) or resistant Gram-negative rods.
- If MRSA infection is considered likely and the patient is very sick, add IV vancomycin 1 g × 2 daily (assuming normal renal function) given over at least 100 min while awaiting culture results.
   A urine sample was obtained from this patient. Microscopy found it to contain 1000 WCC/mm^3 and + + bacteria.

Management (Sepsis Six)

1. High-flow oxygen.
2. Blood cultures and consider source control.
3. Intravenous antibiotics.
4. Intravenous fluid resuscitation.
5. Check haemoglobin and serial lactates.
6. Hourly urine output measurement.
   Progress. This severely shocked patient with a clinical risk score of 5 was transferred to ITU. The patient had already been given IV cefuroxime and this was continued. On admission, she was also given a single dose of gentamicin. The following day, both her urine and blood cultures grew an *E. coli* that was susceptible to cefuroxime and gentamicin but resistant to amoxicillin. She made a good recovery.

Remember

Many hospitals have specific guidelines for antibiotic usage: *always check* or get microbiological advice.

In your hospital, do you know the approximate percentage of organisms causing urinary tract infections that are susceptible to commonly used antibiotics?

In many areas, approximately 50% of *E. coli* causing urinary tract infection are resistant to amoxicillin and 20−30% are resistant to trimethoprim. More than 90% are susceptible to cefuroxime, ciprofloxacin and gentamicin. You need to know local resistance patterns.

MENINGOCOCCAL MENINGITIS AND SEPSIS

Case history

An 18-year-old woman is brought into A&E in a 'collapsed' state. The previous day she had apparently been well, apart from symptoms of a minor upper respiratory tract infection. She woke up feeling very unwell and asked her flatmate to call the emergency doctor. The flatmate noted that her friend had a couple of spots on her chest but by the time the doctor arrived she was developing a more widespread petechial rash. The emergency doctor transferred her immediately to hospital after giving her a single dose of benzylpenicillin.

  The patient was febrile with a temperature of 38°C.
  A petechial rash was present (Fig. 1.3).
  The patient was hypotensive and shocked.
  There was minimal neck stiffness.

What do you think is the most likely diagnosis?

This young woman has **fulminant meningococcaemia**, which has a worse prognosis than meningococcal meningitis and usually follows an extremely rapid downhill course.

What should the immediate management be?

Take blood and throat cultures, and then start antibiotics immediately. Give IV benzylpenicillin, initially 2.4 g 4-hourly *or* IV cefotaxime 2 g × 6-hourly *or* IV ceftriaxone 2 g × 2 daily for presumed meningococcal meningitis/septicaemia.

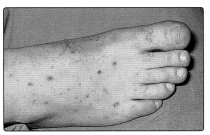

Figure 1.3 Meningococcal rash. (From Fuller, *Neurology Illustrated Colour Text*, with permission.)

Kumar & Clark's Cases in Clinical Medicine

> ### Remember
> The first doctor to see a patient suspected of having meningococcal sepsis or meningitis should immediately give benzylpenicillin IM injection before immediate transfer to hospital.

What investigations should be performed?

Relevant investigations are shown in the box. Other causes of meningitis/septicaemia should be excluded.

> ### Investigations
> - FBC and differential
> - U&Es
> - Liver biochemistry
> - ESR or CRP
> - Blood cultures: always before starting antibiotics
> - Throat swab to look for meningococcal carriage
> - Culture of petechial lesions is sometimes performed
> - Lumbar puncture is not indicated in meningococcal septicaemia

Who should be informed and what further action should be taken?

The consultant (or his/her deputy) in charge of communicable disease control (CCDC) should be informed immediately by telephone if a clinical diagnosis of meningococcal disease is made. Formal notification should then be given in writing. Notification books should be kept on all wards. Rifampicin prophylaxis can then be arranged for any close contacts.

Contacts who should receive prophylaxis

- People who live in the same household as the case or who have lived there in the previous week.
- Sexual partners.
- Work fellows sharing a small office, i.e. an office for two.
- Staff carrying out mouth-to-mouth resuscitation on the patient or 'specialling' the patient, especially in the first 24 h.
- The patient herself at the end of her parenteral therapy.
- School contacts if more than one case in a school.

Once the CCDC has been informed, he/she will usually arrange for chemoprophylaxis (Table 1.1), but might ask the hospital doctor to do this for the patient's relatives.

> ### Remember
> The patient should have rifampicin 600 mg × 2 daily for 2 days after she has finished her parenteral antibiotics to eradicate carriage of *N. meningitidis* from her nasopharynx.

What should you tell people who are taking rifampicin prophylaxis?

- It might interfere with the effectiveness of the oral contraceptive if they are taking this. Hence they should take additional contraceptive measures for the remainder of the cycle.
- Their secretions (e.g. tears) might turn orangey-pink and their soft contact lenses will also be permanently stained unless they remove them!

Table 1.1 Recommended chemoprophylaxis of meningococcal meningitis

Drug	Dosage
First choice	
Rifampicin	
Adults and children over 12 years	600 mg × 2 daily for 2 days
Children 1–12 years	10 mg/kg × 2 daily for 2 days (maximum dose 600 mg × 2 daily for 2 days)
Infants, 12 months	5 mg/kg × 2 daily for 2 days
Other options	
Ciprofloxacin	
Adults	500 mg single dose
Children	Not recommended
Pregnancy/breastfeeding mothers	Not recommended
Ceftriaxone	
Adults	250 mg IM as a single dose
Children, 12 years	125 mg IM as a single dose

Overall management

This patient was treated with intravenous ceftriaxone 2 g IV × 2 daily in the ICU. After a stormy course she made a full recovery. There were no secondary cases.

PSEUDOMEMBRANOUS COLITIS

This is the condition caused by *Clostridium difficile*; a pseudomembrane is seen on sigmoidoscopy.

Case history

A 40-year-old man, who had been on the intensive care unit for 3 weeks with a head injury following a road traffic accident, developed severe diarrhoea. He was on a ventilator and currently was finishing a course of a third-generation parenteral cephalosporin for hospital-acquired pneumonia. According to the nurses, one other patient on the ITU currently also has diarrhoea.

What other questions do you want to ask?

You would want to know:

- What is the diarrhoea like? Are the stools liquid or bloody?
- How long has the patient been on broad-spectrum antibiotics?
- Does any other patient/member of the staff have diarrhoea? (One of the ITU nurses informs you that another patient did have loose stools

and you need to ascertain if this is really the case and if there were any obvious reasons for this.)

What is your differential diagnosis?

This would include:
- Antibiotic-associated diarrhoea, particularly pseudomembranous colitis
- Diarrhoea due to enteral feeding
- Other bacterial causes, e.g. *Salmonella* spp., *Shigella* spp., *Campylobacter* spp., *E. coli* 0157; these are less likely because the patient has not been eating, but could occur as a result of cross-infection
- Viral gastroenteritis.

What investigations would you perform?

You would need to send a stool from the patient to the microbiology laboratory (and also from any other patient/staff member with diarrhoea) for microscopy, culture and sensitivity. If several patients/members of staff are affected, stools should also be sent to the virology department to look for a viral aetiology, e.g. small round viruses. In addition, you would specifically need to request an examination for *C. difficile* (toxin) − the organism responsible for the toxin of pseudomembranous colitis. Do a sigmoidoscopy to look for the typical pseudomembrane seen in pseudomembranous colitis and exclude inflammatory bowel disease by rectal biopsy.

The patient was thought, on clinical grounds, to have pseudomembranous colitis. This was later confirmed by the microbiology department, which found the stool to be positive for *C. difficile* toxin.

> **Remember**
>
> Culture of *C. difficile* itself in a stool is insufficient evidence that a patient has pseudomembranous colitis; only toxin-producing strains cause this.

How would you manage the patient?

The patient should be isolated in a side room, if possible, to prevent cross-infection. You need to ensure that the patient is adequately hydrated. In patients with antibiotic-associated diarrhoea, any broad-spectrum antibiotics that the patient is taking should be stopped if it is at all possible. If it is not feasible to do this, try to change to a narrow-spectrum agent (discuss with microbiology). Specific first-line therapy for pseudomembranous colitis is oral metronidazole 400 mg × 3 for 7−10 days. Oral vancomycin 125−250 mg × 4 for 7−10 days is used if there is no response to metronidazole. Fidaxomicin 200 mg is also effective.

Note: you don't need to check vancomycin levels in patients receiving oral vancomycin because it is not systemically absorbed.

Normally, metronidazole is tried first because there is a worry that use of oral vancomycin might predispose to the development of vancomycin-resistant enterococci in the gastrointestinal tract; in some parts of the world, enterococcal vancomycin resistance is becoming a major problem. Installing a faecal transplant from a healthy donor restores normal flora and eradicates *C. difficile* infections.

Progress. This patient initially responded to metronidazole but after 8 days his diarrhoea returned (up to 30% of cases relapse); he was switched to vancomycin, to which he responded.

He was eventually weaned from the ventilator and made a good physical recovery but with impaired cognitive function.

Remember

Prevention

Infection control relies on:

- Responsible use of antibiotics
- Hygiene, which should involve all health workers, as well as patients and relatives
- Washing hands thoroughly using soap and water, which is essential as alcohol disinfectants don't kill *C. difficile* spores
- Hospital cleaning of surfaces, which should be performed regularly to try to reduce transmission from fomites
- Isolation of patients with *C. difficile*.

FOOD POISONING: *E. COLI* O157

Enterohaemorrhagic *Escherichia coli* (EHEC)

EHEC (usually serotype O157:H7, and also known as verotoxin-producing *E. coli*, or VTEC) is a well-recognised cause of gastroenteritis in humans. It is a zoonosis usually associated with cattle, the organism being found in the intestines of herbivores. There have been a number of major outbreaks (notably in Scotland and Japan) associated with contaminated food. Run-off water from where cattle have been grazing is used in irrigation and therefore salads and vegetables are a source of infection, as well as milk and underdone beef, e.g. hamburgers.

EHEC secretes a toxin (Shiga-like toxin 1), which affects vascular endothelial cells in the gut and in the kidney. After an incubation period of 12–48 h it causes diarrhoea (frequently bloody), associated with abdominal pain and nausea. Some days after the onset of symptoms the patient may develop thrombotic thrombocytopenic purpura or haemolytic uraemic syndrome (HUS). This is more common in children, and may lead to permanent renal damage or death. Treatment is mainly supportive: there is evidence that antibiotic therapy for gastroenteritis might precipitate HUS by causing increased toxin release.

Case history

A 15-year-old girl is admitted to hospital with bloody diarrhoea; her parents and her three siblings are well. They have apparently all eaten the same food during the last week, except on a single occasion when the patient ate a beefburger cooked at a local party. The mother remembers that it looked rather raw inside. The girl had eaten chicken at least three times during the previous week. She looked slightly dehydrated and had a temperature of 37.8°C. Her abdomen was soft but generally tender, and bowel sounds were increased.

What is the differential diagnosis in this patient?

Infectious gastroenteritis with bloody diarrhoea due to:

- *Campylobacter* spp. (chicken the likely source)
- *E. coli* O157 (beef the likely source)
- *Shigella* spp.
- *Salmonella* spp.
- Onset of inflammatory bowel disease.

Investigations

Should include:
- FBC, including platelets
- U&Es (*E. coli* O157 can cause HUS)
- Blood culture
- Stools for microscopy, culture and sensitivity
  Full clinical details should be put on the form accompanying the stool

Remember

- Most laboratories routinely look for *E. coli* O157 in people with bloody diarrhoea.
- Abdominal X-rays and sigmoidoscopy might also be required if inflammatory bowel disease is considered a likely diagnosis.

What would your initial management be?

The patient should be admitted to the MAU and put into excretion–secretion isolation (assuming a probable infective aetiology). Ensure adequate hydration. Oral/IV antibiotics can have a place in treating severe infections due to *Salmonella* spp., *Campylobacter* spp. and *Shigella* spp.; they should not be used in infections caused by *E. coli* O157. The disease should be notified to the CCDC both by telephone immediately and in writing when the diagnosis has been made. Rapid notification is required if the patient works in the food industry or with the very young, the elderly or the immunosuppressed.

Progress. This patient had E. coli O157 and didn't develop HUS. She made an uneventful recovery.

Information

FEATURES OF HAEMOLYTIC URAEMIC SYNDROME (HUS)
- Intravascular haemolysis with red cell fragmentation (microangiopathic haemolysis)
- Thrombocytopenia
- Acute kidney injury
  Mortality is high in the elderly; treatment is by plasma exchange, with some patients requiring haemofiltration dialysis.

TYPHOID

This is the typical form of enteric fever and is caused by *Salmonella typhi*. Enteric fever is an acute systemic illness with fever, headache and abdominal discomfort.

Case history

A 35-year-old Asian male presents with a 1-week history of fever, headache, a dry cough and constipation. He is resident in the UK and has just returned from a 6-week holiday in Bangladesh, where he was visiting relatives. He works as a chef in a local restaurant. While he was away, one of the relatives he was staying with had a high fever and severe diarrhoea.

On examination, the patient had a fever of 39.5°C with a pulse rate of only 85/min. Examination of the cardiovascular, respiratory and central nervous systems was unremarkable.

The abdomen was slightly tender.

- FBC, routine chemistry, CXR and blood cultures taken
- FBC shows a slight leucopenia
- Gram-negative rods are seen in a film of the blood cultures taken after 24-h incubation

What is the most likely diagnosis?

S. typhi (this was later confirmed as being the definitive diagnosis).

How would you manage this patient?

The patient should be nursed in a side room with excretion–secretion precautions used (consult your local infection control manual). The control of infection officer should be alerted, as should your local CCDC, as soon as a definite diagnosis is made. Your CCDC should be alerted immediately by telephone and also via the formal notification book, which should be available on every ward. This is particularly important because this patient is a food handler. If the patient subsequently develops diarrhoea, adequate fluids are required to avoid dehydration. Pending antibiotic sensitivity testing, the patient should be commenced on ciprofloxacin 500–750 mg × 2 daily for 10 days.

N.B. Cefuroxime, although frequently used for treating Gram-negative sepsis, is not effective against *S. typhi*, which is an intracellular pathogen.

Remember

Ciprofloxacin is extremely well absorbed and so can be given by the oral route 500 mg 12-hourly as long as the patient is not vomiting. After starting ciprofloxacin the patient began to feel better very quickly but it took 3–6 days for the temperature to settle.

Progress. The patient was discharged after 6 days, feeling well and with no fever. He needed a follow-up appointment to ensure that he does not become a carrier of *S. typhi*. He must remain away from his job as a food handler until he is known to have negative stool cultures for *S. typhi*.

MALARIA

Case history

A 20-year-old student returns from a 6-week backpacking tour of Africa. Two weeks after his return he goes to A&E complaining of fever, headache and malaise of 7 days' duration.

On examination, the patient is thin and febrile with a temperature of 38°C. There are no other abnormal findings.

What further questions do you want to ask this man?

It is essential — as always — to acquire a full and detailed history. Particular note should be taken about exactly where the patient has travelled, what vaccinations he had prior to his trip, whether he took anti-malarial prophylaxis regularly, and, if so, what he took. Did he remember being bitten by any insects? Did he have close contact with anyone who was obviously unwell? What sort of food did he eat? Did he have unprotected sex with any strangers while travelling?

Differential diagnosis is shown in Box 1.3.

Kumar & Clark's Cases in Clinical Medicine

> **Box 1.3** Causes of febrile illness in travellers returning from the tropics
> and worldwide
>
> Low/mid income countries (LMICs)
>
> - Malaria
> - Schistosomiasis
> - Dengue
> - Tick typhus
> - Typhoid
> - Tuberculosis
> - Dysentery
> - Hepatitis A
> - Amoebiasis
>
> Specific geographical areas (see text)
>
> - Histoplasmosis
> - Brucellosis
>
> Worldwide
>
> - Influenza
> - Pneumonia
> - Upper respiratory tract infection
> - Urinary tract infection
> - Traveller's diarrhoea
> - Viral infection
> - Sexually transmitted diseases
>
> WHO advises that fever occurring in a traveller 1 week or more after entering a
> malaria risk area and up to 3 months after departure is a medical emergency.

Remember

Just because someone has been travelling, it does not mean that they can't have a common type of infection such as influenza, a common cold or a sexually transmitted infection (STI). Holidays are notorious for people picking up STIs.

Investigations

Start with simple, cheap and relatively non-invasive investigations whenever possible. Perform other investigations as appropriate, depending on symptoms, signs and results of initial investigations, e.g. imaging (CT scan, ultrasound or MRI), aspiration or needle biopsy.

Investigations

- FBC
- Routine blood chemistry
- Urine analysis
- Blood cultures
- Stool cultures
- CXR
- Thick and thin blood films for malarial parasites: × 3
- Store blood for serology and take a second sample 2 weeks later

Diagnosis

Thick and thin blood films showed that this patient had **malaria** with a 5% parasitaemia. His malaria was due to *Plasmodium falciparum.* This is a serious infection and requires immediate emergency treatment in an HDU/ITU.

How would you manage the patient?

P. falciparum is resistant to chloroquine. Artesunate 2.5 mg/kg IV is very effective and is first-line therapy. Alternatively, patients with this disease should be commenced on IV quinine sulfate 20 mg/kg infused over 4 h, followed by 10 mg/kg infused over 4 h 8-hourly, until the switch to oral therapy (quinine salt 600 mg 8-hourly) can be made. Total dose is for 7 days. Both treatments are followed by a single dose in adults of 3 tablets of pyrimethamine with sulfadoxine (Fansidar). Doxycycline 200 mg once daily for 7 days can be used as an alternative to pyrimethamine and sulfadoxine. IV quinine might potentiate hypoglycaemia and patients taking it should have their blood sugar monitored regularly. Ideally, they should also be on cardiac monitors.

Progress. This young man made a full recovery. He admitted that he had not taken his malaria prophylaxis regularly.

SHINGLES

Varicella zoster virus causes a primary infection – chickenpox, usually in children.

The virus remains latent in dorsal root and cranial nerve ganglia, and reactivation results in shingles.

Case history

A 75-year-old man presents to his GP with severe right-sided chest pain for the previous 2 days. In the past 24 h he has noted a rash on the right side of his chest, in the distribution of T5–T6.

What do you think the likely diagnosis is?

Shingles.

What question would you like to ask the patient?

Have you had chickenpox?

Remember

Not everyone who has antibodies to varicella zoster virus remembers having the primary disease.

All people over the age of 65 years should have prophylactic varicella inoculation.

What investigations might you perform?

The disease is usually diagnosed clinically. It can be confirmed by examination of the vesicular fluid under an electron microscope to look for herpes virus. Serology can also be performed.

How would you manage the patient?

This patient requires admission to hospital (see later). He should be nursed in a side room and only by nurses who are known to have antibodies against varicella zoster virus. If he were to remain at home, he must avoid contact with people who have no history of having had chickenpox.

As the patient has had the rash for less than 3 days he should be commenced on aciclovir. Alternative anti-viral agents active against varicella zoster virus include famciclovir or valaciclovir. The usual adult dose of aciclovir for treatment of shingles is 800 mg $\times$ 5 daily by mouth or 5 mg/kg $\times$ 3 daily if given intravenously.

Remember

- Modification of the dose of aciclovir might be required if the patient has renal impairment.
- Patients should be prevailed upon not to scratch their lesions, as this can predispose to secondary infection. Calamine lotion can help.
- Patients are likely to require analgesia.

Progress. The patient was admitted to hospital because he lives on his own. He was started on oral aciclovir 200 mg $\times$ 5 daily. Twenty-four hours later he developed a high fever. A nurse noticed that one of the lesions had an inflamed area around it.

What do you think has happened? How would you manage the patient?

Secondary infection of the shingles lesions has occurred. The most likely pathogens to cause this are *Streptococcus pyogenes* or *S. aureus*. Swabs should be taken and sent to microbiology for microscopy, culture and sensitivity, and blood cultures should also be taken. The patient was commenced on IV benzylpenicillin (active against *Strep. pyogenes*) and IV flucloxacillin (active against *S. aureus*), and switched to oral therapy after 3 days. His infected area settled, but on discharge after 6 days he still had a painful area of shingles on his chest with some new lesions. His aciclovir was therefore continued for 10 days.

He was also given amitriptyline 10 mg at night for pain. He remained unwell for 3 weeks, but after 2 months his pain had settled and he made a full recovery.

Information

Ophthalmic herpes is infection of the 1st division of the Vth nerve and can lead to corneal scarring and secondary panophthalmitis. **Ramsay Hunt syndrome** is due to herpes infection of the geniculate ganglia. It causes a facial palsy with vesicles on the pinna of the ear. **Post-herpetic neuralgia** is a burning, continuous pain in the area of the previous eruption. It is common in the elderly and accompanied by depression. It is difficult to treat.

EPSTEIN–BARR VIRUS

This causes an acute febrile illness, usually in teenagers or young adults, which is known as infective mononucleosis (glandular fever). It is transmitted by saliva or aerosol.

Case history

A 19-year-old college student presents to his doctor with a 1-week history of severe sore throat, fever and extreme fatigue.

On examination, the patient is found to have a fever of 38.8°C, and cervical, axillary and inguinal lymphadenopathy.

The tonsils appear enlarged and the pharynx erythematous; palatal petechiae are present.

The spleen is just palpable.

What is the likely diagnosis in this patient?

The most likely diagnosis in a person of this age with a short history of fever, malaise, general lymphadenopathy and severe sore throat is infectious mononucleosis (glandular fever).

Streptococcal sore throats can mimic infectious mononucleosis clinically, although hepatosplenomegaly and inguinal and axillary lymphadenopathy will be absent.

Cytomegalovirus infections and toxoplasmosis also present in a similar fashion, although the sore throat is usually less severe. Viral hepatitis can also sometimes present with fever, lymphadenopathy, malaise and an atypical lymphocytosis. HIV seroconversion can also present as a glandular-fever-like illness. Lymphomas and leukaemia occasionally present in this way.

How would you confirm the diagnosis?

A full blood count should be performed. In over two-thirds of patients this will show a mononuclear lymphocytosis with atypical lymphocytes. A mild neutropenia is frequently present and platelet counts are commonly slightly decreased. Serum aminotransferases are usually raised.

Heterophile antibodies that agglutinate sheep red blood cells (the Paul—Bunnell test) usually become positive during the second week of infection.

The Monospot test (a rapid screening test) will be positive in glandular fever in 85% of cases. In addition, Epstein—Barr virus-specific antibodies can be looked for in Paul—Bunnell-negative 'glandular fever' or in atypical cases, but these tests are generally not performed. Ask your local virology laboratory for further details, if required.

Treatment

This is generally supportive. Contact sports should be avoided while splenomegaly is present. Aspirin helps relieve the sore throat and reduce fever. Occasionally, the tonsils can be so swollen that airway obstruction seems imminent: in these cases a short course of steroids is helpful, usually commencing with approximately 60 mg prednisolone/day in individual cases and stopping within 1—2 weeks. Corticosteroids are also indicated in cases with marked thrombocytopenia, haemolysis or CNS involvement.

Remember

About 90% of patients with infectious mononucleosis who are given ampicillin or amoxicillin will develop a rash.

If the diagnosis is unclear, if it is suspected that the patient might have a sore throat due to *Strep. pyogenes* or if a secondary streptococcal infection is suspected, the patient should be commenced on IV benzylpenicillin (if in hospital) pending culture and serology results. If the patient is not admitted, high-dose oral penicillin is an alternative.

Prognosis. This student's sore throat and fever settled after 5—6 days but he still felt unwell for a further 3 weeks.

CORONAVIRUS

SARS, MERS and SARS-CoV-2, see p. 333.

Further reading

Pyrexia of unknown origin

WHO. Infectious diseases. http://www.who.int/topics/infectious_diseases/en

Meningococcal meningitis and sepsis

Quagliarello V. Dissemination of *Neisseria meningitidis*. *New England Journal of Medicine* 2011; **364**: 1573—1575.

The returning traveller

WHO guidelines. www.who.int/topics/infectious_diseases/en/
WHO. Treatment of malaria. www.who.int/malaria/publications/atoz/9789241549127/en/

Shingles

Cohen JL. Herpes zoster. *New England Journal of Medicine* 2013; **369**: 255—263.

General information

British Infection Association. britishinfection.org
Centers for Disease Control and Prevention (USA). www.cdc.gov

Sexually Transmitted Infections 2

HIV/AIDS

Case history

A 35-year-old European man is newly diagnosed as HIV-positive. He was tested because he had been feeling generally unwell over a 6-month period and had lost weight. He presents with a persistent cough, which has developed and worsened over the preceding 2 weeks.

On examination, he has a temperature of 39°C, his pulse is 100/min and he has a respiratory rate of 20/min.

There are signs of oral candidiasis. He is on no regular medication. You are the medical trainee on acute take.

What are the likely diagnoses and the immediate management?

Pneumocystis jiroveci pneumonia commonly has an insidious onset, often with worsening shortness of breath and deteriorating exercise tolerance; the cough is usually non-productive.

- Examination of the chest can yield few signs other than tachypnoea and tachycardia. Fine inspiratory crackles might be heard.
- The CXR is often normal or shows little, although bilateral perihilar interstitial shadowing with a bat-wing appearance is the characteristic abnormality.
- High-resolution CT of the lungs shows a characteristic ground glass appearance, even when there is little to see on the plain CXR.
- Oxygen saturation characteristically falls on exercise. Arterial blood gas analysis might show hypoxia with a normal carbon dioxide and pH.
- The diagnosis is made on broncho-alveolar lavage.

The introduction of highly active anti-retroviral therapy (ART) in HIV-infected people has led to a significant decline in *Pneumocystis* infection and it is most commonly seen in those not previously recognised as HIV-infected. *Pneumocystis* infection occurs most frequently in the context of significant immunosuppression, when the CD4 count is <200 cells/mm^3. There may be clinical markers of poor immune function, such as candidiasis, as in this patient.

Primary prophylaxis (co-trimoxazole is first-line) is recommended in those who are aware of their HIV status, if their CD4 count falls into this range. This intervention alone has reduced the incidence of *Pneumocystis* infection in HIV-infected populations. *Pneumocystis* pneumonia is an AIDS-defining diagnosis.

How would you treat this patient?

IV co-trimoxazole (trimethoprim 15 mg/kg per day plus sulfamethoxazole 75 mg/kg per day) is the preferred first-line treatment, although a significant proportion of patients will develop allergy. IV pentamidine or dapsone plus pyrimethamine are also used.

Treatment is given for 3 weeks. Systemic corticosteroids (IV methylprednisolone 40 mg × 4 daily for 5 days) are added in severe cases (PO$_2$ <8 kPa).

Patients with *Pneumocystis* infection can develop respiratory failure and require ventilatory support. Pneumothorax is a further complication of *Pneumocystis* infection.

If the organism is not cleared by treatment, secondary prophylaxis (usually co-trimoxazole) is recommended. This can be withdrawn later if the patient starts ART and the CD4 count remains consistently >200 cells/mm^3.

Initiation of therapy in a patient not already on ART should be discussed with a specialist physician.

What other chest conditions are associated with HIV?

Tuberculosis

Tuberculosis is caused by *Mycobacterium tuberculosis (MTB)*, which has a high pathogenicity. It can develop relatively early in the course of HIV infection. It is particularly common in those who have lived in areas of the world with a high incidence of MTB, e.g. sub-Saharan Africa. Pulmonary infection presents with a cough (usually productive) and chest pain, but, in the context of HIV infection, presentation is often insidious and non-specific, with fever, sweats, malaise and weight loss. History of contact with MTB should always be sought, along with details of any previous anti-tuberculous therapy, because in such patients there is a risk of multidrug-resistant tuberculosis (MDRTB). There might be generalised lymph node enlargement or hepatomegaly in addition to signs in the chest. In some cases, pulmonary infection is coupled with CNS involvement — either TB meningitis or tuberculoma. The chest radiological changes are few and are frequently atypical, showing lower zone changes without cavitation. Other radiological findings include hilar lymphadenopathy, pleural effusion or lobar consolidation.

In patients with HIV, the usual immunological reactions to MTB might be blunted or absent, making diagnosis more difficult. Mantoux tests are rarely helpful because immunosuppressed patients don't produce a normal delayed hypersensitivity reaction. Granuloma formation can be compromised, leading to atypical histological changes. Sputum smears may be negative in up to 50% of those with culture-proven TB. Urine lipoarabinomannan (LF-LAM) is detected in some patients with active TB, providing a result in 30 min. The sensitivity of the test is low but is higher in HIV patients with low CD4 cell counts. Diagnosis relies heavily on clinical suspicion backed by positive cultures from, for example, sputum, broncho-alveolar lavage, blood, bone marrow and lymph nodes, as appropriate.

Treatment of TB in HIV-co-infected patients presents specific challenges and requires input from a specialist physician. Treatment is similar to that for HIV-negative patients, although intermittent and short-course regimens are not advised.

Therapy should be initiated with four drugs — isoniazid, rifampicin, pyrazinamide and ethambutol — for 2 months. Once sensitivities are confirmed, pyrazinamide and ethambutol can be withdrawn and the other two drugs continued for 4 months, although this might be extended in some circumstances. The drug–drug interactions between anti-retroviral and anti-tuberculous medications are complex and are a consequence of enzyme induction or inhibition. There are interactions between rifampicin derivatives and the protease inhibitor class of anti-retroviral agents, leading to an increase in rifampicin toxicity and reduced protease efficacy. The non-nucleoside reverse transcriptase class also interacts variably with rifampicin, requiring dose alterations. Additionally, there are overlapping toxicities between ART regimens and anti-tuberculous drugs: in particular, hepato-toxicity, peripheral neuropathy and gastrointestinal side-effects.

Bacterial chest infection

Several respiratory infections are more common in patients with HIV infection: in particular, *Streptococcus pneumoniae, Haemophilus influenzae* and *Moraxella catarrhalis*. The onset is usually rapid, with a productive cough. Signs of consolidation occur and radiological changes of consolidation or infiltration might be present. Diagnosis is based on sputum and blood cultures, and management is with appropriate broad-spectrum antibiotics (e.g. cefotaxime).

Other infective conditions

Cytomegalovirus, *Cryptococcus neoformans, Aspergillus fumigatus, Histoplasma capsulatum* and *Nocardia asteroides* can all cause fever, cough and dyspnoea in association with advanced HIV infection. The clinical signs and radiological findings are usually non-diagnostic. The diagnosis depends on broncho-alveolar lavage.

Malignancy

The incidence of **Kaposi's sarcoma** (KS) has declined significantly since the widespread introduction of ART. This is a vascular tumour associated with human herpes virus type 8 (HHV8). Although most commonly found on the skin, KS can infiltrate the lungs to cause cough and shortness of breath. On examination, other KS lesions are usually found on the skin or in the mouth, but in rare cases the lungs alone may be involved.

Radiological changes are of diffuse lung infiltration, often with a nodular appearance. Pleural effusion might be present. Lesions are visualised on bronchosocopy. Treatment is with systemic chemotherapy. ART should be initiated if the patient is not already on treatment.

Non-Hodgkin lymphoma can also cause lung infiltration. Patients additionally present with systemic 'B' symptoms. On examination, lymphadenopathy and splenomegaly might be found. Hilar lymphadenopathy seen on the CXR and CT scan indicate widespread lymph node enlargement in the chest and abdominal cavities. The diagnosis is made on the histological appearance of lymph node biopsy. Such lymphomas are often aggressive. Treatment is with chemotherapy (see *Kumar and Clark's Clinical Medicine*, 10th edn, Ch. 17).

How would you manage an HIV-positive patient with chest problems?

The differential diagnosis in an HIV-infected patient presenting with respiratory symptoms is wide. There is considerable advantage in establishing a specific diagnosis rather than treating symptoms empirically. Factors that have an impact on diagnosis and management include clinical presentation, level of immunosuppression of the individual, lifetime exposure to infective agents and current medication.

Remember

IN HIV-INFECTED PATIENTS
- Common conditions can have unusual presentations.
- Uncommon conditions occur more frequently.
- Many different conditions can present in similar ways — clinically and radiologically.
- Standard investigations that depend on an intact immune system will not be useful.
- A tissue or culture diagnosis is frequently required.
- Pathology is related to:
  - The degree of immunosuppression
  - The virulence of the organism
  - The microbiological repertoire to which an individual has been exposed
  - The multiple pathology that is frequently encountered
  - The medication that the patient is taking.

Assessment

- Full history and examination, including details of travel, previous infections, previous or existing HIV-related pathology, current surrogate marker data (if known), current therapy, including anti-retroviral drugs and anti-microbial prophylaxis.
- Assessment of the degree of immunosuppression by looking for clinical signs such as oral candidiasis, hairy oral leukoplakia and seborrhoeic dermatitis. Look for pathology in all systems, including examination of the mouth and fundi.
- Chest X-ray, exercise oximetry, blood gases, blood cultures, sputum examination for acid-fast bacilli (AFB), and microscopy, culture and sensitivity. Full blood count, liver and renal function.

Treatment

If the patient is clinically immunosuppressed, has a previous AIDS-defining illness or is known to have a CD4 count $<200/mm^3$ *and* has chest X-ray abnormalities, desaturates on exercise or has a hypoxic blood gas picture suggestive of *Pneumocystis* infection, institute therapy pending bronchoscopy. Organisms will still be found several days into treatment.

Remember

- Drug allergies
- Bone marrow suppression with high-dose co-trimoxazole
- Hypotension/hypoglycaemia with IV pentamidine
- CD4 counts and HIV viral load measurements are altered in the face of any acute infection and might not accurately reflect the underlying situation.

  If the patient has a history of TB or of exposure to TB, or has clinical and radiological findings consistent with TB, isolate and investigate. Don't initiate empirical anti-tuberculous therapy without an expert opinion, as this will have long-lasting and far-reaching consequences for the patient and for future management.

If the patient has a sputum smear that is positive for AFB or has culture-proven TB, isolate and start anti-tuberculous therapy with four drugs. Notify and seek expert opinion.

If the patient has clinical or radiological signs of bacterial infection, institute therapy with broad-spectrum antibiotics, e.g. amoxicillin or azithromycin.

Remember

If the patient does not respond as detailed:
- Reconsider the diagnosis
- Suspect multiple pathology.

Further reading

Melhuish A, Lewthwaite P. Natural history of HIV and AIDS. *Medicine* 2018; **46**: 356–361.
Yarchoan R, Uldrick JS. HIV associated cancer and related diseases. *New England Journal of Medicine* 2018; **378**: 1029–1045.
British HIV Association. bhiva.org
World Health Organisation. who.int/hiv/pub

FEEDING THE PATIENT

Case history

A surgical colleague phones you to ask about parenteral nutrition for a 70-year-old man who had an oesophago-gastrectomy 5 days previously. Postoperative care had been straightforward and no prior provision for parenteral nutrition had been made. It now seems likely that he has an anastomotic leak.

What should you advise?

Parenteral nutrition is never an emergency therapy. It can always wait until expert advice is available next day. You say that you will bring your consultant along the following morning.

Remember

- It is better to predict (if possible) whether some form of supplementary nutrition is likely to be required **before** an event.
- Over 10% of patients in hospital are said to be malnourished.

How do you assess the nutritional state?

This can be done simply by looking at the patient! Does he/she look malnourished? Other parameters that can help are:
- Weight loss >10%
- Serum albumin <35 g/L
- Serum transferrin <1.5 g/L
- Body mass index (BMI) = weight (kg) ÷ height (m^2); the normal range is 18.5–24.9.

An evaluation of the nutritional status can be done using the MUST criteria (Fig. 3.1).

Patients for whom nutrition will be necessary

- All severely malnourished patients on admission to hospital
- Moderately malnourished patients who are not expected to eat for 3–5 days because of their illness
- Normally nourished patients not expected to eat for 7–10 days.

Always feed enterally rather than parentally if possible

Information

STANDARD ENTERIC DIET PROVIDING 8.4 MJ PER DAY (2000 KCAL)
Energy
- Carbohydrate as glucose polymers (49–53% of total energy)
- Fat as triglycerides (30–35% of total energy)

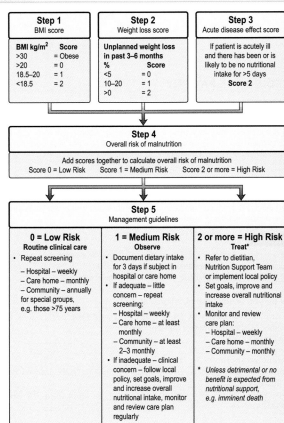

Figure 3.1 Malnutrition Universal Screening Tool (MUST). BMI, Body Mass Index. (Reproduced with permission from the British Association for Parenteral and Enteral Nutrition [BAPEN]: www.bapen.org.uk.)

Nitrogen
- Whole protein (10–14 g of nitrogen/day)

Other
- Additional electrolytes, vitamins and trace elements.

This provides
Ratio of energy kJ: nitrogen : g = 620 : 1 (ratio of energy kcal: nitrogen : g = 150 : 1).
  Osmolality = 285–300 mOsmol/kg.
  See current national formularies for ready-made formulations.

Methods of feeding enterally

- By mouth
- By fine-bore nasogastric tube (check position with pH paper; if in doubt, X-ray. Feeding tubes are usually placed endoscopically)
- Percutaneous endoscopic gastrostomy (PEG; refer to gastroenterologist for insertion) for prolonged period, i.e. >30 days.

Methods of parenteral nutrition

- **Peripheral nutrition.** This is the initial preferred option. Peripheral cannulas are inserted into the mid arm vein. Each catheter will last 5 days and the procedure has fewer complications than a central venous catheter.
- **Central nutrition.** A cannula is inserted via an infra-clavicular approach into the subclavian vein in theatre. Infusions include nitrogen for protein synthesis, calories, electrolytes, vitamins and trace elements. Complications include sepsis, thrombosis, pneumothorax and embolism. Most hospitals have nutrition teams to advise on the nutritional regimens that are required.

Remember

Monitor carefully with:
- Daily plasma electrolytes
- Daily glucose
- Weekly assessments of nutritional status.

Progress. This patient was not suitable for enteral nutrition because of his gastrointestinal surgery; thus parenteral nutrition was appropriate.

He was started with peripheral nutrition via a mid arm cannula. However, after 5 days it was felt that he required longer-term nutrition and a central catheter was inserted. The anastomotic leak settled on conservative management and he was able to return home on soft foods 4 weeks later.

Further reading

BAPEN. Information on parenteral and enteral nutrition. www.bapen.org.uk
European Society for Parenteral and Enteral Nutrition. Guidelines. www.espen.org
Malone A. Clinical guidelines from the American Society for Parenteral and Enteral Nutrition: best practice recommendations for patient care. *Journal of Infusion Nursing* 2014; **37**: 179–184.
National Institute for Health and Care Excellence (NICE). Guidelines for nutritional support. www.nice.org.uk/guidance/cg32

Gastroenterology 4

VOMITING

Vomiting centres are located on the lateral reticular formation of the medulla. They are stimulated by chemoreceptors trigger zones on the floor of the 4th ventricle and also by vagal afferents from the GI tract.

Causes of vomiting are shown in Box 4.1.

Case history

A 70-year-old man was admitted with a 2-week history of repeated vomiting. He had lost more than 6 kg in weight. He had recently developed colicky abdominal pain and constipation without passage of wind.

On examination, his abdomen was distended and he was tender in the epigastrium.

You call for surgical advice. The surgeon, in addition to your findings, notes that there are increased bowel sounds. The patient's hernial orifices and rectal examination show no abnormality.

Box 4.1 Causes of vomiting

- Any GI disease
- Infections:
  - Viruses (influenza, norovirus)
  - Bacterial (pertussis, urinary infection)
- CNS disease:
  - Raised intracranial pressure
  - Vestibular disturbance
  - Migraine
- Metabolic:
  - Uraemia
  - Hypercalcaemia
- Diabetic ketoacidosis
- Drugs:
  - Antibiotics
  - Chemotherapy
  - Digoxin
  - Immunotherapy
  - Incretins
  - Levodopa
  - Opiates
- Reflex:
  - Myocardial infarction
  - Biliary colic
- Psychogenic
- Pregnancy
- Alcohol excess

Remember

Non-gastrointestinal (GI) causes are possible: a full examination is therefore necessary. *Note:* look at the fundi for papilloedema.

Investigations

- Haematological:
  - FBC, ESR, CRP
- Radiological:
  - Abdominal X-ray (AXR)
  - Chest X-ray (CXR)
- Biochemical:
  - Electrolytes
  - Urea/creatinine/eGFR
  - Liver biochemistry
  - Calcium
  - Amylase
- **CXR:** Normal. Look for evidence of air under the diaphragm (perforation), signs of pneumonia, hilar mass (tumour).
- **AXR:**
  - **Normal**. With a history of this length, a normal X-ray would suggest that large or small bowel obstruction is unlikely. High obstruction in the GI tract, i.e. in the oesophagus or stomach, is possible. Investigate for non-GI causes (metabolic, neurological — exclude brainstem lesion), occasionally severe depression.
  - **Abnormal**. Might show evidence of small or large bowel obstruction or gastric distension.

  In this patient, the AXR showed small bowel obstruction (Fig. 4.1). The ***differential diagnosis*** is shown in the Information box.

Information

SMALL INTESTINAL OBSTRUCTION: DIFFERENTIAL DIAGNOSIS
- Adhesions (80% in adults)
- Hernia
- Crohn's disease
- Intussusception
- Obstruction due to extrinsic involvement by cancer

Management

The ultimate goal is to relieve obstruction. In the interim:
- Infuse glucose/saline to maintain electrolyte balance (with additional K^+ 20 mmol/L).
- Insert nasogastric tube (on continuous drainage).
- Contact surgeons, await instruction as to further investigations (such as CT scan to localise obstructive lesion).

  Progress. At operation, a carcinoma of the ascending colon was found and resected.

HICCUPS

Hiccups are due to involuntary diaphragmatic contractions with closure of the glottis. They are very common and usually not sinister, even if persistent.

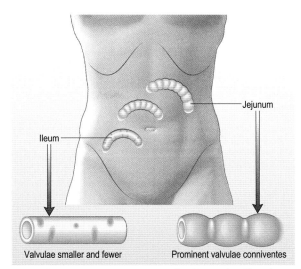

Valvulae smaller and fewer   Prominent valvulae conniventes

Figure 4.1 Small bowel obstruction, showing dilated loops of small bowel.

Case history

You are called by the surgical registrar because he is concerned that a 70-year-old man has had continuous hiccups for 48 h, along with a fever, malaise and right hypochondrial pain. Ten days ago he had been admitted with intestinal obstruction (see case earlier), and a laparotomy for a carcinoma of the ascending colon had been performed. This is a classic situation for a **subphrenic abscess** occurring post surgery in an elderly person.

How would you investigate?

Check Hb, WCC and liver biochemistry. An urgent ultrasound was performed and confirmed the diagnosis of a subphrenic abscess. Blood cultures were taken, as the patient was febrile.

Treatment and prognosis of the abscess

He had drainage under ultrasound control and antibiotics were started. The bacteria causing abscesses are usually *Bacteroides* spp. and/or *Escherichia coli* and he was therefore treated with ciprofloxacin and metronidazole. His hiccups were controlled with chlorpromazine 50 mg as necessary.

Other causes of hiccups

- Metabolic, e.g. uraemia
- Neurological, e.g. brainstem tumour
- Other abdominal pathology
- No pathological cause.

WEIGHT LOSS

Weight loss is often a perceived symptom by patients that needs to be verified. It is a general symptom, which can reflect disease in any part of the body.

Always make sure that the patient has a sufficient calorie intake for his/her requirements, bearing in mind the amount of exercise taken. In a young female, think of anorexia nervosa.

Reduced calorie intake can be caused by intentional dieting but can also be a symptom of generalised disease due to anorexia.

Case history

A 40-year-old man has been admitted with a fever, tremor and 10 kg weight loss. He has previously been counselled for alcohol misuse.

What should you do?

You need to consider a number of diagnoses and this might be helped by additional history and examination:

- Hyperthyroidism: check for symptoms and signs of hyperthyroidism (see p. 411).
- Alcoholic liver disease (see p. 67).
- Malnutrition: check by asking the patient's family. Perhaps there is a psychiatric history?
- Underlying cancer, particularly lung, bowel and pancreas.
- Biochemical investigations: should help determine underlying metabolic or renal disease.
- Malabsorption: often causes anorexia, contributing to weight loss.

This patient had no signs of chronic liver disease but did admit to recurrent episodes of upper abdominal pain radiating through to his back. These tended to occur on Monday, following his weekend binges. This suggests **pancreatic disease** resulting from his heavy alcohol intake.

What initial investigations are appropriate?

- FBC, liver biochemistry, calcium, blood alcohol
- Plain X-ray of the abdomen for pancreatic calcification
- Abdominal ultrasound to assess the pancreas for cysts and potential masses.

This patient was admitted in a malnourished, hyperdynamic state due to **acute alcohol withdrawal** (see p. 67). Treat this initially and investigate the pancreas later.

Further investigations

- CT scan of the pancreas
- MRCP (magnetic resonance cholangiopancreatography): this is non-invasive and of value in assessment of the pancreas and biliary tree
- ERCP (endoscopic retrograde cholangiopancreatography) to delineate the biliary and pancreatic ducts (if MRCP is unavailable)
- Endoscopic ultrasound: can help define pancreatic cysts and masses

Progress. This man was treated initially with benzodiazepine and IV thiamine (p. 67) and made a good recovery from his acute withdrawal state. Further investigations showed chronic pancreatitis; he was referred to the Liver clinic.

DYSPHAGIA

Dysphagia is difficulty in swallowing. It is an immediate, obstructive sensation during the passage of liquid or solid through the pharynx or oesophagus.

Case history

A 55-year-old patient has been referred urgently because of acute dysphagia. She gave a history of reflux for years and increasing dysphagia for 6 months. She had been eating an orange, which became lodged in her gullet and all efforts to dislodge it were unsuccessful. The underlying diagnosis is likely to be **food bolus obstruction** on an already present oesophageal stricture.

What should you do?

Refer the patient for an urgent endoscopy. The endoscopy findings were of a stricture in the mid-oesophagus with no obvious malignant lesion. Biopsies were taken and the stricture dilated.

Remember

Submucosal cancer can look like a benign lesion.

Unfortunately, this woman developed severe chest pain immediately after the dilatation and surgical emphysema could be felt in her neck. Clinically, an oesophageal tear is suspected.

A CXR, with a water-soluble contrast agent orally, confirms an oesophageal rupture.

Diagnosis

The underlying cause is more likely to be **oesophageal cancer** because careful dilatation of benign lesions rarely causes a tear.

Initial management

- Nil by mouth
- IV line for fluids
- Antibiotic prophylaxis
- Surgical referral.

Small tears in a peptic stricture can resolve in a few days with conservative management. Large tears generally need surgery in a dedicated thoracic unit. Endoscopic stenting is used initially for tears in malignant lesions but, again, surgery may be required.

Biopsies later confirmed a **squamous carcinoma**.

Management will include assessment for surgery with:

- Blood count, liver biochemistry
- CXR
- ECG
- Respiratory function tests
- Abdominal ultrasound, CT scan to assess operability
- Endoscopic ultrasound: an accurate way of staging lesion and any local lymph nodes
- PET scan: to look for distant metastases.

Discussion should take place at an MDT to decide on the patient's treatment.

As investigations showed no distant metastases, surgery with neo-adjuvant (preoperative) and adjuvant (postoperative) chemoradiation treatment was given.

CONSTIPATION

This is the infrequent passage of stools (<3 per week) with straining and the passage of hard stools.

Your trainee doctor asks you what she should prescribe for an elderly man who has not opened his bowels for 5 days. The patient, who was previously well and active, had been admitted a week ago with a chest infection. Rectal examination revealed a loaded colon with no local lesion.

Should this patient be investigated?

Not initially because it seems likely that constipation is due to immobility. Colonic investigation may be necessary if there is no improvement.

Treatment

- Initially, the patient will require a laxative to 'get things moving'. Glycerol suppositories are useful. Oral magnesium sulphate, an osmotic purgative, is effective and cheaper than the more usually prescribed osmotic laxative lactulose.
- Don't use stimulant laxatives.
- Stop 'constipating' drugs if possible.
- Faecal impaction might require digital extraction, followed by small-volume phosphate enemas.
- Advise the patient about high-fibre diets and fluid intake.

Information

CAUSES OF CONSTIPATION

- Simple/idiopathic
- Intestinal obstruction
- Colonic disease, e.g. carcinoma
- Painful anal conditions
- Drugs, e.g. codeine, iron, verapamil, tricyclic anti-depressants, opiates
- Hypothyroidism, hypercalcaemia
- Depression
- Immobility

DIARRHOEA

Increased frequency of defecation, even in a previously fit patient, can produce dehydration and *severe* electrolyte depletion. Diarrhoea can also be a recurrent problem in patients with established gastrointestinal disease.

What should you do in a case of diarrhoea presenting in A&E?

In the history, ascertain whether the patient has eaten suspect food or travelled overseas. Check for drug history, e.g. antibiotics. Ask about accompanying symptoms, e.g. abdominal pain, weight loss. It is essential to:

- Establish history of onset
- Determine frequency, consistency, content of stool, presence of blood
- Determine the state of hydration and electrolyte balance

- Send stool for culture, parasites (ova or cysts) and *Clostridium difficile* toxin assay (if the patient has previously been hospitalised or been on antibiotics)
- Perform a rectal examination; sigmoidoscopy (if bloody diarrhoea) should be done by the gastroenterology team
- Take blood cultures in severe cases with a temperature
- Do a plain AXR.

LIKELY PATHOGENS CAUSING DIARRHOEA

- Bacteria (50%):
  - *E. coli*
  - *Campylobacter* spp.
  - *Salmonella* spp.
  - *Shigella* spp.
- Viruses (1% but seldom produce severe diarrhoea in adults):
  - Rotavirus
  - Norovirus
- Protozoa:
  - *Giardia intestinalis*
  - *Entamoeba histolytica*
  - *Cryptosporidium*
- Helminths (e.g. *Strongyloides*)
- In some cases no pathogens or multiple pathogens are found (20–50% of cases)

Management

This will depend on the case scenario (see later) but most diarrhoeal illnesses are self-limiting and short-lived; 1–10% might persist for a month. Identification of the pathogen will determine specific therapy (see Ch. 1).

Case history (1)

A 24-year-old returned from travelling for 3 months, during which he passed through several countries. He was fairly well when he came home but after 3 days developed severe diarrhoea, which has now been present for 2 weeks.

On admission to the MAU he is dehydrated and has lost over 5 kg in weight.

What immediate action would you take?

- FBC, U&Es, liver biochemistry.
- Send stools for ova, cysts and culture.
- Rehydration with oral glucose/electrolyte solutions initially. IV fluids are usually not necessary.
- Vomiting might need to be treated with an anti-emetic (metoclopramide 10 mg × 3 daily).

Diagnosis

This is not acute diarrhoea with a viral/bacterial cause, as the patient didn't have diarrhoea when he returned to the UK. Viral/bacterial diarrhoea usually starts in the country where the infection occurred and generally clears up within 7 days. Possible causes are shown in the Information box.

Information

CAUSES OF NON-ACUTE DIARRHOEA IN A RETURNING TRAVELLER

- Giardiasis
- Cryptosporidiosis
- Amoebiasis
- Tropical sprue (SE Asia, Caribbean)
- Schistosomiasis
- Strongyloidiasis

Stool samples showed no abnormal findings.

Progress. Giardiasis is very likely in this patient. Treatment with metronidazole 2 g a day for 3 successive days was given, with dramatic improvement.

Case history (2)

A 30-year-old, white, Caucasian, female patient presented with a 2-week history of passing 6–10 motions a day. The stools were loose and contained blood. She felt tired and had lost about 5 kg in weight.

On admission to the MAU she was not dehydrated but had a fever and was very lethargic.

What is the differential diagnosis?

- Infective diarrhoea. Send specimens for microbiological testing.
- First presentation of inflammatory bowel disease (most likely in this woman).

Inflammatory bowel disease (IBD)

In any case of persistent diarrhoea presenting in A&E in developed countries, IBD is a possible cause. A previous history of intermittent diarrhoea or recurrent abdominal pain is often present. In lower/mid income countries, infective causes are more likely and must be excluded.

What general measures should you take?

- Acute diarrhoea (for more than 2 weeks) is usually not infective.
- Take blood for FBC, ESR, CRP, U&Es, liver biochemistry.
- Check a plain AXR for the presence of stool, mucosal oedema, bowel dilatation or perforation.
- Sigmoidoscopy: the presence of an inflamed, friable mucosa with loss of vascular pattern or patchy inflammation indicates IBD. Take a rectal biopsy.
- Stool cultures (*N.B.* Infective gastroenteritis must always be ruled out). *C. difficile* toxin assay — 4 stool specimens (90% sensitivity).

In this patient you have ruled out infective gastroenteritis, as three stool cultures were negative. Taking into account the history and the sigmoidoscopic finding, you presume this must be IBD. Her Hb was 100 g/L and CRP 84 mg/L.

Acute colitis is associated with diarrhoea, abdominal pain, fever and systemic disturbance. There is blood in the stools in ulcerative colitis but Crohn's disease patients only have bloody diarrhoea with Crohn's colitis. To assess severity, check the factors shown in Table 4.1.

Always look for the presence of:

- Toxic dilatation: colon >5 cm in diameter and mucosal islands on plain AXR (Fig. 4.2).
- Perforation (on AXR).

Table 4.1 Findings in a severe attack of ulcerative colitis

Findings	↓/↑	Results
Hb	↓	<100 g/L
Albumin	↓	<30 g/L
Fever	↑	>37.5°C
Stool frequency	↑	>6/day
ESR	↑	>30 mm/h
Pulse rate	↑	>90 bpm
Platelets	↑	
WCC	↑	

How would you manage this acute situation?

- IV fluids with glucose/saline.
- IV therapy with steroids (IV hydrocortisone 100 mg × 4 daily), followed by oral therapy (prednisolone 40 mg per day) if the patient improves.
- IV antibiotics (metronidazole/cephalosporin).
- Further management: refer to gastroenterologists; consult GI surgeons.

Remember

In acute severe ulcerative colitis, at 3 days post treatment, a CRP >45 mg/L or stool frequency >8/day has an 85% chance of needing a colectomy.

Progress and management. There was no response to treatment at 3 days (see Information box). The patient was started on infliximab 5 mg/kg as 'rescue therapy' to avoid immediate colectomy. Ciclosporin 2 mg/kg/day is an alternative.

This patient responded to infliximab and is being followed closely in the colitis clinic. She is continuing on infliximab therapy on a protocol, lasting up to 46 weeks.

Does this patient have Crohn's disease or ulcerative colitis?

Both can produce acute colitis. The differentiation is by colonoscopy and histological appearance (Table 4.2).

Information

Crohn's disease
- Affects any part of the GI tract, from mouth to anus
- 70% of cases affect the terminal ileum
- Can be controlled but not cured

Kumar & Clark's Cases in Clinical Medicine

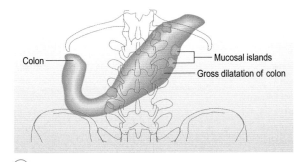

(a)

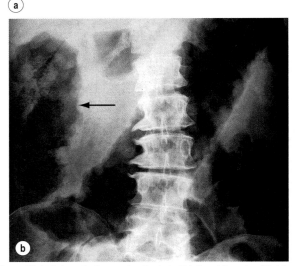

(b)

Figure 4.2 (a) Schematic diagram showing toxic dilatation of the colon; (b) plain abdominal X-ray showing toxic dilatation in ulcerative colitis. Arrow shows mucosal island.

Ulcerative colitis
- Confined to colon
- Cured by colectomy
- Can affect the rectum alone (proctitis); sigmoid and descending colon (left-sided colitis); or the whole colon (extensive colitis)

Both
- Extra-GI manifestations, e.g. pyoderma gangrenosum (Fig. 4.3 and Box 4.2)

Table 4.2 Differentiating between Crohn's disease and ulcerative colitis

Histological findings	Crohn's disease	Ulcerative colitis
Inflammation	Deep (transmural), patchy	Superficial (mucosal) continuous
Granulomas	++	Rare
Goblet cells	Present	Depleted
Crypt abscesses	+	++

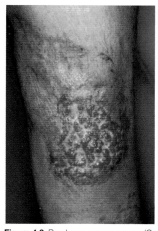
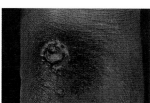

Figure 4.3 Pyoderma gangrenosum. (Courtesy of Dr David Paige.)

ABDOMINAL PAIN

Most diseases of the GI tract are associated with abdominal pain but pain can also be referred to the chest or back. The characteristics of the pain can help in the diagnosis.

Case history

A 40-year-old man presents with epigastric and central abdominal cramping pain. For 48 h the pain has been continuous, severe and associated with vomiting. The pain does not radiate but is getting worse by the hour. ***On examination***, he has a temperature of 38°C and a pulse rate of 98 bpm. He has tenderness across the upper abdomen but no other signs. His bowel sounds are normal. He has no alteration of bowel habit and reports no weight loss.

Box 4.2 Extra-gastrointestinal manifestations of inflammatory bowel disease

- Eyes:
  - Uveitis
  - Episcleritis, conjunctivitis
- Joints:
  - Type I (pauci-articular) arthropathy
  - Type II (polyarticular) arthropathy
  - Arthralgia
  - Axial spondyloarthritis
  - Inflammatory back pain
- Skin:
  - Pyoderma gangrenosum (see Fig. 4.3)
- Liver and biliary tree:
  - Sclerosing cholangitis
  - Fatty liver
  - Chronic hepatitis
  - Cirrhosis
  - Gallstones
- Nephrolithiasis
- Venous thrombosis

Immediate investigations

- Haematological: Hb, WCC, ESR
- Biochemical: U&Es, liver biochemistry, amylase
- Radiological: initial AXR for obstruction; CXR in acute pain for intestinal perforation.

Management

Develop the management plan to include:
- Symptomatic relief
- Information for patient and relatives
- Further investigations (endoscopy, ultrasound, CT and MRI as necessary to exclude perforation, obstruction, stones, calcification, cancer and ascites)
- Consultation with surgical colleagues.

In this case, abdominal pain situated in the epigastrium and central abdomen, and of the severity described, is always due to organic disease. Your differential diagnosis should include the following:
- An acute surgical cause:
  Aortic aneurysm dissection
  Appendicitis (even occasionally with upper abdominal pain)
  Perforation
  Intestinal obstruction.
- Acute pancreatitis:
  Severe pain
  Often associated with heavy alcohol use, gallstones, viral infection (e.g. mumps)

↑Serum amylase ($>5 \times$ normal)

Gastric retention and vomiting

Ultrasonographic changes and contrast-enhanced dynamic CT (best investigation) show pancreatic swelling, necrosis and peripancreatic fluid collection.

Remember

ACUTE PANCREATITIS: ASSESSMENT OF SEVERITY AND POOR PROGNOSIS (FIRST 48 H): (GLASGOW PROGNOSTIC CRITERIA)

- Age >55 years
- Blood glucose >10 mmol/L
- Serum urea >16 mmol/L
- Serum calcium <2 mmol/L
- Serum LDH >600 U/L
- PaO_2 <8 kPa
- WCC $>15 \times 10^9$/L
- Serum albumin <30 g/L
- Serum AST >200 U/L

N.B. More than 3 positive factors during the first 48 h suggest **severe acute pancreatitis** and a poorer prognosis.

Symptom relief

Symptom relief depends on diagnosis. Use anti-spasmodics (hyoscine $20-40$ mg $\times 4$ daily). Minor analgesics (paracetamol) can help and NSAIDs are useful in some cases. When prescribing opiates (morphine, codeine), remember that they can increase constipation and cause spasm in the sphincter of Oddi. Give anti-emetics (metoclopramide 10 mg $\times 2$ daily or prochlorperazine 5 mg $\times 2$ daily) as necessary.

Patient information

This depends on diagnosis but should be delivered to both patients and relatives sensitively and with an understanding of underlying pathology.

Diagnosis and progress. In this case, the 40-year-old patient turned out to have **acute pancreatitis**, with a serum amylase of 1000 units. He quickly settled by being kept nil by mouth and having IV fluids. The aetiology was never established but was thought perhaps to have been viral.

GASTRO-OESOPHAGEAL REFLUX DISEASE (GORD)

Gastro-oesophageal reflux occurs normally. GORD occurs when the anti-reflux mechanism fails, allowing acidic gastric contents to make prolonged contact with the oesophageal mucosa.

Case history

A 48-year-old man was admitted with severe epigastric pain radiating up into his chest. He thought he had had a heart attack (see p. 270).

What investigations would you do on admission?

It is critical to exclude life-threatening conditions, such as myocardial infarction, pulmonary embolism and pneumothorax, before labelling such pain as due to reflux.

- FBC, liver biochemistry, serum amylase
- ECG, repeated after 1 h
- CXR
- Cardiac markers, e.g. serum troponins and creatine kinase

In this patient, two ECGs, CXR and cardiac markers (e.g. creatine kinase, troponins) were normal. Additional features in the history included:
- Long history of reflux (GORD)
- Burning nature of the pain
- Flatulence
- A relationship of the present pain to previous similar pain
- A food-related element
- Exacerbation of pain with drinking hot liquids.

Features of gastro-oesophageal reflux
- Burning pain produced by bending, stooping or lying down
- Pain seldom radiates to the arms
- Pain precipitated by drinking hot liquids or alcohol
- Pain relieved by antacids.

Features of myocardial ischaemia
- Gripping or crushing pain
- Pain radiates into neck, shoulders and both arms
- Pain produced by exercise
- Pain accompanied by breathlessness.

A diagnosis of **GORD** was made in this patient from the history.

Progress and management. The patient was given liquid Gaviscon (10 mL) and a proton pump inhibitor (PPI, e.g. lansoprazole 30 mg × 2 daily for 6 weeks, reducing to 10 mg) to control the symptoms. Endoscopy will need to be performed in this man in view of his age.

Remember

- Reflux can be difficult to diagnose, and although it is often associated with a hiatus hernia, more formal investigation might be necessary, e.g. endoscopy followed by oesophageal pH, impedance and pressure monitoring if necessary.
- At endoscopy, assess the degree of oesophagitis and check for Barrett's oesophagus (including biopsies).

BARRETT'S OESOPHAGUS

This occurs as a result of long-standing reflux. It consists of columnar epithelium with intestinal metaplasia extending upwards into the lower oesophagus and replacing normal squamous epithelium. Barrett's oesophagus (even a short segment <3 cm) is pre-malignant for **adenocarcinoma**. Risk factors for progression are male sex, age >45 years, length of segment >8 cm, early age of onset and duration of symptoms of GORD, the presence of ulceration and stricture, and a family history. Dysplasia is patchy and biopsies from all four quadrants (every 2 cm) of the Barrett's segment must be performed. There is no evidence that treatment with PPIs or surgery leads to Barrett's regression. Patients without dysplasia don't require **surveillance**. Low-grade dysplasia requires regular endoscopic surveillance. High-grade dysplasia is treated with radiofrequency ablation using the HALO system, but endoscopic ablation therapy or laser is also used.

PEPTIC ULCER DISEASE

Case history (1)

In the clinic you see a 40-year-old man with epigastric pain that has been present on and off for a number of years. The doctor's letter indicates that the man has been a regular attender and has received antacids, H_2 receptor antagonists and a PPI at some time over the last 5 years. Recently, the patient was found to have *Helicobacter pylori* antibodies in his serum and was given eradication therapy.

What should you do?

The history of intermittent epigastric pain is highly suggestive of peptic ulcer disease and you note there are no alarm features in the history. The patient has been given *H. pylori* eradication therapy but the GP has not indicated the drugs that were used. The patient remembers taking two different tablets for 1 week. You ask about smoking (which delays ulcer healing) and also take a drug history. There is no history of NSAID or aspirin use.

Remember

ALARM FEATURES
- Weight loss
- Anorexia
- Dysphagia
- Protracted vomiting
- Haematemesis or melaena

In the absence of alarm features it is reasonable to try a PPI if the history is suggestive of reflux, e.g. heartburn worse on bending.

What would you do next?

You would need to establish whether the patient has had successful *H. pylori* eradication.

Tests for *H. pylori*
- Stool antigen test (current infection)
- Antral biopsy: either for histology or for *Campylobacter*-like organism (CLO, urease) testing (for current infections)
- Urea breath tests (for current infections) measuring $^{13}CO_2$ (Fig. 4.4)
- Serological IgG antibodies (useful in the community but testing does not distinguish between past or current infections).

This patient's urea breath test is positive, indicating continuing *H. pylori* infection.

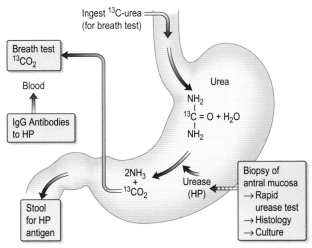

Figure 4.4 Metabolism of urea by *Helicobacter pylori* (HP), showing the different tests that are available for the detection of *H. pylori*.

Treatment of *H. pylori* infection

Patients with peptic ulcer disease who are *H. pylori*-positive should be given combination eradication therapy:

- Clarithromycin 500 mg × 2 for 1 week
- Amoxicillin 1 g × 2 daily for 1 week
- Omeprazole 20 mg × 2 daily for 2 weeks.

With increasing resistance to clarithromycin, quadruple therapy is now being used, as in this patient. He was given lansoprazole 30 mg × 2, tri-potassium di-citrato bismuthate 120 mg × 4, tetracycline 500 mg × 4 and metronidazole 500 mg × 3 – all daily for 2 weeks.

Progress. This patient has had no further problems since his quadruple therapy and a stool antigen test was negative for *H. pylori*.

Case history (2)

You are asked by the cardiologists to see a man with epigastric pain. He has been admitted for urgent percutaneous coronary intervention (PCI). He is already on aspirin 75 mg daily. He has had many similar episodes of pain over the years. Approximately 10 years ago, he had an endoscopy and was told that he had an ulcer and given Zantac. He points with one finger to his epigastrium as the site of his pain.

This is a classic history of duodenal ulcer disease.

What should you do?

As the PCI is tomorrow, you recommend that he is given a PPI, e.g. omeprazole 20 mg × 2 daily, and referred to Gastroenterology outpatients.

The cardiology specialist registrar would like to put the patient on anti-platelet therapy post PCI and is worried that he has an ulcer. This is a problem of balancing the risks. As placement of the coronary stent is urgent, they will have to go ahead with anti-platelet therapy with a cytoprotective PPI. The ideal situation for this man would be to perform endoscopy prior to PCI, and if an ulcer is present, to heal his ulcer before the intervention. He should have a stool *H. pylori* antigen checked and, if this is positive, should receive *H. pylori* eradication therapy.

After reassessment with the consultant cardiologist, it is decided that the PCI is still urgent and will go ahead, despite its risks, which are fully discussed with the patient.

How do you investigate a patient with a suspected ulcer in the community?

- Under 45 years of age: *H. pylori* serology. If positive, give eradication therapy. If negative, treat symptomatically.
- Over 45 years: patients with new dyspepsia and those with alarm symptoms (e.g. anorexia, weight loss) should be referred for endoscopy (cost-effective).

Remember

- *H. pylori* serology can remain positive, even after successful eradication of *H. pylori*.
- Current *H. pylori* infection can be detected by the urea breath test (see Fig. 4.4), endoscopy (urease test, histology or culture) and detection of stool antigen (cost-effective).

Case history

A 40-year-old woman was seen in the A&E department with a sprained ankle. She was sent home with a strapped ankle and given diclofenac to take for the pain. There was no history of indigestion. Ten days later she is brought in by ambulance, having vomited blood. The bleeding was thought to be related to the NSAID therapy.

On examination, she was not shocked and there are no signs of chronic liver disease. She had stopped bleeding and an endoscopy was performed in the next 24 h.

A bleeding ulcer, with a fresh adherent clot, was seen on endoscopy; it was injected with adrenaline (epinephrine) 1:10 000 and a heater probe was also used. A biopsy was taken for *H. pylori*.

A bleeding ulcer might have certain stigmata that suggest that rebleeding is likely to recur (see Remember box).

Gastric cancer does not usually cause an acute GI bleed; it is more likely to produce anaemia from chronic blood loss.

Remember

STIGMATA OF A RECENT BLEED FROM AN ULCER ON ENDOSCOPY
- Spurting vessel
- Prominent vessel
- Fresh adherent clot

Progress. The *H. pylori* test was positive, indicating chronic peptic ulcer disease. The haematemesis was precipitated by the NSAIDs.

Discharge policy

The patient's age, diagnosis on endoscopy, co-morbidity, and the presence or absence of shock should be taken into consideration. In general, patients under the age of 60, as well as older patients who are haemodynamically stable and have no stigmata of recent haemorrhage on endoscopy, can be discharged within 24 h.

Note: All shocked patients need careful observation in hospital. Check your own hospital's guidelines.

IRON DEFICIENCY ANAEMIA

Case history

A 40-year-old, female, globe-trotting managing director was found at routine screening to have an Hb of 80 g/L with an iron-deficient appearance on the film.

She admitted to some ankle swelling and increased breathlessness of recent onset. Examination was unhelpful.

FBC, film and low serum ferritin confirmed **iron deficiency**.

What do you do?

- Exclude all obvious causes of bleeding:
  Heavy periods
  Rectal bleeding
  Recurrent nose bleeds.
- If there is no obvious menorrhagia, you can assume that the anaemia is due to GI disease. Malabsorption: coeliac disease is still very under-diagnosed.
- The patient travels abroad a lot and could have a bowel infestation. Remember that hookworm is the most common cause of iron deficiency anaemia worldwide.
- Occult bleeding from the GI tract is common and can be confirmed by haemoccult testing. This is totally unnecessary, however, in a patient with iron deficiency because if there is no history of blood loss, blood can then be lost only from the GI tract.

Information

FAECAL OCCULT BLOODS
- Of no use in males or post-menopausal females with iron deficiency anaemia and no other cause for bleeding
- Useful for screening populations for colonic cancer

What additional investigations are appropriate?

- Rectal examination is mandatory to exclude rectal cancer, and a proctoscopy to exclude piles.
- Gastroscopy: peptic ulcer, gastric cancer and GORD can certainly occur in this age group. Also do a duodenal biopsy for coeliac disease (Fig. 4.5).

Remember

COELIAC DISEASE
- This is increasingly recognised worldwide and has an incidence of <1 : 100 in many countries. Certain areas of the world are said to have a higher incidence, e.g. Ireland and Italy.

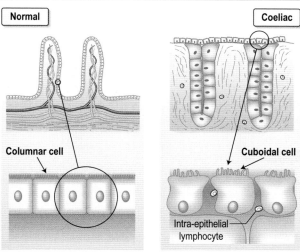

Normal | Coeliac

Columnar cell

Cuboidal cell

Intra-epithelial lymphocyte

Figure 4.5 Small intestinal mucosa showing normal villi with normal columnar cells, compared to coeliac mucosa showing subtotal villus atrophy, crypt hyperplasia, lamina propria inflammation and an increase in intra-epithelial lymphocytes.

- HLA-DQ2 and HLA-DQ8 are present in 90–95% of coeliac patients.
- Malabsorption of iron, as well as increased iron loss, can occur. There might be other deficiencies as well, e.g. calcium and folic acid.
- A history of steatorrhoea can be missed, unless a detailed stool history is taken (*Note:* many patients don't have steatorrhoea or any gastrointestinal symptoms).
- Coeliac serology with anti-endomysial and anti-tissue transglutaminase (the target antigen for the endomysial antibody) antibodies should be checked. A serum IgA must be performed, as these are IgA in vitro tests. Deaminated gluten peptide (DGP) testing is now available. These tests have a high sensitivity and specificity.
- Diagnosis is confirmed by biopsy of duodenal/jejunal mucosa.
- Treatment is with a gluten-free diet.

If gastroscopy is unhelpful, full colonic assessment is necessary. The best investigation is colonoscopy, which will allow full assessment of the colon; biopsy, polypectomy and laser treatment of angiodysplasia can be performed as appropriate.

If the above investigations are negative, you have a problem. A small minority of patients fall into this category and the host of further investigations, performed with advice from the GI unit, will include:

- Small bowel MRI
- Capsule endoscopy
- Enteroscopy
- Meckel's scan
- Angiography: preferably performed when a patient is bleeding, and in this patient unlikely to be helpful
- Laparotomy with possibly simultaneous on-table endoscopy.

Progress. This patient turned out to have menorrhagia due to fibroids, despite initially denying heavy periods.

Remember

- If there is iron deficiency anaemia in a post-menopausal female or any male with no obvious cause of blood loss, there must be a GI cause.
- Few patients have an inadequate iron intake in developed countries.

RECTAL BLEEDING

Rectal bleeding is characterised by the passage of fresh blood rectally, as opposed to either occult loss, when blood can be detected only by laboratory testing, or melaena (see p. 63).

Case history

An 80-year-old woman was admitted in a shocked state after having passed 'a great deal' of fresh blood from her rectum. She gave no other history, and prior to the incident had just returned on her bicycle from doing the shopping. Abdominal examination was normal.

How would you manage the patient initially?

- Establish an IV infusion and give 0.9% saline.
- Check Hb and U&Es.
- Group and cross-match blood.
- Insert a CVP line.
- Transfuse blood.
  The patient stabilised and had no further bleeding.

Additional examination

Additional investigations must include a rectal examination, proctoscopy and rigid sigmoidoscopy.

Proctoscopy

This will allow the diagnosis of haemorrhoids and an anal fissure. These are the most common causes of rectal bleeding, but rarely — if ever — cause torrential blood loss. Features of bleeding from an anorectal lesion are:

- Passage of blood after a motion, and not mixed with it
- Blood dripping into the pan
- Blood just on the paper
- Anal pain, particularly with an anal fissure.

Flexi-sigmoidoscopy

This will determine the presence of colitis and might show a lesion, e.g. carcinoma. If local anorectal disease is excluded, other causes include:

- Cancer
- Diverticular disease
- Colitis
- Angiodysplasia
- Polyps
- Ischaemia.

Progress. In this patient, sigmoidoscopy showed that the blood was coming from above the limit of the scope. Colonoscopy showed a bleeding polyp; this was excised.

Remember

Even in the presence of severe diverticular disease, a polyp and carcinoma can be the cause of the bleeding and must be excluded by colonoscopy.

FAMILY HISTORY OF COLON CANCER

Case history

A doctor phones to discuss a possible referral to the Gastroenterology clinic. He has just seen an anxious, 32-year-old woman, whose mother has recently died of colonic cancer. The patient has just discovered that her maternal aunt died of a similar complaint. The doctor emphasises that the patient herself has no GI symptoms.

What should you advise?

The patient needs to be seen by a gastroenterologist with a view to a full discussion of the pros and cons of having a colonoscopy.

Family cancer syndromes include:

- **Familial adenomatous polyposis:** multiple polyps are found throughout the colon and upper small bowel. All patients should be screened after age 12 years because *all* will develop colon cancer unless the colon is removed.
- **Hereditary non-polyposis cancer of the colon (HNPCC)** (Box 4.3): this accounts for 5–10% of colon cancers; the average age of diagnosis is 45 years. Cancers are mainly in the right-hand side of the colon.

A flexible sigmoidoscope can only reach 60–70 cm up the colon, where approximately 60% of cancers occur (Fig. 4.6).

The gastroenterologist advises a colonoscopy for this patient, which she agrees to have after full discussion.

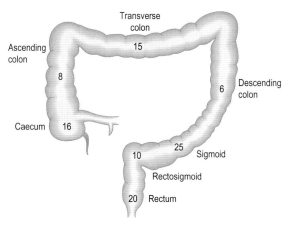

Figure 4.6 Distribution of colorectal cancer (%).

> **Box 4.3** Diagnostic criteria for hereditary non-polyposis colon cancer (HNPCC)
>
> Modified Amsterdam criteria
>
> - One individual diagnosed with colorectal cancer (or extra-colonic HNPCC-associated tumours) before age 50 years
> - Two affected generations
> - Three affected relatives, one a first-degree relative of the other two
> - Familial adenomatous polyposis should be excluded
> - Tumours should be verified by pathological examination
>
> Bethesda guidelines
>
> - Colorectal cancer diagnosed in patient who is younger than 50 years
> - Presence of synchronous, metachronous colorectal, or other HNPCC-associated tumours, irrespective of age
> - Colorectal cancer with the MSI-H histology diagnosed in a patient who is younger than 60 years
> - Colorectal cancer diagnosed in one or more first-degree relatives with an HNPCC-related tumour, with one of the cancers being diagnosed under age 50 years
> - Colorectal cancer diagnosed in two or more first- or second-degree relatives with HNPCC-related tumours, irrespective of age
>
> MSI-H, microsatellite instability — high.

Remember

RISKS FOR DEVELOPMENT OF COLON CANCER
- Normal: 1 : 50
- With a first-degree relative: 1 : 17
- With an elderly first-degree relative: 1 : 30

Progress. This patient's colonoscopy showed a 2 cm polyp, which was fully excised. Histologically, it was a tubular adenoma. She was asked to return for a surveillance colonoscopy in 3 years' time, and was told that she would need continuous follow-up in view of the family history.

FUNCTIONAL BOWEL DISEASE

Case history

A 30-year-old woman is in the A&E department with severe lower abdominal pain. She is rolling around in agony but the surgical registrar has found no evidence of serious disease. He has already examined her fully and investigated her with routine blood tests and an AXR, all of which are normal. Her boyfriend is aggressive and insisting that something must be done. The A&E doctor is looking for help.

What do you do?

- Retake the history, bearing in mind the possibility of this being irritable bowel syndrome (IBS).

- Re-examine the abdomen: think again of all the causes of an acute abdomen (see Information box).
- Review the investigations.

The history strongly supports the diagnosis of IBS. Remember that the pain can be very severe and real to the patient, even though it is related to life events, i.e. the pain is not just 'all in the mind'.

Management

This can be very difficult, particularly because relatives often feel unable to cope. The situation needs to be calmed down with strong reassurance and pain relief (e.g. NSAID and anti-spasmodics). Refer the patient to Gastroenterology outpatients.

Information

Acute abdominal pain of sudden onset
- Perforation, e.g. duodenal ulcer
- Rupture, e.g. aneurysm
- Torsion, e.g. ovarian cyst

Acute abdominal pain of gradual onset
- Inflammatory conditions, e.g. appendicitis, back pain

Think of
- Pancreatitis
- Ruptured aortic aneurysm
- Renal tract disease

Further reading

Diarrhoea

Friedman S. Tofacitinib for ulcerative colitis — a promising new step forward. *New England Journal of Medicine* 2017; **376**: 1792–1793.

Lamb CA, Kennedy NA, Raine T, et al. BSG consensus guidelines on management of inflammatory bowel disease in adults. *Gut* 2019; **68**: suppl 3.

Abdominal pain

Forsmark CE, Vege SS, Wilcox CM. Acute pancreatitis. *New England Journal of Medicine* 2016; **375**: 1972–1981.

Peptic ulcer disease

Cook D, Guyatt G. Prophylaxis against upper gastrointestinal bleeding in hospitalized patients. *New England Journal of Medicine* 2018; **378**: 2506–2516.

Editorial. Managing acute upper gastrointestinal bleeding. *Lancet* 2011; **377**: 1048.

Laine L. Upper gastrointestinal bleeding due to a peptic ulcer. *New England Journal of Medicine* 2016; **374**: 2367–2376.

Iron deficiency anaemia

Goddard AF, James MW, McIntyre AS, et al. Guidelines for the management of iron deficiency anaemia. *Gut* 2011; **60**: 1309–1316.

Family history of colon cancer

Sinicrole FA. Lynch syndrome — associated colorectal cancer. *New England Journal of Medicine* 2018; **379**: 764–773.

Liver and Biliary Tract Disorders 5

ABNORMAL LIVER BIOCHEMISTRY

'Liver function tests' are routinely requested.

Serum bilirubin, aminotransferases, alkaline phosphatase, γ-glutamyl transpeptidase (γ-GT) and total proteins are measured. These are, in fact, tests of liver damage (hence the term 'liver biochemistry') rather than actual liver function. Liver function is assessed by serum albumin and the pro-thrombin time.

Case history

A doctor phones you to ask whether a hospital referral is necessary for her patient. The doctor has recently seen a 55-year-old patient for a medical insurance examination for an American bank. She had found no problems with the patient at the time of the examination but the liver biochemistry results have come back abnormal. The tests showed:

- Serum bilirubin: 14 μmol/L
- Serum alkaline phosphatase: 134 IU/L
- AST: 70 IU/L
- ALT: 90 IU/L.

What advice do you give?

These tests suggest intra-hepatic disease and you ask about the patient's alcohol history. The answer is that only occasional alcohol is taken. You suggest that the doctor could arrange the following tests while waiting for an outpatient appointment:

- Repeat liver biochemistry
- Viral markers
- Serum autoantibodies
- Serum ferritin.

These tests will yield a diagnosis in most cases.

The doctor asks whether an ultrasound would be helpful

No. This is not the pattern of biliary or pancreatic disease.

You arrange to see the patient with your consultant in outpatients. At outpatients the history is again unhelpful. There is no history of:

- Blood transfusions
- Previous hepatitis
- IV drug use
- Sexual promiscuity.

On examination, you notice a few spider naevi. The liver is not palpable.

The results of the tests performed by the doctor are now available (Table 5.1). HCV antibodies indicate **HCV infection** (chronic hepatitis) and the patient will require HCV RNA, liver biopsy and treatment with anti-viral therapy.

Armed with the HCV result, you discuss IV drug use with your patient, who then admits to the very occasional use of IV drugs in her twenties.

Although this patient didn't have HBV, you need to know the significance of HBV markers (Table 5.2).

Progress. This patient was referred to the Liver clinic. Her HCV RNA showed 45 000 IU/mL viral load with genotype I infection. Direct-acting

Table 5.1 Further investigations into the cause of abnormal liver biochemistry

Test	Result	Implication
Repeat liver biochemistry	Similar to earlier	
Hepatitis A	IgG-positive IgM-negative	Patient has been infected with HAV in the past or immunised. This virus does *not* cause chronic liver disease
HBsAg	Negative	See later
HCV antibodies	Positive	
Autoantibody screen	Negative	Positive titres usually found in autoimmune hepatitis
Serum ferritin	110 µg/L	This excludes hereditary haemochromatosis

Table 5.2 Significance of viral markers in hepatitis B

Markers	Significance
Antigens	
HbsAg	Acute or chronic infection
HbeAg	Acute hepatitis B Persistence implies: Continuous infectious state Development of chronicity
HBV DNA	Implies viral replication Found in serum and liver Levels indicate response to antiviral treatment
Antibodies	
Anti-HBs	Immunity to HBV; previous exposure; vaccination
Anti-HBe	Seroconversion
Anti-HBc	
IgM	Acute hepatitis B (high titre) Chronic hepatitis B (low titre)
IgG	Past exposure to hepatitis B (HBsAg-negative)

From Feather A, Randall D, Waterhouse M, eds. *Kumar and Clark's Clinical Medicine, 10th edn.* Edinburgh: Elsevier, 2020; Box 34.9.

anti-viral agents are now the standard of care in the treatment of chronic HCV infection.

She was treated with glecaprevir–pibrentasvir once daily for 8 weeks, her liver biopsy showing no evidence of cirrhosis.

She had a sustained virological response and continues to be followed up in the Liver clinic.

JAUNDICE

Jaundice is detected clinically when the serum bilirubin is greater than 50 μmol/L (3 mg/dL).

Case history (1)

A 45-year-old woman has been admitted to the MAU with deep jaundice. She gives a history of two episodes of severe abdominal pain, which had lasted for about half an hour. She has lost her appetite and consequently lost some weight.

Abdominal examination is unhelpful; there were no signs of chronic liver disease.

The blood tests showed a raised serum bilirubin, an ALT of 50 U/L and a high alkaline phosphate of 410 IU/L. You order an ultrasound examination of the liver and biliary tree, as you suspect that she has gallstone disease (Fig. 5.1).

Investigations

- Blood count, liver biochemistry
- Liver function (INR and albumin)
- Abdominal ultrasound
- Viral markers to exclude hepatitis causing intra-hepatic cholestasis

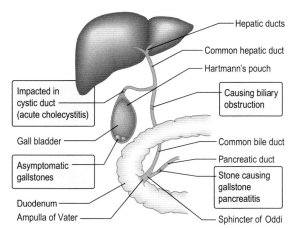

Figure 5.1 Clinical presentation of gallstones.

- Hepatic ducts
- Common hepatic duct
- Hartmann's pouch
- Causing biliary obstruction
- Impacted in cystic duct (acute cholecystitis)
- Gall bladder
- Asymptomatic gallstones
- Duodenum
- Ampulla of Vater
- Common bile duct
- Pancreatic duct
- Stone causing gallstone pancreatitis
- Sphincter of Oddi

Ultrasound in extra-hepatic obstruction can show:
- Dilatation of the intra-hepatic biliary tree
- Dilatation of the common bile duct
- Gallstones in the gall bladder
- Gallstones in the biliary tree
- A pancreatic mass
- Metastatic liver disease.

In this patient, the ultrasound showed gallstones in the gall bladder and a dilated common bile duct. Provided this patient's clotting is satisfactory, the next procedure should be an ERCP. This would enable better visualisation of the system and would allow a gallstone that is causing the obstruction in the common bile duct to be removed. A sphincterotomy would need to be performed beforehand and the stone could be removed with a basket or a balloon. If the stone is very large, it can be crushed and the debris removed. In an elderly patient, stent insertion to maintain drainage is an option.

Progress. In this patient the stones were cleared from the common bile duct at ERCP and this was followed by a laparoscopic cholecystectomy.

Remember

- Cholangitis often accompanies gallstones obstructing the biliary tree and urgent duct drainage should be performed. Antibiotics (e.g. ciprofloxacin 500 mg × 2 daily for 7–10 days) should be given.
- The residual stones are removed endoscopically when the patient has recovered.

Case history (2)

A 78-year-old man is admitted with marked jaundice. He was previously fit and well but the ultrasound arranged by his doctor showed a dilated biliary system with the probability of a pancreatic mass.

An endoscopic ultrasound and/or CT scan should be performed to assess the possibility of operability, although this is rare.

An ERCP with placement of a stent through the stricture enables drainage and is the usual treatment. This makes the patient feel a lot better, as well as relieving the jaundice. This was performed in this man.

Jaundice without pain is quite common with carcinoma of the pancreas but with gallstones there is usually a history of biliary pain accompanying the jaundice.

A similar obstruction could equally well be related to an obstruction higher up in the duct system, perhaps due to a cholangiocarcinoma. This could arise in pre-existing sclerosing cholangitis, although this would usually occur at a younger age.

Complications of ERCP sphincterotomy (complication rate 8–12%)

- Bleeding (severe in 2%).
- Perforation.
- Acute pancreatitis (5%).
- Cholangitis.

Case history (3)

A 20-year-old woman is admitted in a confused state and deeply jaundiced. She has recently returned from India, where she had been trekking; she had had a major argument with her boyfriend. A subconjunctival haemorrhage was noticed on examination.

This patient is critically ill with fulminant hepatic failure and it is essential to stabilise her as soon as possible.

A central venous line was inserted, and as her haemoglobin was very low, she was given 2 units of red blood cells. The clotting studies give an indication of the degree of damage to her liver, and will be useful for daily follow-up. It is also necessary to make sure that the patient's potassium and blood sugar are satisfactory, and whether replacements are necessary.

Investigations

- Hb
- Clotting studies and albumin
- Liver enzymes
- Blood sugar
- U&Es

This woman's investigation showed a bilirubin of 130 μmol/L, ALT 900 IU/L, AST 785 IU/L, alkaline phosphatase 109 IU/L, albumin 34 g/L, INR 2.2, indicating **severe hepatocellular damage**.

Further management

This patient is liable to infection and intravenous antibiotics are required after blood cultures have been taken.

Remember

Hepatic encephalopathy should be treated with a low-protein diet and rifaximin.

It is essential to try to establish the cause of this patient's jaundice. This might be hepatitis A or hepatitis E – both are endemic causes of hepatitis in India and often follow an initial respiratory type of illness; they can occasionally cause fulminant liver damage. A paracetamol overdose is also a possibility, as her boyfriend said that she was very upset when they returned to the UK.

Further investigation

- Viral markers for the above causes.
- Paracetamol levels.

These must be obtained urgently. Other investigations would include the following, if no cause has been found:

- Autoantibodies
- Copper studies
- Alpha-1 anti-trypsin levels.

In this case, the patient's relatives arrive and say they have found empty containers labelled 'paracetamol 500 mg tablets' in her bedroom.

The patient might well stabilise at this stage but a close eye will need to be kept on her for potential infections, particularly with opportunistic organisms. It is reasonable to give acetylcysteine in the initial management of such comatosed patients, whether or not the paracetamol blood level is high.

This patient's clinical condition deteriorated, with an early warning score (NEWS) of 5. She became increasingly drowsy and confused, and developed a flapping tremor and fetor hepaticus. Her investigations now showed a serum bilirubin of 320 µmol/L, ALT 3800 U/L, AST 4200 U/L and serum albumin 32 g/L, with an INR of 3.62. Urgent advice was sought from the nearest Liver unit.

CRITERIA FOR TRANSFER TO A SPECIALISED UNIT
- INR 3.0
- Presence of hepatic encephalopathy
- Hypotension after resuscitation with fluid
- Metabolic acidosis
- Prothrombin time (s) > interval (h) from overdose (in paracetamol cases)

You arrange for transfer. In specialised units, 70% of patients with paracetamol overdose and grade IV encephalopathy survive. Factors that indicate a poor prognosis with paracetamol overdose (without transplantation) are:
- Arterial pH <7.3 *or*
- Serum creatinine >300 µmol/L
- Prothrombin time >100 s
- Grade III–IV encephalopathy.

Progress. This woman was seriously ill with acute hepatic failure. She survived with supportive therapy, and transplantation was not necessary.

ACUTE LIVER DISEASE

Case history

A medical student turns up in A&E with jaundice. He is very worried that he has gallstones and might need surgery. He has never seen jaundice outside a surgical ward.

How do you approach this situation?

First, you point out that gallstones are rare in a young person and that viral hepatitis is, by far and away, the most likely diagnosis. You quickly ascertain that he has been previously immunised against hepatitis B and only drinks beer after rugby. He denies IV drug use. Your thoughts now turn to how he acquired hepatitis A. There is no clue from the history:
- No contacts with jaundice
- No prodromal features
- No travel abroad.
   On examination, apart from jaundice, there are no other abnormal signs.
   Take blood for:
- Liver biochemistry
- HAV IgM (to indicate acute HAV infection).
   You tell him to go back to his student flat, be careful with his personal hygiene and return in 2 days for his results (Table 5.3).
   Oops! HAV IgM-negative! You realise that although hepatitis A is very, very common in such a situation, there are other causes. You had omitted to take a careful drug history from someone you knew.
   Progress. This student turned out to have glandular fever (Epstein–Barr virus infection), which can occasionally present with jaundice.

Table 5.3	Test results in acute liver disease	
Test	**Result**	**Implication**
Serum bilirubin	70 μmol/L	
AST	300 IU/L	
ALT	280 IU/L	}Compatible with acute hepatitis
Alkaline phosphatase	140 IU/L	
HAV IgM	Negative	

ASCITES

Ascites is fluid within the peritoneal cavity due to sodium and water retention, e.g. cirrhosis or heart failure, or secondary to malignant deposits.

Case history (1)

A 45-year-old woman presents with ascites gradually increasing over 2 weeks.

Examination shows no abnormality outside the abdomen.

Determining the cause of the ascites is essential to developing a management plan and she is admitted to the MAU.

Investigations

- Liver biochemistry
- FBC
- INR and serum albumin
- Ascitic tap — for white cell count, culture, protein, malignant cells

Information

PARACENTESIS (ASCITIC TAP)

- Obtain the patient's consent after explaining the procedure.
- Percuss the dull area in the right iliac fossa.
- Clean the skin and inject local anaesthetic (1% lidocaine) into the skin using an orange needle.
- Insert a 21-gauge needle (green) on a 20 mL syringe into the fluid.
- Withdraw approximately 20 mL.
- Withdraw the needle and apply a dressing.

Ascitic fluid

The ascitic protein concentration, as well as the serum : ascites albumin gradient (SAG), helps differentiate a transudate (<5 g/L or SAG >11 g/L) from an exudate (>25 g/L or SAG >11 g/L).

In this case, a high ascitic protein (>25 g/L) suggests tumour or infection.

Malignant cells were present; further imaging with ultrasound and abdominal and pelvic CT were performed to determine the tumour site.

Diagnosis. In this patient, the age and sex suggested an **ovarian malignancy** and this was confirmed.

Progress. She was referred to the Gynaecology department for further management.

Case history (2)

A 45-year-old man has attended his doctor on many occasions with alcohol-related problems. He is sent to A&E with a swollen abdomen. He admits to drinking 60–80 units per week for 20 years.

On examination, he is not jaundiced but he does have spider naevi, liver palms, Dupuytren's contractures and testicular atrophy, as well as gross ascites and pitting ankle oedema.

What should you do?

Investigations

- Liver biochemistry
- FBC
- Serum albumin and INR
- Urea, creatinine, eGFR and electrolytes

An ascitic tap is necessary to rule out infection and malignancy, even though he has **chronic liver disease**.

Ascitic fluid showed 25 cells/mm^3 and protein content of 23 g/L, with a SAG of <9 g/L, i.e. a transudate.

- A transudate (<25 g/L) indicates cirrhosis without any complication.
- In a patient with known liver disease, a high WCC and high protein levels suggest infection (spontaneous bacterial peritonitis).

Ultrasound of the liver and spleen is now performed. It shows splenomegaly (portal hypertension) and an irregular liver with fat, indicative of cirrhosis.

Immediate management

- Bed rest.
- Salt restriction.
- Daily weights and U&Es.
- Start diuretics – spironolactone 100 mg/day (increasing gradually to 400 mg/day) to obtain a weight loss of 500 g/day.
- If there is an inadequate response to these measures, introduce furosemide 40–120 mg/day.
- Give thiamine 25–50 mg daily.
  The patient *must* stop drinking.

Subsequent management

It may be necessary to perform a liver biopsy to confirm the cause of cirrhosis, but only after the ascites is removed. If it is impossible to do a percutaneous liver biopsy, then biopsy can be undertaken through the jugular vein under X-ray control.

Progress. This patient was referred to the Alcohol Dependency Unit after resolution of his ankle swelling and ascites. He may require liver transplantation and should be referred to a Liver unit for assessment. He continues to abstain from alcohol but at present does not fit the criteria for transplantation (MELD – Model for End-stage Liver Disease – Score 7).

Remember

Liver disease with few cutaneous or other signs of liver disease can occur, particularly in chronic hepatitis C.

HAEMATEMESIS AND MELAENA

Haematemesis is vomiting blood. Melaena is the passage of black, tarry stools, usually from a lesion proximal to the right colon.

Case history

A 70-year-old man was admitted, having vomited blood this morning. His stools have been loose and black (melaena).

On initial assessment he looked pale and was shocked, with a tachycardia of 110 bpm and a BP of 80/60 mmHg.

An IV cannula was immediately inserted, blood taken for Hb, U&Es, clotting, and grouping and cross-matching for 4 units. He was initially given fluid replacement with a colloid and transferred to ITU after qSOFA assessment.

Resuscitation

- IV access.
- CVP assessment.
- Fluid replacement (initially with colloid).
- Blood transfusion.
- O_2 for shocked patients.

Remember

Hb <100 g/L, urea ↑, postural hypotension present, pulse rate 110 bpm. This patient is severely compromised and needs urgent treatment.

The gastroenterologists and surgical teams were informed. He was admitted to the high-dependency unit and a CVP line was inserted.

Many hospitals have MDTs and protocols. Keep the patient nil by mouth until the bleeding has stopped. Causes of upper gastrointestinal bleeding are shown in Fig. 5.2.

A further history of this man revealed that he had had a high alcohol intake of 70 units/week for many years. He had no history of long-term dyspepsia and didn't take NSAIDs, including aspirin.

On examination, he had signs of chronic liver disease with spider naevi and gynaecomastia. His liver was 4 cm palpable and he had splenomegaly.

Remember

SHOCK
- Pallor
- Cold nose
- ↓ Systolic BP.

Common causes of a GI bleed

- Peptic ulcer.
- Gastric erosions.
- Oesophageal varices.

Management

The patient's Hb was returned as 90 g/L and the urea was raised at 10 mmol/L. A blood transfusion was started to resuscitate him (Fig. 5.3).

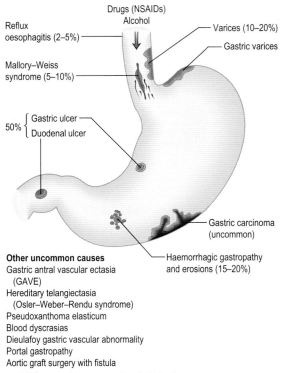

Figure 5.2 Causes of upper gastrointestinal bleeding.

On improvement, he had an endoscopy, which showed oesophageal varices, and these were banded (Fig. 5.4). On return to the ward, he had a further haematemesis 4 h later. Vasoconstrictor therapy was given.

Vasoconstrictor therapy

The main use of this is for emergency control of bleeding while waiting for endoscopy and in combination with endoscopic techniques. The aim of vasoconstrictor agents is to restrict portal inflow by splanchnic arterial constriction.

- **Terlipressin.** This is the only vasoconstrictor shown to reduce mortality. Dose is 2 mg 6-hourly, reducing to 1 mg 4-hourly after 48 h if a prolonged dosage regimen is used. It should not be given to patients with ischaemic heart disease. The patient will complain of abdominal colic, will defecate and have facial pallor owing to the generalised vasoconstriction.

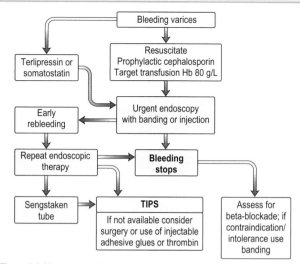

Figure 5.3 Management of gastrointestinal haemorrhage due to oesophageal varices. TIPS, transjugular intra-hepatic portosystemic shunt.

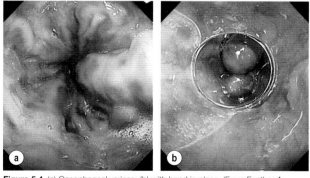

Figure 5.4 (a) Oesophageal varices; (b) with band in place. (From Feather A, Randall D, Waterhouse M, eds. *Kumar and Clark's Clinical Medicine*, 10th edn. Edinburgh: Elsevier, 2020; Fig. 34.24, courtesy of Dr Peter Fairclough.)

- **Somatostatin.** This drug has few side-effects. An infusion of 250–500 μg/h appears to reduce bleeding but has no effect on mortality. It should be used if there are contraindications to terlipressin.

Balloon tamponade with a Sengstaken—Blakemore tube can be used if the bleeding continues. Use the gastric balloon only initially, but if the bleeding is not controlled, inflate the oesophageal balloon, remembering that continuous inflation leads to oesophageal damage. It has serious complications and should be left in situ for only 24 h.

If these measures fail, a transjugular intra-hepatic portosystemic shunt (TIPS) might be required; this is often used as the treatment of choice for gastric varices.

Progress. Unfortunately, this patient continued to bleed, despite a repeat endoscopy with injection of the varices. A Sengstaken—Blakemore tube was put in place and he was therefore referred urgently to a Liver unit for TIPS insertion.

Remember

Erosions can bleed profusely and be very difficult to control.

LIVER FAILURE

Case history

A 60-year-old female has been a known user of alcohol for the past 20 years. She is admitted because of a deterioration in her health, with confusion and the development of ascites.

Further history indicates that she stopped drinking some 2 months ago and suffered no withdrawal symptoms.

On examination, you wonder whether she has liver failure.

What signs indicate liver failure?

- Jaundice.
- Ascites/portal hypertension (splenomegaly).
- Hepatic encephalopathy:
  - Hepatic flap
  - Fetor hepaticus
  - Constructional apraxia.
- Signs of chronic liver disease, e.g.:
  - Spider naevi
  - Gynaecomastia
  - Dupuytren's contracture
  - Liver palms.

If there is no risk of bleeding, concentrate on determining the level of encephalopathy:

- Grade 1: disorientated
- Grade 2: confused
- Grade 3: comatose
- Grade 4: unconscious.

Early signs can be demonstrated by asking the patient to copy a five-pointed star.

Information

Portosystemic encephalopathy (PSE) is a neuropsychiatric syndrome that occurs in cirrhosis. The blood bypasses the liver via collaterals, allowing 'toxic' metabolites to pass directly to the brain. The nature of these 'toxins' is unclear but they appear to be related to ammonia. Treatment is aimed at reduction of protein breakdown in the gut and rifaximin therapy.

Immediate management

- Measure electrolytes and blood sugar, liver function and liver biochemistry.
- Perform an ascitic tap to rule out infection (see p. 61).
- Institute a low-protein and low-salt diet.
- Give parenteral thiamine.
- Establish an infusion of 5% glucose (10% if blood sugar is low).
- Start diuretic therapy (see ascites).
- Use purgatives: lactulose $10-20$ mL $\times 3$/day to produce $2-3$ stools a day.
- Determine presence of infection both in ascites (ascitic tap) and systemically (blood culture), and treat.

Further management

Monitor daily:
- Weight (see ascites)
- Conscious level (GCS score)
- Liver biochemistry and coagulation
- Electrolytes and blood sugar.

Progress. This woman's condition improved dramatically and she was ready for discharge from hospital after 10 days. She was referred to the Alcohol Dependency Unit and regular follow-up was arranged at the Liver clinic.

EXCESS ALCOHOL USE

Case history

A 45-year-old man presents with a history of excessive alcohol intake for 10 years since his marriage failed. He has sought help from counselling services but has been unable to remain sober. His presenting symptoms were of collapses in the street and home — the most recent collapse was witnessed and reported as epileptic.

Neurological examination shows that he is conscious and aware of his surroundings but confused (GCS 13). He has nystagmus and ataxia when asked to walk. ***Examination of his legs*** shows diminished sensation to light touch, pinprick and vibration below the knees. Ankle jerks are absent.

This man has two features of excess alcohol consumption.
1. Central findings: Wernicke–Korsakoff syndrome. This is sometimes reversible with parenteral thiamine therapy.
2. Peripheral neuropathy: usually not reversible on alcohol abstinence or vitamin therapy.

Management

Start IV vitamins immediately; parenteral vitamin B and C should be used for the first 3 days. *Note:* Serious, allergic adverse reactions can occur. Give injections slowly and know how to treat anaphylaxis. Thiamine 100 mg $\times 3$ daily should be given orally throughout the admission.

Information

Epilepsy occurs in 3–10% of patients who have alcohol dependence associated with:
- Alcohol intoxication
- Alcohol withdrawal
- Hypoglycaemia.

A full history and examination must be undertaken to exclude:
- Neurological damage (central, peripheral)
- Hepatic damage/signs of liver failure
- Use of other drugs.

Further treatment

- Withdraw all alcohol.
- Sedate: use benzodiazepines in adequate doses to produce sedation but beware of respiratory depression.
- Keep under supervision.
- Don't mix sedatives.
- Reduce benzodiazepines slowly over the next 5 days, observing resolution of signs of withdrawal:
  - Sweating
  - Shaking
  - Vomiting
  - Agitation
  - Hallucination.
- Don't use anti-epileptics.

Further management

Seek help from agencies dealing with alcohol and drug use for assessment and further management. Following abstinence, give acamprosate 666 mg × 3 daily. This drug acts by enhancing GABAergic inhibition.

Lesser degrees of damage than in the case described can occur in excess alcohol use and must always be assessed in all patients attending hospital. These findings are commonly hidden and should be sought using a non-judgemental interviewing style.

Additional biochemical tests can help to determine the physical damage produced by alcohol (MCV, triglycerides, uric acid, γ-GT).

Remember

There are many initiating factors for alcohol excess. It produces damage in many areas of function — financial, social, psychological and physical — and all need addressing.

Progress. This man was discharged from hospital with regular attendance at the Alcohol Dependence Unit. His attendance became erratic and he started drinking again.

CHOLECYSTITIS

Case history

A 28-year-old man presents to the A&E department with right hypochondrial pain. This has been persistent, increasing in severity over the last 3 days.

On examination, there is right hypochondrial tenderness. In view of his age and general good health he is sent home after surgical review, given paracetamol and told to see his doctor for follow-up.

Two days later a rather concerned doctor phones A&E to say that the patient's pain has persisted and the tenderness is marked. You ask him to send him back to A&E. *On examination*, you confirm the doctor's findings of marked tenderness in the right hypochondrium. He has a temperature of 37.8°C.

What should you do now?

Given the persistence of pain and the second referral by his doctor, admit the patient to the MAU. Do the blood tests shown in the investigations box.

- FBC
- U&Es
- Liver biochemistry
- Serum amylase
- Blood culture in view of pyrexia

One hour later your trainee doctor phones you to say the patient's WCC is 19 000. Clearly, he has an infection and you tell your trainee to organise an urgent ultrasound while you call the surgical registrar. The surgical registrar recognises the patient he discharged 2 days ago. You discuss possible diagnoses. The ultrasound scan (Fig. 5.5) shows:

- Gallstones in the gall bladder
- Sonographic Murphy's sign
- Gall bladder wall thickening
- Peri-cholecystic fluid.

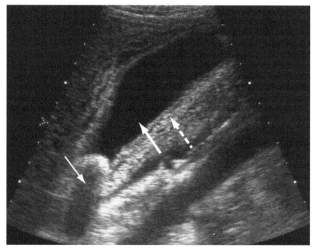

Figure 5.5 Ultrasound scan in a patient with acute cholecystitis. There is a stone (casting an acoustic shadow – thin arrow) impacted in the gall bladder neck, with a distended gall bladder (thick arrow), and thickening and oedema of the gall bladder wall (dashed arrow). (From Kumar P, Clark M, eds. *Kumar and Clark's Clinical Medicine*, 9th edn. Edinburgh: Elsevier, 2017; Fig. 15.4.)

Diagnosis

Remember

- Acute appendicitis: but the site of pain is a bit high.
- Acute cholecystitis: but the patient is 28 years old and a man.
- A localised perforation and other mischief run through your mind.

The diagnosis is **acute cholecystitis.** The surgical specialist registrar starts antibiotics (a cephalosporin, e.g. cefuroxime), nil by mouth and IV fluids. He books the patient for a laparoscopic cholecystectomy in 2 days' time.

Remember

Gallstones can occur at any age and not necessarily in fair, fat, fertile females of 40! Always think of appendicitis in a young patient with acute pain. Ultrasound/CT scans are invaluable in making the diagnosis.

Progress. A successful laparoscopic cholecystectomy was performed with no complications.

Further reading

Abnormal liver biochemistry

Zeuzem S, Foster GR, Wang S, et al. Glecaprevir-pibrentasvir for 8 or 12 weeks in HCV genotype 1 or 3 infection. *New England Journal of Medicine* 2018; **378**: 354–369.

Jaundice

Kindler HL. A glimmer of hope for pancreatic cancer. *New England Journal of Medicine* 2018; **379**: 2463–2464.

Ascites

Lucey MR. Liver transplantation for alcoholic liver disease. *National Review of Gastroenterology and Hepatology* 2014; **11**: 300–307.

Moore KP, Wong F, Gines P, et al. Management of ascites in cirrhosis. Report on the consensus conference of the International Ascites Club. *Hepatology* 2003; **38**: 258–266.

Haematemesis and melaena

BSG (British Society for Gastroenterology). UK guidelines for the management of variceal haemorrhage in cirrhotic patients. www.bsg.org.uk/clinical-resource/uk-guidelines-for-the-management-of-variceal-haemorrhage-in-cirrhotic-patients/

Jalan R, Hayes PC. UK Guidelines on the management of variceal haemorrhage in cirrhotic patients. *Gut* 2000; **46** (Suppl 3–4): III1–III5.

Haematology and Oncology 6

MICROCYTIC AND MACROCYTIC ANAEMIA

Definition of anaemia

Anaemia is present when the level of haemoglobin in the blood is below the normal range (NR). The NR varies at different ages and between men (130–180 g/L) and women (115–155 g/L).

Remember

An accurate result depends on a correctly taken blood sample:
- Avoid prolonged venous occlusion.
- Don't take the sample from an arm with an IV infusion.
  If the haemoglobin concentration does not fit the clinical picture, take another sample.

Assessment

The impact of anaemia on an individual is variable and will depend on:
- The degree of anaemia
- The speed of onset
- Age
- Cardiovascular reserve.
  Symptoms are non-specific and clinical signs easily overlooked:
- Tiredness, lack of energy
- Shortness of breath on exercise
- Palpitations
- Ischaemic pain.

Investigations

The **classification of anaemia** (Fig. 6.1) is based on the mean corpuscular/red cell volume (MCV; NR 76–96 fL).

Further investigation is determined by whether the anaemia is microcytic (<76 fL), macrocytic (> 96 fL) or normocytic.

Case history (1)

A 45-year-old woman of African origin presents to the A&E department with chest pain that is thought to reflect cardiac ischaemia.

On examination, she looked well. CVS examination showed a pulse of 82/min, a blood pressure of 140/80 and no abnormal signs. General examination was normal.

Investigations:
- Hb 99 g/L
- MCV 59 fL
- Red cell distribution width (RDW) 14%
- WCC 6.4×10^9/L
- Platelets 273×10^9/L

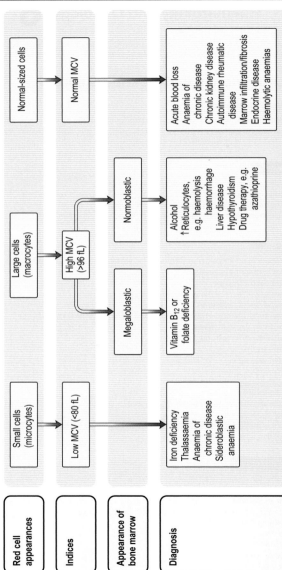

Figure 6.1 Classification of anaemia. MCV, mean corpuscular volume.

- ESR 10 mm/h
- Anisocytosis, poikilocytosis +
- Target cells + +

  These are the features of a microcytic anaemia.

What is the reason for her anaemia and is it relevant to her presentation?

The first thing to exclude is iron deficiency, commonly due to uterine or gastrointestinal bleeding. Iron deficiency is unlikely in this patient:

- Very low MCV with only moderate anaemia
- Minimal variation in red cell size (anisocytosis) and shape (poikilocytosis)
- The serum ferritin (30 µg/L) was normal, indicating normal tissue stores of iron. (*Note:* ferritin can be high because it is an acute-phase protein that rises whenever the ESR or CRP is elevated.)

The anaemia of chronic disorder, a form of functional iron deficiency, is also unlikely without an obvious underlying illness and a normal ESR.

Remember

- Ferritin is an acute-phase protein. Iron deficiency can therefore be difficult to diagnose in the presence of inflammatory disease, and tissue iron stores might need to be examined directly by bone marrow aspiration.
- Serum transferrin receptor assay does differentiate between these conditions.

A common cause of a microcytic anaemia in patients of certain ethnic groups is β-thalassaemia trait. This is common in people from Africa, the Mediterranean, the Middle East, India and SE Asia.

Characteristically, β-thalassaemia trait results in a marked microcytosis with only a moderate anaemia, as shown in this patient. In addition, the RDW is normal. (*N.B.* It is high in iron deficiency.)

Beta-thalassaemia trait is confirmed by measuring HbA_2, which is normally <3.4% of total haemoglobin.

Progress. The HbA_2 in this patient was 5.2%, confirming a diagnosis of β-**thalassaemia trait**.

Patients are asymptomatic and require no treatment. *Note:* Don't give iron. The anaemia is not contributory to this patient's cardiac ischaemia. The patient was referred to the Cardiac department for investigation and management of her chest pain.

Remember

The anaemia of β-thalassaemia trait is:
- Life-long
- Stable.

Iron deficiency anaemia

Iron deficiency anaemia (Fig. 6.2 and see p. 71) responds to treatment with oral iron supplements: ferrous sulphate 200 mg × 3 daily (or all in one dose) for 6 months. It is essential to give a full course of treatment. Lower the dose if GI symptoms occur. Parenteral therapy is required only rarely. The cause of iron deficiency is almost always blood loss and the cause *must* be determined.

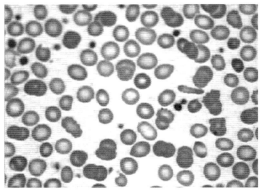

Figure 6.2 Typical blood film in chronic iron deficiency anaemia. Note the pale red cells with pencil (elongated) cells.

Other causes include:
- Poor diet
- Multiple pregnancies
- Regular blood donation.

Case history (2)

An 81-year-old woman presents to the A&E department with recent-onset congestive cardiac failure.

On examination, she is mildly jaundiced and anaemic. Her pulse was 88/min, BP 120/90. She had signs of heart failure with a raised venous pressure, a third heart sound, basal crackles and marked lower leg oedema.

Investigations:
- Hb 32 g/L
- MCV 121 fL
- WCC 1.5×10^9/L
- Platelets 64×10^9/L
- Anisopoikilocytosis + + +
- Hypersegmented neutrophils present

The findings indicate a severe macrocytic anaemia with a moderate neutropenia and thrombocytopenia. The diagnosis could be **pernicious anaemia**.

Vitamin B_{12} or folate deficiency impairs DNA synthesis and affects all rapidly dividing cells, particularly in the bone marrow, resulting in pancytopenia when severe. The anaemia is slow to develop and elderly patients, in particular, often don't present until very late.

Avoid blood transfusion, if at all possible, because there is a risk of volume overload and acute left ventricular failure.

Make a precise diagnosis by measuring serum vitamin B_{12}, serum and red cell folate:

- In vitamin B_{12} deficiency the serum vitamin B_{12} concentration is always reduced; in folate deficiency the red cell folate concentration is always reduced.
- Severe vitamin B_{12} deficiency can be associated with a low red cell folate and a normal or high serum folate. Vitamin B_{12} is the co-factor in the reaction that cycles 5-methyl-tetrahydrofolate. This allows folic acid to be retained within the cells.

Remember

Drugs and rare metabolic defects can result in megaloblastic anaemia with normal vitamin levels:
- Methotrexate induces functional folate deficiency.
- Transcobalamin II deficiency results in intracellular vitamin B_{12} deficiency (but is very rare).

Bone marrow aspiration (not generally necessary since modern analysers can provide rapid vitamin B_{12} levels):
- Confirms megaloblastic erythropoiesis
- Documents pre-treatment iron stores
- Excludes other conditions – myelodysplasia, acute leukaemia and aplastic anaemia – all of which can present with a macrocytosis and pancytopenia.

Causes

- **Folate deficiency?** Nutritional deficiency is almost always a factor in any cause of folate deficiency, whether this is due to increased requirements (e.g. myelofibrosis, haemolysis) or to excess alcohol use. In malabsorption, e.g. coeliac disease, there is also poor dietary intake of folate.
- **B_{12} deficiency?** Most cases of vitamin B_{12} deficiency are due to malabsorption, either gastric (because of intrinsic factor deficiency) or intestinal (due to small bowel disease). Pernicious anaemia (antibodies against intrinsic factor) is the most common cause.

Additional investigations

- Intrinsic factor antibody assay (positive in 50% of patients with pernicious anaemia).
- Anti-tissue transglutaminase antibodies and/or jejunal biopsy (to exclude coeliac disease).
- Barium meal and follow-through (to exclude small bowel disease, e.g. Crohn's disease); in a woman of this age, only after the other causes have been excluded.

Many patients with moderate vitamin B_{12} or folate deficiency have a normal haemoglobin with a raised MCV. Vitamin assays should be performed if the clinical picture is suggestive of a deficiency.
- GI disease or surgery, including glossitis, malabsorption or diarrhoea
- Neurological disease, including visual loss, a peripheral neuropathy or evidence of demyelination
- Psychiatric disorders, including dementia, confusion or depression
- Malabsorption or restricted diets, including vegans and those with anorexia nervosa

- Alcohol excess
- Infertility
- Autoimmune endocrine disease
- Family history of pernicious anaemia
- Drug therapy, particularly anti-convulsants.

Diagnosis. This patient had megaloblastic anaemia secondary to severe vitamin B_{12} deficiency.

Pernicious anaemia

- Serum B_{12}: 25 ng/L (NR 160–960 ng/L).
- Serum folate: 14.6 µg/L (NR 4.0–18.0 µg/L).
- Red cell folate: 86 µg/L (NR 160–640 µg/L).

Management

Whenever possible, treat with one haematinic only. In this patient, treat with hydroxocobalamin 1000 µg IM daily for 3 days, total 5–6 mg over 2 weeks then 1000 µg every 3 months for life.

> **Remember**
>
> Never give folate alone because, although it might partially correct the blood abnormalities associated with vitamin B_{12} deficiency, it will also cause the B_{12} level to drop even further and might precipitate severe neuropathy.

Do FBCs with reticulocytes and U&Es initially daily (in a severely anaemic patient – as in this case) to look for:

- Hypokalaemia, which can occasionally develop 1–2 days post therapy
- Reticulocyte count, which starts to increase 2–3 days after treatment and reaches a peak on days 5–7
- Hb concentration, which often falls further before starting to rise.

Stay calm! Avoid blood transfusion. Failure of the reticulocyte count and haemoglobin to rise in the predicted manner might be due to:

- Incorrect diagnosis and/or treatment: review laboratory data
- Coexistent iron deficiency: check iron stores, e.g. ferritin levels
- Intercurrent infection: review patient – chest infection, urinary tract infection?
- Coexistent hypothyroidism.

> **Remember**
>
> Pernicious anaemia is an autoimmune disease; 1–2% of patients will also develop thyroid disease. Gastric cancer is also slightly more common (1–3% of cases).

The majority of patients with vitamin B_{12} deficiency have vitamin B_{12} malabsorption and require life-long treatment with vitamin B_{12}.

Treatment. Hydroxocobalamin 1000 µg IM every 3 months is given but high doses of vitamin B_{12} (2 mg) daily by mouth are also effective.

Nutritional deficiency of vitamin B_{12} is rare and confined to vegans.

Anaemia due to folic acid deficiency

These patients need 6 months' treatment with folic acid 5 mg daily after the cause (e.g. coeliac disease, see p. 48) has been defined and treated. Folic acid is ineffective, however, in the treatment of methotrexate toxicity, when folinic acid 15 mg IV daily is given.

HAEMOLYTIC ANAEMIA

Haemolytic anaemias are caused by increased destruction of red cells in two sites: intravascular or extravascular.

Case history

A 60-year-old woman presents with a history of feeling tired and exhausted for the last week. She is normally well but is under the care of the haematologists with chronic lymphocytic leukaemia (CLL). She knows all about the condition, having been diagnosed 4 years ago. She is not on any treatment but is under regular follow-up.

On examination, she is clinically jaundiced, with cervical lymphadenopathy and a just palpable spleen.

Investigations:
- Hb 68 g/L
- MCV 90 fL
- WCC 30×10^9/L
- Platelets 172×10^9/L
- Reticulocytes 18.8%
- Anisopoikilocytosis + +
- Polychromasia + +
- Spherocytes present
- Lymphocytosis with smear cells.

She has a normocytic anaemia with a raised white cell count and a reticulocytosis.

A normocytic anaemia can be due to:

- Acute blood loss
- Lack of erythropoietin – chronic kidney disease
- Bone marrow infiltration, e.g. carcinoma
- Haemolysis.

The patient described is anaemic and jaundiced with splenomegaly, suggesting a haemolytic anaemia. To confirm this you need to demonstrate:
- Increased red cell production
- A reduced red cell lifespan.

Increased red cell production

- Reticulocytosis: reticulocytes are immature red cells newly released from the bone marrow. They are larger than mature red cells, contain mRNA and appear polychromatic on standard blood films.
- Bone marrow aspiration: erythroid hyperplasia.

Remember

Cortisol, androgens and thyroxine are all required for optimal erythropoiesis.

Reduced red cell lifespan

- Acholuric jaundice: unconjugated hyperbilirubinaemia, urobilinogen but no bilirubin in the urine.

- Abnormal red cell morphology: this might also indicate the specific cause of the haemolytic anaemia (see later).
- Demonstrated directly by radioactive isotope studies: reduced survival of ^{51}Cr-labelled autologous red cells (performed only if the diagnosis of haemolysis is in doubt).

There are many specific causes of haemolysis. The diagnosis can often be made by review of the blood film. Speak to the Haematology medical staff.

Features of haemolysis on blood film

- Spherocytes: autoimmune haemolytic anaemia, hereditary spherocytosis, *Clostridium welchii* septicaemia, extensive burns.
- Red cell fragments: leaking mechanical heart valve, disseminated malignancy.
- Sickled cells: sickle-cell anaemia, sickle-cell–HbC disease.
- Bitten-out red cells: glucose-6-phosphate dehydrogenase deficiency, unstable haemoglobin, oxidative drug therapy, e.g. dapsone.
- Malaria parasites.

Investigations

- Antibody screen and direct anti-globulin test (DAT): in autoimmune haemolytic anaemia autoantibodies to red cell membrane antigens are present in serum and on the red cell surface
- Urinary haemosiderin: positive in chronic intravascular haemolysis, such as paroxysmal nocturnal haemoglobinuria (PNH, very rare) and leaking mechanical heart valves
- Flow cytometry with antibodies against CD55 and CD59 antigens for PNH
- Glucose-6-phosphate dehydrogenase assay: common enzyme deficiency in particular ethnic groups (African, Mediterranean, SE Asian)

This patient had a strongly positive DAT with anti-IgG (see Fig. 6.13). The antibody eluted from her red cells was also present free in her serum and didn't have any easily definable antigen specificity. She therefore has autoimmune haemolytic anaemia (AIHA) due to an IgG red cell autoantibody active at 37°C. AIHA can be primary or secondary. This patient is known to have CLL, and has lymphadenopathy and a lymphocytosis with small, mature lymphocytes. Her AIHA is secondary to the underlying CLL; 10–15% of patients with CLL develop AIHA.

Diagnosis. Autoimmune haemolytic anaemia (secondary to underlying CLL).

Management

- Start oral prednisolone 60 mg/day. This usually produces a remission. Corticosteroids reduce the production of antibodies and also destroy antibody-coated red cells.
- Blood transfusion is necessary if the Hb continues to fall. Compatibility testing is complex because the autoantibody interferes with the cross-match; the laboratory could carry out autoabsorption studies to exclude additional alloantibodies. Transfuse slowly.
- Refer the patient to her consultant in Haematology to discuss further management.

AIHA can develop acutely with a rapid fall in Hb. This patient has a short history. Check the Hb concentration at least once a day.

Progress. This patient went into remission on the steroids. Steroids are effective in about 80% of cases. The haematologists gradually reduced her steroids over 3 months and she was started on azathioprine. A year later, her CLL became active and she is now on rituximab and fludarabine.

SICKLE-CELL DISEASE

Case history

An 18-year-old female of African origin came to A&E with severe pains in her right leg, left hip, chest and back. She was well known to many of the staff, as she had attended on many occasions with **painful sickle crises.** She had been out all night at a club.

The examination should initially be brief until adequate pain control has been achieved.

Investigations

Performed in the MAU, and aimed at assessing the severity of the crisis and determining any treatable cause:
- FBC plus reticulocytes
- U&Es
- Liver biochemistry.
  Compare values with normal steady-state values, which should be in the patient's notes. Remember that many nucleated red cells can result in an erroneously high WCC count:
- MSU
- Blood cultures
  Infection is a frequent precipitant of a painful crisis:
- O_2 saturation on air (see Information box)
- Group and save

Questions to ask patients presenting with sickle-cell crises

Distribution of pain? Any bone tenderness?
- Lumbar back pain can be particularly severe.
- Rib, sternal or thoracic vertebral pain can impair respiratory effort and predispose to the acute chest syndrome.

Any precipitating factors?
- Exposure to cold/skin chilling (might apply to this patient).
- Dehydration (could also apply to this patient).
- Hypoxia.
- Infection.

A low O_2 saturation might reflect acute lung pathology, e.g. pneumonia or the acute chest syndrome, or chronic sickle-cell-related lung damage.

CXR and arterial gases are indicated only if there is:
- Rib, sternal and thoracic vertebral pain
- Signs of consolidation
- Tachypnoea (> 25/min)
- O_2 saturation $<80\%$ on air or $<95\%$ on maximal supplementary O_2.

Any fever?
- Fever $\pm$ leucocytosis can indicate an underlying infection but is also compatible with ischaemic tissue necrosis secondary to intravascular sickling alone.

Any hepatosplenomegaly?
- Splenomegaly is unusual in adults with HbSS or HbS/β^0 thalassaemia; splenic atrophy is more common.
- A larger spleen than normal for the patient (ask the patient or parents/consult medical notes) might indicate acute splenic sequestration.

Compliance with hyposplenic prophylaxis?
- Patients with HbSS and HbS/β^0 thalassaemia have severe hyposplenism and are susceptible to overwhelming sepsis, particularly with *Streptococcus pneumoniae*.
- Prophylaxis includes penicillin V 500 mg $\times 2$ daily and vaccination with polyvalent pneumococcal, Hib and meningococcal vaccines.

Treatment of acute painful sickle-cell crises

Analgesia
Morphine/diamorphine
- 0.1 mg/kg IV/SC every 20 min until pain controlled, *then*
- 0.05–0.1 mg/kg IV/SC (or oral morphine) every 2–4 h.
- Patient-controlled analgesia (PCA) when pain controlled.

N.B. Ask the patient about previous morphine dosages. Check medical records and discharge summaries. Higher doses may be required in cases who have previously received opioids.

Patient-controlled analgesia (PCA) (example for adults >50 kg)
Diamorphine
- Continuous infusion: 0–10 mg/h.
- PCA bolus dose: 2–10 mg.
- Dose duration: 1 min.
- Lockout time: 20–30 min.

When diamorphine or other parenteral opiates are used, the following parameters must be monitored regularly on an hourly basis:
- Pain score
- Respiratory rate

- O_2 saturation on air
- Analgesia consumption.

Adjuvant oral analgesia
- Paracetamol 1 g 6-hourly
- ± Ibuprofen* 400 mg 8-hourly
- *or* Diclofenac* 50 mg 8-hourly.
  Supplementary analgesia may be provided by:
- Regular oral dihydrocodeine and/or NSAIDs
- TENS (transcutaneous electrical nerve stimulation)
- Acupuncture
- Massage with analgesic rub
- Laxatives (all patients), e.g.:
  - Lactulose 10 mL × 2 daily
  - Senna 2–4 tablets daily
  - Sodium docusate 100 mg × 2 daily
  - Macrogol 1 sachet daily.

Other adjuvants
- Anti-pruritics:
  - Hydroxyzine 25 mg × 2 as required
- Anti-emetics:
  - Prochlorperazine 5–10 mg × 3 as required
  - Cyclizine 50 mg × 3 as required
- Anxiolytic:
  - Haloperidol 1–3 mg oral IM × 2 as required.

Remember

Failure to maintain oxygenation can:
- Exacerbate the painful crisis
- Indicate the development of the acute chest syndrome.

Hydroxycarbamide is useful in increasing HbF. It should be prescribed by haematologists and often takes months to have an effect. It reduces the episodes of pain, the acute chest syndrome and the need for blood transfusions. The overall mortality has also been shown to be reduced.

Supportive measures
- Keep warm: use heat pads.
- Hydration: aim for 3 L/24 h – orally if possible.
- Venous access is often very difficult in these patients; the repeated insertion of IV lines should be avoided to conserve peripheral veins.
- IV hydration is indicated if:
  - Nausea/vomiting is uncontrolled
  - The patient is sedated
  - The serum urea and creatinine are rising.

* Caution advised against using NSAIDs in renal impairment.

Kumar & Clark's Cases in Clinical Medicine

- Oxygenation: aim for O_2 saturation 95%.
- Monitor the Hb concentration daily and transfuse if it falls to 150 g/L. All transfused blood should be matched for minor blood group antigens Kell and Rh (C and e, as well as D antigens).

Remember

Don't use transfusions in this steady-state anaemia, in an uncomplicated painful episode and for minor surgery.

The acute chest syndrome

Most painful sickle-cell crises resolve without complications within 7–10 days. Development of the acute chest syndrome is the most common cause of death in adults with sickle-cell disease.

The syndrome is characterised by:
- Rib, sternal and/or thoracic vertebral pain
- Bilateral basal chest signs with new infiltrates on CXR
- Tachypnoea
- Deteriorating oxygenation
- Falling Hb concentration
- Fever and leucocytosis.

Pathophysiology of acute chest syndrome

- Infection.
- Fat embolism from necrotic bone marrow.
- Pulmonary infarction due to sequestration of sickled red cells.

Treatment of acute chest syndrome

- Exchange blood transfusion to reduce the amount of HbS to <20%.
- Maintenance of oxygenation: this might include, for example, continuous positive airway pressure (CPAP) via a tight-fitting mask, or intermittent positive pressure ventilation (IPPV).
- Aggressive pain relief.
- Intravenous antibiotic therapy.

The majority of patients with a sickle-cell crisis present with severe, acute bone pain secondary to ischaemic bone marrow necrosis. Beware the patient with sickle-cell disease who presents unwell but without pain. Such patients might have other, less common, complications of sickle-cell disease, which can progress very rapidly (Figs. 6.3 and 6.4).

Remember

OTHER COMPLICATIONS OF SICKLE-CELL DISEASE INCLUDE
- Pneumococcal septicaemia
- Splenic sequestration
- Erythrovirus infection associated with marrow aplasia
- Acute folate deficiency.

Progress. This patient's current crisis was more severe than her previous ones and she went on to develop the acute chest syndrome, from which she died.

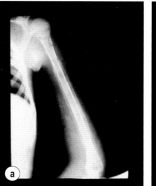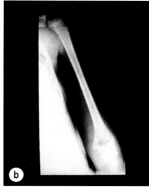

Figure 6.3 (a) Osteomyelitis of the humerus in a sickle patient (pre-treatment). Note the elevation of the periosteum at the distal part of the humerus. (b) The same patient showing normal periosteum following treatment.

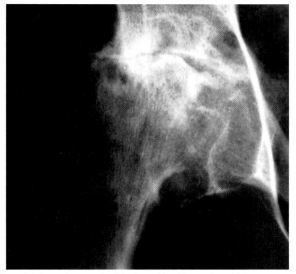

Figure 6.4 Avascular necrosis of the femoral head in a patient with homozygous sickle-cell disease. There is loss of joint space and distortion of the head of the femur and acetabulum.

TYPES OF SICKLE-CELL DISEASE

- Sickle-cell anaemia HbSS.
- Sickle-cell–haemoglobin C disease HbSC.
- Sickle-cell β-thalassaemia.
- Rare compound heterozygotes, e.g. HbSD.

Diagnosis in A&E/MAU

- Information from patient.
- Haemoglobinopathy card.
- Blood count, reticulocyte count and blood film review.
- Serum bilirubin.
- Sickle solubility test (commercial kits are available).
  Later:
- Hb electrophoresis (Fig. 6.5) on cellulose acetate membrane (CAM) at an alkaline pH, *or*
- High-performance liquid chromatography (HPLC).

Typically, the patient will be anaemic with evidence of haemolysis (elevated bilirubin and reticulocyte count). The blood film will show sickled red cells in variable numbers (Fig. 6.6). The sickle solubility test will be positive and CAM electrophoresis or HPLC will confirm the presence of HbS ± HbC or HbD with no HbA (except in HbS/β⁺ thalassaemia).

Beware

- In HbSC and HbS/β⁺ thalassaemia the haemoglobin concentration, reticulocyte count and serum bilirubin can be virtually normal.

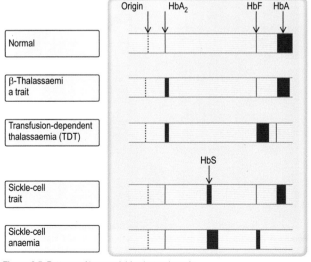

Figure 6.5 Patterns of haemoglobin electrophoresis.

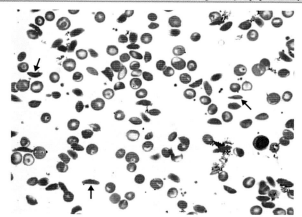

Figure 6.6 Blood film in sickle-cell disease showing numerous sickle-shaped red cells (arrows).

- The sickle solubility test is a qualitative test only and will be positive in any individual where the amount of HbS is >10%. This will include both sickle-cell trait and sickle-cell disease.

ELEVATED HAEMOGLOBIN (POLYCYTHAEMIA)

Case history (1)

A 70-year-old man was admitted with breathlessness, wheeze, fever and cough productive of sputum. As a long-standing smoker he suffers bouts of bronchitis but is otherwise in reasonable health.

On examination, he was not breathless at rest. Pulse was 82/min with no evidence of cardiac failure. Auscultation of the chest showed scattered wheeze and a few crackles at both bases. Peak flow was 350 L/min.

Initial investigations showed Hb 230 g/L, packed cell volume (PCV) 0.62, WCC 12×10^9/L, a mild neutrophilia and platelets 200×10^9/L.

Case history (2)

In the next bed a 54-year-old man has been admitted with chest pain and a suspected myocardial infarct. His general health is reasonable but he has developed severe night sweats and has lost 7 kg over the last 3 months. He denies smoking cigarettes and does not have any previous history of chest problems.

On examination, he looked well. Pulse and BP were normal. There were no abnormal signs in the cardiac or respiratory system.

Investigations show his Hb was 220 g/L with PCV 0.58, WCC 20×10^9/L and platelets 600×10^9/L. LDH was 740 U/L.

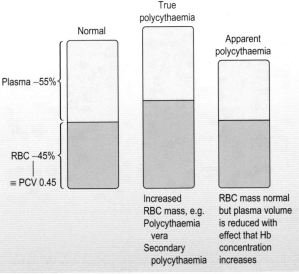

True
polycythaemia

Normal

Apparent
polycythaemia

Plasma ~55%

RBC ~45%

≡ PCV 0.45

Increased
RBC mass, e.g.
Polycythaemia
vera
Secondary
polycythaemia

RBC mass normal
but plasma volume
is reduced with
effect that Hb
concentration
increases

Figure 6.7 Alteration of haemoglobin in relation to plasma. PCV, packed cell volume; RBC, red blood cells.

These two cases both have elevated Hb but is their cause the same?

Haemoglobin (in red blood cells) is required for oxygen transport and, like most things, too much Hb has serious consequences and needs appropriate management (Fig. 6.7).

How to visualise the Hb level:

- Hb is expressed as a concentration, i.e. g/L blood but blood = plasma + solids (red blood cells mainly). Thus Hb level must be related to the level of the plasma.

Preliminary management

- Ensure that there are no hyperviscosity symptoms or signs:
  - Confusion
  - Visual disturbance
  - Peripheral circulatory disturbance.
- Ensure that the patient is adequately hydrated.
- Treat infection (if present).
- Identify correctable causes, e.g. chronic hypoxia.

Having made sure that the patients are stable, the next step is to determine the cause of the high Hb concentration. Before carrying out extensive investigation, it is sensible to contact the Haematology team, who will either advise on further tests or take over each patient's care.

CONDITIONS IN WHICH HB MIGHT BE HIGH

- Primary proliferative polycythaemia (polycythaemia vera, PV)
- Secondary to an underlying hypoxic state: raised Hb serves a purpose:
  - Chronic lung disease
  - Cyanotic heart disease
- Inappropriately high level of erythropoietin production: raised Hb serves no purpose:
  - Renal cell carcinoma
  - Uterine tumours
  - Cerebellar haemangioblastoma
- Relative/apparent polycythaemia:
  - Where the plasma component is reduced with the effect that Hb concentration rises, e.g. dehydration, associated with obesity, hypertension, diuretics, smoking

The Haematology registrar advises you to arrange some investigative tests.

Investigations

- Repeat FBC (to check that the result is correct or that the Hb has normalised with some oral/IV fluid). High haematocrit.
- Biochemistry screen: renal function — is it normal? Uric acid — might be high in some types of polycythaemia.
- Blood film: these patients had elevated platelets and WCC — make sure these are normal peripheral blood cells, with no evidence of leukaemia.
- Presence of *JAK2* mutation (see Remember box).
- Bone marrow (see Remember box).
- Erythropoietin levels (normal or low in PV).

Remember

CRITERIA FOR PV

Modified from revised WHO criteria.

Major Criteria

- Hb >185 g/L in men, >165 g/L in women or other evidence of increased red cell volume
- Presence of *JAK2* tyrosine kinase V617F or other functionally similar mutation, e.g. *JAK2* exon 12

Minor Criteria

- Bone marrow biopsy, showing hypercellularity for age with tri-lineage growth (panmyelosis) with prominent erythroid, granulocytic and megakaryocytic proliferation
- Serum erythropoietin level below the reference range for normals
- Endogenous erythroid colony (EEC) formation in vitro*

Diagnosis requires the presence of both major criteria and one minor criterion, or the presence of the first major criterion together with two minor criteria.

---

*EEC is not routinely available but colony formation in the absence of exogenous erythropoietin in vitro is 100% specific and sensitive in patients without previous treatment.

From Tefferi A, et al. Proposals and rationale for revision of the World Health Organization diagnostic criteria for polycythemia vera, essential thrombocythemia, and primary myelofibrosis: recommendations from an ad hoc international expert panel. *Blood* 2007; **110**: 1092. American Society of Haematology.

Kumar & Clark's Cases in Clinical Medicine

For diagnosis of secondary cases

- Blood gases or pulse oximetry (the latter is painless and quite adequate to exclude hypoxia only).
- CXR: emphysema, other lung pathologies.
- Abdominal ultrasound: is the spleen enlarged? Remember renal and uterine causes of polycythaemia.
- Bone marrow: not diagnostic in isolation but gives additional information.
- Erythropoietin levels raised.

  N.B. It is not necessary to carry out blood viscosity and red cell volume studies.

Classic features of polycythaemia vera

- Weight loss, sweats, pruritus (itching is typically much more pronounced after a warm bath) (Fig. 6.8 shows erythromelalgia).
- High Hb and perhaps raised WCC + platelets.
- Splenomegaly ± hepatomegaly.
- Other causes (e.g. hypoxia) excluded.
- Increased red cell mass.
- Plasma volume normal.

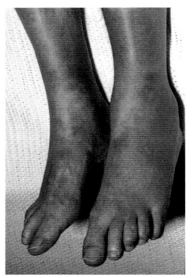

Figure 6.8 Erythromelalgia of the toes. This is a painful complication in which the skin becomes suffused and red, as in this patient.

Secondary polycythaemia

- As for PV, but generally with no hepatosplenomegaly and no thrombocytosis.
- Usually, a secondary cause is found, e.g. cyanotic heart disease, lung disease, renal disease.

Apparent (or relative) polycythaemia

- Red cell mass normal.
- Reduced plasma volume.
- No hepatosplenomegaly.

Management and progress

This is where knowledge of the underlying cause becomes crucial.

Your FIRST patient has secondary polycythaemia due to lung disease

This is a physiological rise in Hb. Reducing the Hb to normal could have serious consequences because the rise in Hb is a compensatory mechanism.

The initial aim is to reduce the Hb to a safe level. Generally, this is achieved by venesection (removal of ~400–500 mL blood) every 2 days. In males the PCV is reduced to <0.5 and in females to <0.45.

All cases of secondary polycythaemia should be treated with venesection and treatment of the underlying cause, if possible. This patient's raised Hb was due to chronic lung disease, with the high Hb due to hypoxia.

Your SECOND patient has polycythaemia vera

(See Remember box above.)

- Venesect 400–500 mL weekly.
- Then control marrow activity with hydroxycarbamide.
- Use targeted therapy with *JAK1* and *JAK2* agonists in patients who don't respond to first-line therapy.

Long-term complications

Up to 30% of patients with PV will develop intense marrow fibrosis and 5% develop acute myeloid leukaemia. The other polycythaemias don't transform.

ELEVATED WHITE BLOOD CELL COUNT

Case history

A 17-year-old boy who has ulcerative colitis was admitted to the MAU because he felt unwell with a headache, sore throat and a temperature. He had also developed diarrhoea but there was no blood in the stools. He was not on steroids but was on azathioprine 100 mg daily.

On examination, his tonsils were enlarged and inflamed; he had palatal petechiae and cervical lymphadenopathy.

Investigations showed an Hb of 124 g/L, MCV 98 fL, WCC 16×10^9/L with abnormal lymphocytes in the peripheral blood. A Monospot test is positive.

Diagnosis: Infectious mononucleosis.

Kumar & Clark's Cases in Clinical Medicine

> ### Box 6.1 Causes of high white blood cell counts
>
> Patients with haematological malignancies likely to have high WCC
>
> - Acute myeloid leukaemia
> - Acute lymphoblastic leukaemia
> - Chronic lymphocytic leukaemia
> - Chronic myeloid leukaemia
> - Lymphoma
> - Other infiltrations: myeloma, myelofibrosis
>
> Situations in which a reactive high WCC occurs
>
> - Infection
> - Corticosteroid therapy
> - Brisk GI tract bleeding
> - 'Stress', e.g. postoperative
> - Post splenectomy

There are many causes of a raised WCC (Box 6.1) and there is overlap with haematological malignancies, many of which present with WCC elevation. As a non-specialist confronted with a patient who has an elevated WCC, the key question for you is: does this elevation represent a haematological malignancy or is it reflecting some other process?

A thorough history and examination will usually allow you to determine the cause of the elevated WCC. 'Alert' features suggesting a possible malignant cause include:

- Ill patients
- Those with bleeding/bruising
- Fever
- Enlargement of liver or spleen, or lymphadenopathy
- Weight loss
- Lymphocytes or bizarre/abnormal cells on blood film.

Is it glandular fever or acute leukaemia?

The atypical lymphocytes seen in this patient with infectious mononucleosis can be confused with leukaemic blasts because the lymphocytes are large, often have nucleoli and resemble lymphoblasts. Specific tests, such as the Monospot, help confirm the diagnosis of infectious mononucleosis. In general, the haematology department will advise on further investigation, e.g. cell marker analysis to exclude leukaemia.

Progress. This patient quickly improved, with no significant flare-up of his colitis. He was sent home after 72 hours, continuing on azathioprine.

Remember

If in doubt, contact the Haematology staff. Early intervention in a patient with acute leukaemia is advised, and if you are not confident that the WCC rise is 'benign', seek expert help. There is less urgency if there is:

- A patient who is obviously well
- Isolated WCC only (Hb/platelets normal)
- Obvious infection
- Simple neutrophilia.

ELEVATED PLATELET COUNT

Case history

A 75-year-old woman was admitted with acute ischaemia of the toes in both feet.

On examination, she was found to have dusky skin on both feet, with evidence of early gangrene in the toes. FBC showed normal Hb, WCC 18×10^9/L (neutrophilia) and platelet count 1500×10^9/L.

Other significant features in this patient:

- Evidence of weight loss
- Splenomegaly 4 cm below the costal margin.

You need to decide whether the marked elevation of the platelet count is likely to be *reactive* to some underlying process/disorder, or whether she has a *primary* marrow disorder, because the management is dictated by the underlying cause.

Why does the platelet count rise in a reactive manner?

In simplistic terms, any acute stress (bleeding, operative surgery, severe infection) causes intense marrow activity with elevation of white cells and platelets in a non-specific way.

Reactive thrombocytosis does not usually exceed 1000×10^9/L, whereas primary thrombocytosis is often $>1000 \times 10^9$/L, but don't rely on platelet count alone. A reactive thrombocythaemia will resolve when the underlying problem, e.g. infection, is treated.

Immediate action

- Contact the haematologist.
- Check end organs — are they threatened?
  - Look at the fundi: vascular occlusion?
  - Extremities: too late at this point because there is vascular damage to the feet in this patient
  - Renal function.
- Is there a secondary (reactive) cause?
  - Infection
  - Bleeding
  - Malignancy (breast, lung, bowel)
  - Autoimmune rheumatic diseases.

If none is obvious, check again for splenomegaly, as was found in this case.

If platelets are raised and there is splenomegaly, then the cause is likely to be a myeloproliferative disorder.

Diagnosis. This patient has a myeloproliferative disorder.

Is there a test that will confirm a primary bone marrow pathology?

Unfortunately not. The *JAK2* tyrosine kinase mutation is present in only 50% of cases (see polycythaemia vera). Bone marrow trephine biopsy can help because increases in the numbers of megakaryocytes (the cells that make platelets; Fig. 6.9) with clustering favour a diagnosis of essential thrombocythaemia (ET), but often it is a diagnosis of exclusion. Blood film examination may show marked variation in size and shape of the platelets (platelet

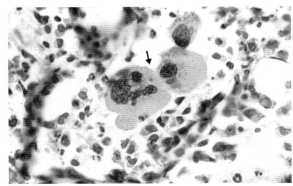

Figure 6.9 Bone marrow in essential thrombocythaemia: clusters of megakaryocytes (from which platelets bud off) are seen in the centre of the field (arrow).

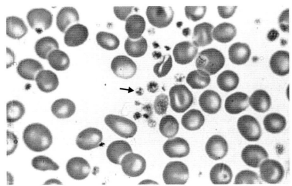

Figure 6.10 Large numbers of platelets (small purple cells, arrow) in the blood film of a patient with essential thrombocythaemia.

anisocytosis; Fig. 6.10) in primary thrombocythaemia – but this is not diagnostic.

Information

MYELOPROLIFERATIVE DISORDERS ASSOCIATED WITH THROMBOCYTOSIS
- Primary (essential) thrombocythaemia
- Polycythaemia vera
- Chronic myeloid leukaemia (CML)
- Myelofibrosis

Management

- Low-dose aspirin 75–300 mg/day (or dipyridamole if aspirin contraindicated).
- Plateletpheresis (using cell separator) if organ function is threatened and a rapid reduction in platelet count is needed.
- Oral hydroxycarbamide (e.g. 2–3 g per day for 2–3 days, dropping thereafter to 500 mg/day) to suppress bone marrow production of platelets (but beware neutropenia if dose too high). Suggested regimen: 10–30 mg/kg/day. Anagrelide and busulfan are also used.

Complications

- Primary thrombocythaemia: generally indolent course but might transform to polycythaemia myelofibrosis in ~5% (occasionally transforms to acute myeloid leukaemia).

Progress. This patient was referred to the Vascular Surgery department, which carried out Doppler and duplex imaging of her peripheral arteries but found no lesion amenable to surgery.

GLUCOSE-6-PHOSPHATE DEHYDROGENASE DEFICIENCY

Definition

Glucose-6-phosphate dehydrogenase (G6PD) is an enzyme in the hexose-monophosphate pathway. It is responsible for generating NADPH, which is the reduced form of nicotinamide adenine dinucleotide phosphate. In the red cell, NADPH is a major source of reduction in the potential required to maintain the iron atoms of haemoglobin in the ferrous state and to prevent membrane lipid peroxidation.

Case history

A 30-year-old Nigerian man was brought to A&E, having collapsed in the street. He had returned from a 3-month holiday in Nigeria 6 days previously. Two days before admission he had developed central colicky abdominal pain and diarrhoea; 1 day before admission he began to feel weak and noticed his urine was discoloured red.

On examination, he was pyrexial (37.8°C), anaemic and jaundiced. There was no hepatosplenomegaly.

Dipstix testing of urine was negative for bilirubin but positive for urobilinogen and blood. Urine microscopy revealed no red cells.

Investigations:
- Hb 54 g/L
- MCV 91 fL
- WCC 15.8 × 10⁹/L
- Platelets 249 × 10⁹/L
- Reticulocytes 11.61%.

Blood film showed polychromasia, irregularly contracted and bitten-out red cells. There were no malaria parasites or Heinz bodies.

The patient has a normocytic anaemia with a reticulocytosis, suggesting **acute hae-molysis or haemorrhage.**

Polychromasia refers to the appearance of reticulocytes, or immature red cells, when stained by using standard stains.

The appearance of the red cells is compatible with oxidative red cell damage. It is unusual to see Heinz bodies when patients have a functional spleen.

Differential diagnosis

Malaria is a common cause of haemolysis in patients returning from the tropics. Other evidence to suggest acute intravascular haemolysis is shown in Table 6.1.

Hb electrophoresis on CAM and agar gel demonstrates sickle-cell trait but no other structural Hb variant. Sickle-cell trait does not result in a haemolytic anaemia.

The negative isopropanol stability test excludes an inherited, unstable Hb variant.

The negative DAT (or Coombs' test) excludes immune-mediated red cell destruction.

G6PD was assayed by two methods that confirmed G6PD deficiency. The most common G6PD variant in individuals of African descent is G6PD A$^-$.

Remember

- G6PD deficiency will be present in all (homozygous) males who carry an affected X chromosome.
- Heterozygous females will have a dual population of red cells.
- Because X chromosome inactivation is random (lyonisation), some heterozygous females will demonstrate clinical G6PD deficiency.

Deficiency of G6PD arises from a large number of different mutations in the *G6PD* gene, the majority of which are point mutations resulting in single amino-acid substitutions. G6PD deficiency is widespread in many tropical and subtropical populations where malaria was, or is, endemic. Frequencies of 20% of the population in Southern Europe and Africa, and 40% in SE Asia and the Middle East have been reported.

G6PD deficiency can present as:
- Neonatal jaundice
- Chronic haemolytic anaemia
- Acute haemolytic anaemia.

An acute haemolytic crisis is the most common presentation, and most affected individuals are asymptomatic until this happens. Acute haemolysis

Table 6.1 Evidence to show intravascular haemolysis

Test	Result
Serum bilirubin	65 μmol/L
Serum haptoglobins	Undetectable
Serum LDH	587 U/L
Schumm's test	Positive

Table 6.2 Drugs that commonly cause acute haemolysis in patients with G6PD

Type	Example
Anti-malarials	Primaquine
	Pyrimethamine
	Chloroquine
	Quinine
Sulfonamides	Sulfasalazine
	Dapsone
	Co-trimoxazole
Other anti-bacterials	Nitrofurantoin
	Nalidixic acid
	Quinolones, e.g. ciprofloxacin
Analgesics	Aspirin ($>$ 1 g per day)
Miscellaneous	Vitamin K analogues
	Naphthalene
	Probenecid
	Dimercaprol
	Methylene blue

occurs when an exogenous factor imposes an extra oxidative stress, which overwhelms the limited supply of NADPH in the red cells. Acute haemolysis can be precipitated by:

* Infection
* Drugs
* Fava beans (as either lightly cooked food or a pollen).

Many drugs (Table 6.2) have been implicated in attacks of acute haemolysis in susceptible individuals.

Remember

* Some drugs (e.g. primaquine, aspirin and vitamin K) can be given safely in reduced doses.
* Some agents (e.g. dapsone and naphthalene) in sufficient amounts will cause haemolysis in individuals with normal levels of G6PD.

Favism is a form of severe, acute, intravascular haemolysis, often with massive haemoglobinuria, precipitated by exposure to fava beans (*Vicia faba*) in individuals with G6PD deficiency. It is most common in children, following the ingestion of fresh, raw beans. Haemolysis is probably precipitated by divicine, a glucoside constituent in fava beans, which generates free oxygen radicals when oxidised.

Diagnosis of G6PD deficiency

Clinical features

- Sudden onset.
- Severe malaise and pallor often with fever and abdominal pain.
- Dark urine.
- Jaundice.

Laboratory features

Blood count:

- Normocytic anaemia
- Reticulocytosis
- Bitten-out irregularly contracted red cells.

The spleen 'bites out' Heinz bodies, which are aggregates of oxidised methaemoglobin, from affected red cells.

Features of intravascular haemolysis

- Decreased haptoglobins.
- Increased LDH.
- Haemoglobinaemia.
- Haemoglobinuria.
- Positive Schumm's test due to methaemalbumin.

One of the isoenzymes of LDH is found in high concentrations in red cells and is released in red cell damage.

Rapid depletion of haptoglobin with the formation of methaemalbumin is typical of intravascular haemolysis. In the absence of other scavenging serum proteins, excess haem binds to albumin and the ferrous iron is subsequently oxidised to ferric iron to give methaemalbumin and a positive Schumm's test. The cause of the intravascular haemolysis in this patient was established by further tests (Table 6.3).

Haemoglobinuria might result in acute kidney injury, particularly in adults – monitor urine output, urea and creatinine.

Table 6.3 Test results confirming the cause of intravascular haemolysis

Test	Result
Haemoglobin electrophoresis	HbA + HbS
Direct anti-globulin test (DAT)	Negative
Isopropanol stability test	Negative
G6PD assay	1.9 IU/gHb

Assessment of G6PD activity

- Qualitative screening test, e.g. cresyl blue decolorisation test.
- Quantitative enzyme assay by spectrophotometry.

Treatment

- Stop any drug that could have precipitated the acute haemolysis.
- Search for and treat any infection.
- Monitor Hb concentration twice daily until stable.
- Bed rest; urgent blood transfusion may be required in severe cases.
- Patient education:
  - Issue G6PD deficiency card and information leaflet.
  - Discuss avoidance of specific drugs and fava beans.
  - Offer family screening.

What had precipitated a haemolytic crisis in this man with G6PD deficiency?

This was initially obscure. He denied any drug ingestion but, on repeated questioning, admitted drinking approximately 50 mL of an oily liquid that he had obtained from his church in Nigeria, where it was used for anointing the faithful. When he produced the bottle, it smelt strongly of mothballs, and ultraviolet spectrophotometry confirmed the presence of naphthalene. Naphthalene is well known to cause acute haemolysis. It was first described in the 19th century after the introduction of β-naphthol to treat hookworm infestations. Many cases of affected infants have been described where the naphthalene was used as a moth repellent in clothes. The presence of G6PD deficiency greatly increases sensitivity to the oxidative red cell damage mediated by naphthalene.

Progress. The patient's Hb concentration didn't fall any further but rose slowly, reaching 92 g/L 7 days later. The reticulocyte count peaked at 17.4% on the fifth day, and the jaundice had resolved by 14 days. Re-assay 6 weeks later confirmed G6PD deficiency.

BLEEDING DISORDERS

These can be due to inherited or acquired causes. They are due to haemolysis (either intra- or extra-vascular) or disorders of coagulation. Always take a good history and use your common sense, as illustrated in the case here.

Kumar & Clark's Cases in Clinical Medicine

You are phoned by a surgical specialist registrar, who is asking for your advice. He has just finished a bilateral hernia repair on a 50-year-old man and the right side is bleeding briskly. The patient has required a transfusion with 2 units of blood in the last 30 min. The surgeon tells you that the surgery has gone well and wants you to sort out his clotting.

What do you think about this case?

This patient is most likely to be **bleeding from a surgical cause**: 2 units in 30 min is far in excess of what you would expect to give in a patient with a clotting disorder, and he is bleeding from only one of the repair sites, not both. Best to advise the registrar to find the bleeding vessel!

Although this might seem like a somewhat silly example, it shows that not all bleeding is due to abnormal clotting. Look at the whole picture before jumping in with fresh frozen plasma (FFP).

Inherited bleeding disorders

You are far more likely to see acquired bleeding disorders than inherited ones. Inherited disorders are uncommon, but must be identified.

Remember

Management of inherited disorders is complex: always seek specialist support.

How can I identify the inherited disorders?

Most inherited disorders of any severity present in childhood, and hence most, if not all, patients will be able to tell you about their problem. They should carry a medical card with them, identifying the problem and their haematology consultant. It should be easy to sort out these patients and get in touch with the appropriate specialist. Always take any suggestion of an inherited bleeding disorder seriously (Figs. 6.11 and 6.12).

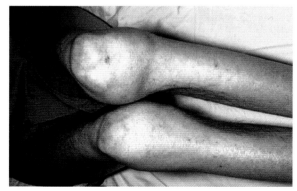

Figure 6.11 Gross arthritis in a patient with haemophilia (inherited factor VIII or IX deficiency).

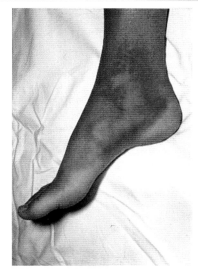

Figure 6.12 This patient with haemophilia A has bled into his foot (note the discoloration of the foot below the medial malleolus).

How can I identify milder forms?

Milder inherited disorders might not present until later in life and usually do so after surgery or other interventions.

Acquired bleeding disorders

As mentioned, these are far more common than inherited problems and are usually seen in particular clinical settings. These common scenarios will be outlined later. Most acquired disorders involve multiple and complex defects of coagulation.

Investigation of a suspected bleeding disorder

Should I check the clotting in everyone who bleeds?

Probably, although this is not absolutely necessary; however, it is best to have a low threshold. A normal set of results might help you be more secure that you are not overlooking something. Remember, though, always to take a full history and family history to try to identify any underlying inherited coagulation defect. For example, if a patient:

- Had excessive bleeding after a previous haemostatic challenge, e.g.
  - Operation
  - Dental extraction
  - Trauma
- Needed a previous blood transfusion for bleeding
- Gave a family history of bleeding
- Had epistaxis, easy bruising.

Kumar & Clark's Cases in Clinical Medicine

What should I request?

You request a basic coagulation screen:

- FBC to check platelet count
- Prothrombin time (PT)
- Activated partial thromboplastin time (APTT).

Remember

Even a 2-second prolongation might indicate an inherited clotting problem of significance and should be investigated more fully.

These are the minimum number of tests to start with. If you really want to check that a clotting disorder exists, then the following should also be performed:

- Fibrinogen level
- Thrombin time (TT).

These tests form your baseline investigations or screening tests.

Acquired disorders are relatively easy because clotting times are usually notably prolonged.

There is a whole range of specialist investigations for the complete study of a coagulation disorder: it is best to seek specialist advice.

Case history (2)

You are called to see a patient in A&E, who is bleeding excessively from a dental extraction. The doctor in A&E thinks that the patient has liver disease and asks you for some help. There is nothing in the history to indicate what the liver problem might be and the patient denies excess alcohol consumption.

On examination, you notice spider naevi, liver palms and splenomegaly. You agree that the excess bleeding is probably due to liver disease.

Bleeding in liver disease

This causes widespread coagulation and bleeding problems. Always be aware that significant liver dysfunction can result in a potentially severe bleeding disorder. The components of liver-related bleeding are:

- Reduced synthesis of coagulation factors: the liver is the source of all coagulation factors (apart from factor VIII).
- Associated vitamin K deficiency: coagulation proteins might be synthesised but will not be active because of vitamin K deficiency.
- Thrombocytopenia: frequently secondary to splenomegaly from portal hypertension.
- Chronic low-grade disseminated intravascular coagulation (DIC): see p. 102.
- Abnormal fibrinogen synthesis: in liver disease, excess sialic acid residues are added to fibrinogen and hence an acquired dysfibrinogenaemia occurs. The classic laboratory defects would be:
- PT prolonged due to decrease in factor II, V, VII or X
- APTT prolonged due to decrease in all factors
- TT prolonged due to abnormal fibrinogen
- Fibrinogen degradation products (FDPs) increased (due to failure to remove from circulation ± chronic DIC).

CAUSES OF VITAMIN K DEFICIENCY
- Biliary obstruction
- Oral warfarin anti-coagulant
- Liver disease
- Malabsorption states
- Inflammatory bowel diseases (with ileal resection)

Management

- Give 10 mg vitamin K daily IV for 3 days.
- For acute bleeding give 10–20 mL/kg FFP to replace all coagulation proteins.
- If the fibrinogen level is low or TT prolonged, give cryoprecipitate to supply fibrinogen.

Progress. This man's bleeding stopped with help from the dental surgeons. The patient has been referred to the Liver clinic for investigation and management of his chronic liver disease.

Case history (3)

A 49-year-old man has been on treatment for hypertension for years. His renal function has gradually deteriorated, despite reasonable control of his blood pressure (now 130/80), stopping smoking and taking statin therapy (his present cholesterol level is 3.2 mmol/L).

His GFR is 32 mL/min/1.73m^2. He has recently suffered from bruising around his upper arms and shins.

Diagnosis: chronic kidney disease

Anyone with significantly impaired renal function can have an acquired bleeding disorder. The major cause is toxic metabolites impairing platelet function, as is the case in this patient.

Is the APTT or PT abnormal in renal disease?

No. As mentioned, the major defect is an acquired platelet disorder. The clotting times are usually normal.

Should the bleeding time be measured regularly in patients with renal disease?

No, but remember that renal disease is a cause of an acquired bleeding disorder, and if you are planning surgery on the patient there might be a bleeding problem.

What can we do in renal disease?

There are several approaches to treatment but sorting out the renal problem first is the best option. Dialysis will improve platelet function; this is why few stable dialysed/controlled patients actually bleed. The real risk group is those with a very high serum creatinine/urea.

Other treatments for bleeding include:
- Synthetic vasopressin analogue (desmopressin)
- Cryoprecipitate
- Platelet transfusion.

These are all used in bleeding episodes.

Kumar & Clark's Cases in Clinical Medicine

DISSEMINATED INTRAVASCULAR COAGULATION (DIC)

This is the most complex of the acquired bleeding disorders.

DIC is inappropriate and continued activation of coagulation that leads ultimately to both bleeding and thrombosis.

The initial phase of DIC is thrombosis. This is why DIC is associated with end-organ damage leading to multi-organ failure.

Remember

DIC is always secondary to some other major clinical problem.

Bleeding arises as a secondary phenomenon due to consumption of coagulation factors and platelets (caused by continued activation of clotting) and the activation of fibrinolysis (breaking down any fibrin that is laid down).

Case history (1)

A 29-year-old man is brought to the Trauma Unit with severe injuries to his abdomen and legs as a result of a road traffic accident. Initial examination and CT scanning confirm that he has fractured both femurs and his pelvis. He has fluid in his abdomen on CT, suggesting internal organ damage.

He is resuscitated and taken to ITU, where he needs ventilation, volume replacement and cardiovascular support with inotropes. His leg fractures are stabilised and he undergoes emergency laparotomy with resection of damaged small bowel. He initially improved, but then his renal and liver function deteriorated and he was diagnosed as having multi-organ failure. He was then noted to be bleeding from his laparotomy wound.

What action should you take?

- Always think about DIC in a bleeding patient.
- Try to make the diagnosis.

What are the causes of DIC?

- Infection.
- Obstetric complications (for women).
- Surgery.
- Trauma.
- Malignancy.
- Liver disease.
- Transfusion reactions.

If someone is bleeding and you always think about DIC, you will not go wrong. In many ways, the long list of causes is academic when you first see the patient — but if they have DIC, you must identify the cause.

How do you make the diagnosis?

Send off all the screening tests and FDPs. The pattern is:

- Platelets low: consumption
- PT prolonged: consumption
- APTT prolonged: consumption
- TT prolonged: consumption of fibrinogen and FDPs
- Fibrinogen low: consumption
- FDPs high: breakdown of fibrin.

Why are FDPs measured?

FDPs tell you that fibrin is being broken down. The most specific test is the D-dimer, which tells you that cross-linked fibrinogen has formed and has then been broken down.

How do you manage DIC?

- Treat the underlying disorder.
- Treat the underlying disorder!
- Treat the underlying disorder!!
- Support with FFP, cryoprecipitate and platelets.

Remember

People die from their underlying disorder rather than the DIC per se.

You must aim to treat the underlying disorder! DIC is always secondary. As mentioned, it is due to inappropriate and continued activation of clotting. Until you stop this by treating the underlying problem, it will not get better.

Blood component therapy is purely supportive. Give:
- 10–20 mL/kg FFP + cryoprecipitate
- Platelets
- Blood as required.

Aim to restore the fibrinogen concentration to normal and the PT/APTT to within 4 s of normal.

Progress. Despite all efforts, the patient died.

Case history (2)

A 50-year-old patient has carcinoma of the lung with a prolonged PT, APTT, TT, low fibrinogen and platelet count, and high FDPs, but he is not bleeding.

Does this patient have DIC?

This is the picture of subclinical DIC — laboratory abnormalities but no bleeding. It is seen in chronic DIC, e.g. in liver disease or malignancy. DIC ranges from florid bleeding to abnormalities that are picked up only by laboratory testing.

Remember

People die from their underlying disorder rather than the DIC per se.

Anti-coagulant overdosage

An obvious cause of bleeding. Don't forget to look for warfarin/heparin usage.

Action

Confirm anti-coagulant overdosage by finding a prolonged PT (warfarin) or APTT (heparin). The treatment of bleeding depends on the problem, but in essence:

If due to warfarin: STOP WARFARIN

- Minor bleeding: if INR >6.0. Restart warfarin when INR <5.0; check INR daily. If INR >8.0, give vitamin K 2.5 mg oral or 0.5 mg IV.

- Major bleeding: give prothrombin complex concentrate 50 units/kg or FFP 15 mL/kg; give vitamin K 5 mg IV.

Remember

High PT (due to warfarin) without bleeding usually requires no treatment, apart from stopping warfarin.

If due to heparin: STOP HEPARIN

If bleeding is excessive or uncontrolled:

- Protamine reversal (1 mg IV neutralises 100 units heparin — maximum dose 40 mg). Protamine has no effect on low-molecular-weight (LMW) heparin.
- Seek advice.
- Heparin excess will correct in a few hours.

Remember

Thrombin inhibitors that are being used for anti-coagulation, e.g. apixaban and rivaroxaban, have no antidotes.

Surgical cause

Suspect if there is rapid blood loss at operation. Don't under-estimate the number of times this is forgotten and people chase a medical cause for bleeding when a vessel has a hole in it.

If you have a hole in a vessel, bleeding will not stop until the hole is fixed, however good the coagulation system is.

Remember

Surgical and medical bleeding might coexist. If you correct the coagulation and the patient is still bleeding, think surgical, whatever the surgeon says!

PLATELET DISORDERS

Case history (1)

You are asked to see a 24-year-old woman who is in A&E. She has presented with petechiae scattered over her body. The A&E doctor has found that she has a platelet count of 10×10^9/L. This woman seems very well and tells you that she has had the petechiae for at least a week. She has no other symptoms. She is on the contraceptive pill but is taking no other tablets. She does not smoke and drinks wine (6 units) at the weekend only.

On examination, she has petechiae over her trunk, arms and legs. She has no other abnormal signs.

Investigations:

You note the platelet count and also that all the other parameters in her blood count are normal. She also has normal routine biochemistry.

Remember

Meningococcal septicaemia has a purpuric rash and/or petechiae.

Box 6.2 Causes of thrombocytopenia

Failure of platelet production

Marrow aplasia

Metabolic defects
- Vitamin B$_{12}$/folate deficiency
- Uraemia
- Alcohol excess
- Liver disease

Drugs
- Chemotherapy $\pm$ radiation

Marrow infiltration
- Leukaemia
- Lymphoma
- Myeloma
- Myelofibrosis
- Carcinoma

Decreased platelet survival

Immune
- Immune thrombocytopenic purpura (ITP)
- Systemic lupus erythematosus (SLE)
- Chronic lymphocytic leukaemia (CLL)
- Hodgkin lymphoma
- Drug-related

Infection
- Malaria
- Virus infection

Consumption
- DIC
- Extracorporeal circulation
- Haemolytic uraemic syndrome (HUS)
- Thrombotic thrombocytopenic purpura (TTP)

Loss from circulation
- Splenomegaly
- Massive transfusion

There are multiple causes of thrombocytopenia (Box 6.2). Thrombocytopenia may be the presentation of another disorder rather than a primary platelet disorder. All patients with severe thrombocytopenia (defined as $< 20 \times 10^9$/L, which produces spontaneous haemorrhage) require admission for investigation/ treatment.

Remember

The list of causes (Box 6.2) is not comprehensive and excludes inherited thrombocytopenia or causes that would present in childhood.

Questions that need to be answered immediately

- Does this patient have immune thrombocytopenic purpura (ITP)? Normal Hb, normal WCC, no hepatosplenomegaly or lymphadenopathy.

- Does she have acute leukaemia (see p. 123)? High WCC, abnormal white cells on film, lymphadenopathy, hepatosplenomegaly (occasionally).
- Does she have aplastic anaemia? Low Hb, low WCC, no lymphadenopathy, no hepatosplenomegaly.

The *diagnosis* appears to be **ITP**. You are called back to see the patient 20 minutes later, as she has had a massive haematemesis. You think the diagnosis is ITP because there are no other features to make you think it is aplastic anaemia or acute leukaemia.

Major bleeding in ITP is not common but can be a serious complication. Treatment approaches should be decided by a haematologist.

Management for this patient

- Adequate and secure IV access.
- ABO and Rh(D) group and cross-match 6 units of blood.
- Fluid and blood replacement as appropriate.
- Start high-dose IV immunoglobulin infusion 0.4 g/kg/24 h.
- Platelet transfusion: 2 units immediately.
- Oral prednisolone: 1 mg/kg daily.

Progress. She had no further haematemesis and her platelet count rose to 50×10^9/L on day 5 but remained at that level. After discussion, she was referred for splenectomy, which produced a good response in her platelet count. See page 113 for management of a splenectomised patient.

Learning points

- High-dose immunoglobulin elevates the platelet count by macrophage Fc receptor blockade of the reticuloendothelial system.
- Endogenous platelets usually rise after 24–48 h; the survival of exogenous platelets is improved.
- Platelet transfusion is usually not necessary in ITP, except in the situation of life-threatening haemorrhage, such as in this case.
- 75% of patients respond to oral steroids but the full therapeutic effect may take 2–4 weeks to develop.

Remember

ITP might become chronic and might require long-term treatment ± splenectomy. Romiplostim and eltrombopag, thrombopoietin receptor agonists, are used if splenectomy has no effect.

Case history (2)

You are asked to see a 50-year-old man on a surgical ward, who has come into hospital for an elective hernia repair. He is found on a routine preoperative FBC to have a platelet count of 90×10^9/L. His Hb and WCC count are normal.

This chronic presentation of mild thrombocytopenia is reasonably common. To establish the cause you should systematically go through the causes of thrombocytopenia from an initial clinical history and examination.

Can he go ahead and have his hernia repair?

It might take a while to get to the bottom of his thrombocytopenia. Elective surgery can be performed, as the platelet count is $>80 \times 10^9$/L.

Avoid any NSAIDs as postoperative analgesia; make sure aspirin has not been taken within the last 10 days.

This man was discharged following a successful surgical repair, and 1 week later his platelet count was 96×10^9/L. By 1 month the platelet count was normal. No clear reason for the thrombocytopenia was found but a **viral cause** seemed the most likely.

Case history (3)

A 28-year-old woman has had a D&C for long-standing menorrhagia. It is now 5 days after the procedure and she is still bleeding. She has been back in theatre and no local defect is found. She says she had problems in the past with bleeding after dental extractions. Her PT, APTT and platelet count are normal.

Diagnosis

This is the typical picture of an **inherited platelet disorder**. Severe platelet function disorders present in childhood but milder versions don't usually present until surgery in adulthood. Clues here are bleeding after dental extraction and long-standing menorrhagia.

Management

Assess the extent of bleeding. Treatment options include:
- Tranexamic acid 1 g $\times$ 4 daily if mild bleeding
- Platelet transfusion if severe bleeding.

In a classic platelet function disorder the bleeding time is prolonged, but this test is difficult to perform. If you suspect a platelet function disorder, organise platelet function studies with your haematological laboratory.

Progress. This patient stopped bleeding following a platelet transfusion. She was referred to the Haematology department for follow-up.

THROMBOSIS

Case history (1)

You are asked to see a 24-year-old woman who has had a life-threatening pulmonary embolus. She received fibrolytic therapy (see p. 351) on the ICU. Her condition stabilised and she is now on warfarin following initial treatment with LMW heparin. She wants to know why she has had a pulmonary embolus. She has a family history of deep vein thrombosis (DVT).

Are investigations indicated?

Thrombosis is common, but relatively uncommon under the age of 45 years unless there is a precipitating event (see later). In such patients with a family history, about 50% have a definable underlying prothrombotic state. It is well worth investigating her formally for a prothrombotic state.

Attempt to identify any precipitating event, such as:
- Taking the combined oral contraceptive pill
- Immobility and/or recent surgery/fracture/injury
- Long-haul flight
- Obesity
- Malignancy.

Should she be investigated now or later?

She is on warfarin, which can interfere with thrombotic investigations. Identifying an underlying thrombotic state acutely will not change the immediate management.

Remember

- An abnormal result after an acute thrombosis does not mean an abnormality genuinely exists
- It must be rechecked
- However, a normal result is normal.

She is on warfarin and so formal studies must be delayed. Refer her to a specialist for follow-up and investigation.

What investigations will be requested after stopping warfarin?

Investigations

- Lupus anti-coagulant
- Anti-phospholipid antibody
- Protein C deficiency
- Protein S deficiency
- Anti-thrombin deficiency
- Factor V Leiden
- 3' prothrombin UTR variant
- *JAK2* mutation

These aim to look for an inherited deficiency of natural anti-coagulants, mutations leading to increased thrombin generation or acquired causes of a prothrombotic state.

Progress. This woman has factor Leiden deficiency. She is referred to a specialist for long-term follow-up, counselling and family studies.

Case history (2)

You are asked to see a 70-year-old man who had a DVT after a knee replacement, despite DVT prophylaxis. He has no family history of venous thrombosis. At present he is on rivaroxaban 10 mg daily for 3 months.

Should he be investigated for thrombophilia?

No! At this age and in this setting, it is likely that a DVT has been precipitated by the surgery. The pick-up rate for a significant thrombotic disorder is very low in this setting. When asked to assess the thrombotic status, balance the likelihood of finding a defect against the value of identifying the exact defect.

Case history (3)

You are called to see a 45-year-old man who is being anti-coagulated for acute iliofemoral vein thrombosis with heparin. His APTT remains normal on 28 000 units heparin per 24 h. The dose of heparin has been progressively increased over the last 3 days but his leg swelling is worse.

What do you advise?

The target APTT for heparin for an acute thrombosis is 1.5–2.5 times the mid-point of the NR. The most common reasons for failure are:

- Under-monitoring
- Under-dosing
- Not actually receiving dose of heparin prescribed.

Action

- Ensure prescribed dose is being given.
- Increase dose by 10% per 24 h.
- Recheck APTT in 4 h.
- If still low, repeat 10% increase in heparin dose and recheck at 4-hourly intervals.

Heparin monitoring is notoriously bad in most hospitals. If IV heparin is being used, it should be monitored as follows:

- Check APTT every 4 h until target reached.
- Increase dose in 10% increments.
- Once target APTT reached, repeat at 4 h.
- If APTT is stable, repeat 12-hourly.

Remember

- Outcome is dependent on the effectiveness of anti-coagulation within the first 48 h.
- Heparin resistance is rare; poor heparin control is very common.

For how long should a patient with venous thromboembolic disease be anti-coagulated with warfarin?

The duration and target INRs for various thrombotic conditions are listed in Table 6.4.

Recurrent venous thromboembolism (VTE) is essentially two or more events. The more events there are, the greater the likelihood of recurrence.

Long-term anti-coagulation carries the risk of major haemorrhage (4% per annum) and death ($\sim 0.5\%$ per annum). These must be balanced against recurrence prevention. Complications are far more common in older patients.

Recurrence is much higher in patients anti-coagulated for 6 weeks rather than 6 months.

Remember

- Drug interactions with warfarin
- Need to amend dosage in patients undergoing invasive procedures
- Regular anti-coagulant clinic follow-up

Novel orally active anti-coagulant drugs

A number of orally active direct thrombin and Xa inhibitor drugs (dabigatran, rivaroxaban, apixaban and edoxaban) are being used for prevention and treatment of thrombosis. Such drugs have a much broader therapeutic window than warfarin, and offer the prospect of fixed drug dosing without the need to monitor coagulation. Antidotes are being developed. Andexanet reverses epixaban and rivaroxaban, and idaracizumab is the antidote for dabigatran.

Table 6.4 Duration and target INRs for thrombotic conditions

Condition	Duration	INR target
Uncomplicated DVT	6 months	2.5
Complex DVT	6 months	2.5
Pulmonary embolus	6 months	2.5
Recurrent VTE	Indefinite	2.5; if the recurrent event occurs while taking warfarin, the intensity of anti-coagulation is increased to a target of 3.5
Atrial fibrillation	Indefinite	2.5
Mechanical heart valves	Indefinite	3.5

DVT, deep vein thrombosis; INR, international normalised ratio; VTE venous thromboembolism.

Case history (4)

You are asked to see a 36-year-old woman with an acutely swollen calf. Clinical diagnosis is a distal DVT. She has no complicating problems.

How should she be treated?

Initially, the diagnosis should be confirmed by venous compression ultra-sonography (sensitivity 97% for proximal and 73% for calf veins). An acutely swollen leg has a range of causes:

- DVT
- Ruptured Baker's cyst
- Rupture of head of gastrocnemius
- Acute knee injury
- Haematoma
- Infection (e.g. cellulitis).

Action

If a DVT is confirmed:

- Give SC LMW heparin.
- Warfarinise the patient.

This can be managed in outpatients with good nursing and laboratory support.

If the DVT is complex (i.e. iliofemoral):

- Admit.
- Give IV unfractionated heparin or LMW heparin.
- Warfarinise.

There is an increasing move to outpatient management of VTE.

Dabigatran or rivaroxaban (see earlier) is being used instead of warfarin in some centres.

Case history (5)

You are called about a 36-year-old man with an acute right lower limb ischaemia due to an arterial thrombosis. He has a family history of thrombosis. There has been improvement in the ischaemic area over 24 h. The patient is on IV heparin infusion and is being monitored by the vascular surgeons. In view of the family history, the doctor wonders whether the man should be investigated for thrombophilia. The doctor has already sent off a standard thrombophilia screen (see Investigations box, p. 99) and asks if this is all that you need.

You tell him that thrombophilia is uncommon in arterial disease but there are a number of risk factors for arterial thrombosis. You suggest that he requests:

- Plasma homocysteine
- Lipid profile
- Plasminogen activator inhibitor.

Finding a cause in arterial disease is less likely than in venous thrombosis.

Progress. No evidence of thrombophilia was found in this man, but he is a smoker and his cholesterol was 7.4 mmol/L with risk factors for atherosclerosis. His lifestyle issues were addressed by the cardiac rehabilitation nurse specialist and he was started on a statin.

Case history (6)

You are asked to see a 60-year-old woman with a right leg DVT, who is on unfractionated heparin. She has been in hospital for 5 days and started warfarin therapy 48 h previously. She has now developed a cold, painful leg on the left that is pulseless. You are told that her platelet count has been falling since starting heparin.

What is the most likely diagnosis to consider?

This would be a good picture for **heparin-induced thrombocytopenia with thrombosis (HIT)** of the artery. The classic features are progressive platelet decline and new thrombosis. HIT is a clinical diagnosis and is diagnosed in any patient on heparin whose platelet count falls significantly.

Action

- Stop *all* heparin (including heparin flush).
- Contact a haematologist.
- Alternative forms of anti-coagulation are not required for the DVT in this woman because she is on warfarin, the INR is 2.0 and heparin was about to be discontinued.

HIT is due to an immune induction of anti-heparin/PF4 antibodies, which bind to and activate platelets via an Fc receptor. This results in a pro-thrombotic state with low platelets. There is usually a previous history of heparin exposure.

N.B.

- Fatal thrombosis, both venous and arterial, can arise if heparin is not stopped immediately.
- HIT can occur after SC heparin use. It is becoming increasingly common with use of heparin prophylaxis.

Progress. This woman has left acute ischaemic lower limb and required surgical removal of the thrombus in her popliteal artery. She fortunately made a good recovery, although she still has a swollen, painful right leg (from the DVT) and ischaemic pain in the left leg after exertion.

SPLENOMEGALY, SPLENECTOMY AND HYPOSPLENISM

Case history (1)

A 55-year-old man presented with a 3-month history of discomfort in the left side of his abdomen. The discomfort is present most of the time and now seems to be getting worse.

He has had rheumatoid arthritis for many years, but his condition has stabilised on methotrexate therapy and occasional use of diclofenac for pain in his knees.

On examination, he looks pale and has evidence of rheumatoid arthritis in his hands, with ulnar drift and palmar subluxation of the MCPs. He has rheumatoid nodules in both elbows. Both knees are deformed. Examination of his abdomen shows a large spleen.

Investigations show a normochromic normocytic anaemia with low platelets and a neutropenia.

The diagnosis is **Felty's syndrome** in a patient with rheumatoid arthritis.

Felty's syndrome consists of splenomegaly and neutropenia in a patient with rheumatoid arthritis. A normochromic, normocytic anaemia of chronic disease is usually present, although iron-deficient and rare haemolytic (Coombs'-positive) anaemias are seen. Hypersplenism causing a pancytopenia may occur (see later).

Spleen size can be assessed by abdominal palpation or by imaging, e.g. ultrasound. CT, MRI and PET scans are also used to delineate the cause, e.g. lymphoproliferative disease.

There are many causes of splenomegaly, with the most frequent showing geographical variation. In temperate climates malignant blood diseases, portal hypertension, haemolytic anaemias and infective endocarditis account for most cases, whereas in tropical countries malaria, leishmaniasis and the haemoglobinopathies are prevalent.

Information

CAUSES OF SPLENOMEGALY

- Malignant haematological disease, e.g. acute or chronic leukaemia, malignant lymphoma
- Myeloproliferative disorders, e.g. polycythaemia vera, myelofibrosis (often massive)
- Haemoglobinopathies, e.g. β-thalassaemia major, Hb, H, SC or E disease
- Haemolytic anaemias, e.g. hereditary spherocytosis
- Congestive splenomegaly, e.g. portal hypertension (cirrhosis)
- Inborn errors of metabolism, e.g. Gaucher's disease
- Autoimmune rheumatic disorders: e.g. systemic lupus erythematosus (SLE), rheumatoid arthritis (Felty's syndrome)
- Infections:
  - Viral, e.g. infectious mononucleosis
  - Bacterial (any bacteria), occasionally — remember infective endocarditis
  - Protozoal, e.g. malaria, kala-azar
- Miscellaneous (rare), e.g. amyloid, tropical splenomegaly.

Enlargement of the spleen from any cause can be complicated by **hypersplenism.** This is characterised by:

- Splenomegaly
- Pancytopenia
- Normal or hypercellular bone marrow.

Pathophysiology of hypersplenism

Mature red cells, neutrophils and platelets 'pool', or are trapped, in the sinusoids of the large spleen and prematurely destroyed.

Causes of hyposplenism

- Congenital absence.
- Splenectomy: surgical or by irradiation.
- Splenic atrophy, e.g. coeliac disease, chronic inflammatory bowel disease.
- Splenic infarction, e.g. sickle-cell anaemia (HbSS).
- Splenic infiltration.

Remember

Surgical splenectomy might be carried out because of:

- Trauma
- Treatment, e.g. hereditary spherocytosis, idiopathic thrombocytopenic purpura or myelofibrosis.
  Splenic function can be assessed by:
- Peripheral blood film: look for abnormal red cells:
  - Acanthocytes (spiky red cells)
  - Target cells (like an archery target)
  - Pappenheimer bodies (iron granules)
  - Howell—Jolly bodies (nuclear DNA fragments)
- Differential interference microscopy of blood: increased pitted red cell (red cells with submembrane vacuoles) count
- Radioactive spleen scan (see earlier)

The functional size of the spleen can be assessed by scanning with a scintillation counter following the injection of radiolabelled (^{99m}Tc), heat-damaged, autologous red cells. These cells are removed from the circulation solely by the spleen.

Progress. In this patient with rheumatoid arthritis, Felty's syndrome was confirmed as the cause of the splenomegaly. Over the following year, he developed recurrent infections with a persistent, refractory neutropenia and eventually had a splenectomy.

Case history (2)

A 6-month-old baby boy of Nigerian parents was admitted to A&E, collapsed and unconscious. The family was travelling to the airport by taxi and diverted the car to hospital when the baby became suddenly unwell. Twelve hours before admission the child had been seen at a different A&E department with a short history of poor feeding, irritability and diarrhoea. He was noted to be febrile but not thought to be seriously unwell.

On examination, the child was noted to be pale, with a GCS of 5. He was febrile at 39.5°, with a firm spleen extending to below the umbilicus. Shortly afterwards, the child had a cardiorespiratory arrest and could not be resuscitated. The results of a blood count and blood film taken before death were:

Blood count:
- Hb 24 g/L
- MCV 76 fL

- WCC 30.5×10^9/L
- Platelets 27×10^9/L
- Reticulocytes 7.0%
  Blood film:
- Polychromasia
- Very reduced platelets
- Nucleated red cells
- Occasional elongated sickle cells
- Diplococci both within neutrophils and macrophages, and free in the plasma
  Subsequent investigations demonstrated *Streptococcus pneumoniae* on blood culture.

Diagnosis. Sickle-cell anaemia with pneumococcal sepsis.
Haemoglobin electrophoresis showed:
- HbS: 90%
- HbF: 8%
- HbA$_2$: 1.8%.

Remember

Prevention of pneumococcal sepsis in babies with sickle-cell anaemia is dependent on maternal antenatal haemoglobinopathy. At-risk pregnancies need to be identified and screened:
- Haemoglobinopathy screening of cord blood samples
- Institution of penicillin prophylaxis by 8 weeks of age.

Progress. This baby presented moribund with splenomegaly, severe anaemia and thrombocytopenia. The reticulocytosis/polychromasia and nucleated red cells suggested a haemolytic anaemia. Hb electrophoresis subsequently confirmed sickle-cell anaemia (HbSS). The sickle-cell mutation affects the β-globin gene and only assumes clinical importance 4 months after birth, when β-globin gene activity is suppressed and the β-globin gene activated.

This child's death was due to overwhelming infection with *Strep. pneumoniae*, which was present in enormous numbers in the bloodstream. The thrombocytopenia was almost certainly related to DIC secondary to the bacterial infection. Severe hyposplenism is a characteristic feature of sickle-cell anaemia and is established by 4–6 months. Pneumococcal sepsis secondary to hyposplenism is a common cause of death in children <3 years old with sickle-cell anaemia.

The gross splenomegaly and severe anaemia were due to acute splenic sequestration of sickled red cells within the spleen, which often accompanies pneumococcal sepsis in this age group (see p. 115).

Overwhelming post-splenectomy infection (OPSI) is the most feared complication of hyposplenism.

Remember

- The greatest risk of OPSI following splenectomy is in the first 2 years but the increased risk is life-long.
- The mortality rate with OPSI due to *Strep. pneumoniae* is 50% despite treatment.

Pathophysiology

- Decreased antibody synthesis.
- Decreased phagocytosis of opsonised bacteria.

The major pathogens involved in OPSI

- *Streptococcus pneumoniae* (> 80%).
- *Haemophilus influenzae* type B.
- *Neisseria meningitidis*.

These are all encapsulated bacteria − the spleen is a vital first line of defence against encapsulated organisms. Severe infections in the hyposplenic patient can also occur in malaria and babesiosis (mosquito and tick bites, respectively) and following dog bites with *Capnocytophaga canimorsus*.

Remember

- Following vaccination, check adequacy of antibody response.
- Repeat antibody levels at 5 years post vaccination and give booster doses if appropriate.

Prevention of OPSI

This depends on:

- Identification of the patient at risk
- Education of the patient about the risks of infection, dog bites and tropical travel
- Issue of a 'post-splenectomy' card and leaflet to the patient
- Life-long prophylactic antibiotic therapy, e.g. penicillin V 250 mg × 2 daily
- Vaccination with a pneumococcal polysaccharide conjugate vaccine and the Hib vaccine
- Meningococcal conjugate (ACWY) series and monovalent meningococcal serogroup B vaccine series.

BLOOD TRANSFUSION

The Blood Transfusion department supplies red cells, platelets and plasma products, such as FFP, cryoprecipitate and human albumin.

The efficient and safe provision of blood products depends on good communication between you and the laboratory, and accurate patient identification.

Always

- Provide complete and accurate patient identification on the blood sample and request form.
- Tell the Blood Transfusion department how much of what blood product is required and the urgency of the clinical situation.

Never

- Take blood from more than one patient at a time.
- Pre-label the blood sample tube.

Remember

When you request blood, always make clear the urgency of the clinical situation:
- Very urgent: there is a life-threatening haemorrhage and blood is required in 1–5 min:
  - ACTION: No pre-transfusion compatibility test. The laboratory will issue group 0 Rh (D)-negative blood
- Urgent: blood required in 5–10 min:
  - ACTION: ABO and Rh(D) group on patient sample. The laboratory will issue ABO and Rh(D) group-compatible blood
- Non-urgent: blood required in 30–60 min:
  - ACTION: Full pre-transfusion compatibility test. The laboratory will issue fully compatible blood.

To provide compatible red cells for transfusion, the following procedures are undertaken by the Blood Transfusion laboratory:
- ABO and Rh(D) blood group:
  - Major haemolytic transfusion reactions usually result from the transfusion of ABO incompatible blood.
  - The Rh(D) antigen is very immunogenic and the development of anti-D must be avoided in women of childbearing age.
- Antibody screen: excludes the presence of clinically significant red cell alloantibodies in the patient's plasma. These might result in an acute or delayed haemolytic transfusion reaction.
- Selection of appropriate donor units: wherever possible, blood of the same ABO and Rh(D) group as the patient is selected and will be negative for the appropriate antigen if an alloantibody has been identified.
- Cross-match: the patient's plasma is reacted with the donor red cells in vitro. Incompatibility is indicated by agglutination or haemolysis.

A full compatibility procedure is always completed but this can be retrospective if the clinical demand for blood is urgent.

Case history (1)

You are asked to see a 72-year-old man with myelodysplasia, who receives regular blood transfusions. One unit of blood was given uneventfully but 15 min into the second unit he began to shiver, felt unwell, and developed a pyrexia and tachycardia.

A febrile transfusion reaction to HLA or granulocyte antigens is common in multi-transfused patients but can't be safely distinguished from a haemolytic transfusion reaction due to red cell antibodies without appropriate laboratory tests.

Action

- Stop the transfusion immediately:
  - Replace giving set
  - Keep IV line open with 0.9% saline.
- Check patient identification:
  - Wrist band
  - Compatibility form
  - Compatibility label on unit of blood.
- Take appropriate samples:
  - Blood count
  - Blood cultures

- Blood transfusion sample
- Urine for Hb.
- Take samples and a relevant unit of blood to the laboratory.
- Inform Haematology medical staff of the problem.
- The laboratory will:
  - Check laboratory documentation
  - Repeat ABO Rh(D) group, antibody screen and cross-match on pre- and post-transfusion samples in parallel
  - Carry out a DAT (Coombs' test; see Fig. 6.13) to exclude the presence of alloantibodies on the patient's red cells.

Outcome

The red cell alloantibody was identified.

Diagnosis. Haemolytic transfusion reaction.

Monitor renal function, urine output, Hb concentration and check coagulation screen.

A major ABO incompatibility can be life-threatening, with acute kidney injury and DIC:

- Monitor as above.
- Insert urinary catheter and monitor urine output.
- Give IV fluids to maintain urine output (>1.5 mL/h per kg).
- If urine output is inadequate, insert CVP line and give fluid challenge and diuretics (see p. 209).
- Refer to Renal unit.
- Report to SHOT (Serious Hazards of Blood Transfusion), a confidential enquiry into major blood transfusion errors in the UK.

Progress. An error in the collection of the blood from the laboratory led to the wrong blood being given to this man. The error was reported to the hospital as a serious event. The patient maintained his normal BP and his symptoms settled, requiring no further treatment for this.

A major review of blood transfusion procedures was instituted. Fortunately, with the prompt treatment, this man had no serious problems.

Presentation of other acute complications of blood transfusion

- Non-haemolytic (febrile) transfusion reactions. These are due to the presence of leucocyte antibodies in a multiply transfused person acting against donor leucocytes in red cell concentrate, leading to release of pyrogens. Leucocyte-depleted blood is now used in many countries and so the febrile reaction is not often seen.
- Breathlessness:
  - Acute volume overload
  - Transfusion-related acute lung injury (TRALI): characterised by dyspnoea, fever, cough and lung shadowing on CXR.
- Urticaria or anaphylaxis: reaction to plasma proteins.
- Collapse or hypotension: major ABO incompatibility-infected blood product.
- Cardiac arrhythmia:
  - Hypocalcaemia
  - Hyperkalaemia
  - Rapid transfusion with 'cold' blood.

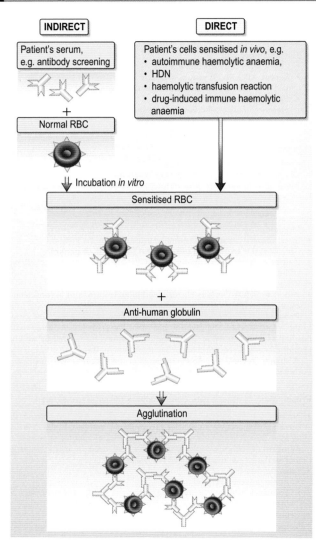

Figure 6.13 Antiglobulin (Coombs') tests. The anti-human globulin forms bridges between the sensitised cells, causing visible agglutination. The direct test detects patients' cells sensitised in vivo. The indirect test detects normal cells sensitised in vitro. HDN, haemolytic disease of newborn, RBC, red blood cell.

There are other longer-term complications of blood transfusion, including:
- Post-transfusion purpura (PTP)
- Viral infection: hepatitis C, hepatitis B, HIV (*Note:* donor blood in many countries checked for these), cytomegalovirus (CMV)
- Iron overload (multiple transfusions)
- Graft-versus-host disease.

Case history (2)

A 64-year-old man with known severe chronic liver disease, who is on the liver transplant list, has been admitted on a number of occasions with haematemesis due to variceal bleeding. Endoscopic banding of the varices has been undertaken and he is on propranolol therapy.

He is admitted on this occasion with a large haematemesis.

On examination, he is cold and pale, with pulse rate of 120/min and BP of 80/50.

He is in hypovolaemic shock and needs urgent resuscitation with fluid and blood, and vasoconstrictor therapy with terlipressin before urgent endoscopy.

Management of massive haemorrhage (Fig. 6.14)

- Communicate nature and urgency of the situation to the laboratory.
- Predict requirements for blood and blood products; always try to think ahead.
- Monitor:
  - Volume replacement
  - Haemostatic parameters
  - Serum calcium: blood is preserved with citrate–phosphate dextrose solution, which chelates calcium.
- Maintain intravascular volume.
- Avoid:
  - Hypovolaemia
  - Acute kidney injury
  - DIC
  - Cardiac arrhythmias.
- Use:
  - Saline/colloid solutions
  - Group O Rh(D) negative blood
  - ABO Rh(D) group-compatible blood until fully compatible blood available.

Remember

Give blood through a blood warmer to minimise hyperkalaemia and cardiac arrhythmias.

Check for failure of haemostasis

- Initially at beginning of emergency.
- Every 5 units of blood given.
- Whenever additional blood products (platelets, FFP, cryoprecipitate) are given.

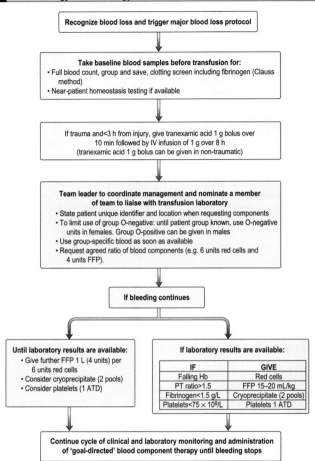

Figure 6.14 Algorithm for the management of major haemorrhage. ATD, adult therapeutic dose; FFP, fresh frozen plasma; PT, prothrombin time. (From Norfolk D. *Handbook of Transfusion Medicine*, 2013. The Stationery Office, with permission. Available at www.transfusionguidelines.com.)

Anticipate haemostatic failure. Check:

- FBC
- PT/INR
- APTT
- Fibrinogen concentration
- FDPs or fibrin D-dimers

Causes of haemostasis failure

- DIC: secondary to hypovolaemic shock with additional liver failure, infection or tissue trauma.
- Dilutional coagulopathy.
- Stored blood depleted of coagulation factors and containing few platelets.

Action

- Request platelets to maintain platelet count $>50 \times 10^9/L$ or if sequential platelet counts are falling progressively.
- Request cryoprecipitate (10 units) if fibrinogen concentration <1.0 g/L.
- Request FFP (10–20 mL/kg) if PT/INR and partial thromboplastin time with kaolin (PTTK) prolonged.

Remember

- FFP takes 30 min to unfreeze.
- Platelets might need to be delivered from Regional Transfusion Centres.

Progress. This man was given 9 units of blood and also balloon tampo-nade, as he was exsanguinating. He could not be resuscitated.

HAEMATOLOGICAL ONCOLOGY

This umbrella term covers a huge range of disorders. Some present dramatically and require urgent treatment; at the other end of the spectrum, there are diseases that are indolent and chronic, often requiring no therapy. You should be able to recognise the low-grade (non-urgent) and high-grade (urgent) disorders, and refer to your Haematology department. (Outside normal hours don't be afraid to talk to the Haematology registrar/consultant on call.)

What main groups of disease are there?

- Leukaemias can be acute (short duration, serious, rapidly fatal if not treated) or chronic. They generally have elevated WCC and other features (see later). These are marrow-/blood-based diseases.
- Lymphomas are lymph node-based, sometimes involving blood and marrow. Some need urgent treatment and others can be sorted out at leisure.
- Myeloma is a low-grade, highly destructive disorder caused by malignant plasma cells, often presenting with bone pain, kidney injury and hypercalcaemia.

Case history (1)

A 63-year-old cleaner is admitted to MAU with pyrexia and cough productive of sputum. Her general health has been reasonable until now.

On examination, she has chest signs suggestive of pneumonia. In addition, she has generalised lymphadenopathy and a three-fingerbreadth spleen. Scarring over her trunk is, she claims, due to shingles 4 months earlier.

An FBC shows mild anaemia (Hb 106 g/L), normal platelets and an elevated WCC of 25×10^9/L. The Haematology technician phones to say that most of the white cells are lymphocytes and there are smear cells on the film.

Remember

A smear cell is an artefact induced by making the blood film (the CLL cells are fragile and burst). There are no smear cells actually circulating in the patient's blood.

What do you need to establish now?

- Whether this is an acute or chronic disease.
- If urgent treatment is required.
- What steps you would need to take to make a diagnosis.

Key features

- Older patient.
- Fairly well.
- Shingles.
- Active infection.
- Lymphadenopathy/splenomegaly.
- High WCC with smear cells.

This must be **chronic lymphocytic leukaemia** (CLL), the most common leukaemia in adults (Fig. 6.15). It is a slowly progressive disorder, and is an

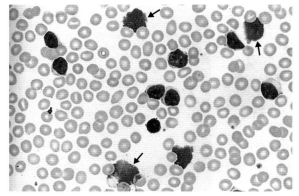

Figure 6.15 Blood film in chronic lymphocytic leukaemia showing numerous smear cells (artefacts; arrows).

incidental finding or presents with an infective complication. Shingles is a fairly common presenting feature.

CLL is a disease mainly of the B lymphocytes (95%, the remaining 5% are T lymphocytes) — determined by checking cell markers. There is a reduction in immunoglobulin synthesis, leading to the infective complications.

Other features

- Possibly, decreased Hb and platelets (depends on disease stage).
- Haemolytic anaemia (red cell autoantibodies).
- Other autoimmune complications.

Management

On day of admission

Start IV antibiotics (e.g. cefuroxime 750 mg × 3, erythromycin 500 mg × 4); rehydrate if necessary. Refer to the Haematology department next day.

The prognosis in CLL is very variable and the disease may remain stable for several years. Many patients (approximately 30%) with CLL never need any treatment at all and lead normal lives.

Long-term treatment

Observation; the patient might require oral chemotherapy at a later stage (e.g. chlorambucil). Rituximab, in combination with chemotherapy, is first-line therapy.

Case history (2)

You are called to see a 43-year-old accountant in A&E. This man went to see his doctor suffering from excessive tiredness. You are presented with an anxious, pale man, who has bruising over his lower limbs and arms. Temperature is 39°C. He is admitted urgently to the MAU, where further examination reveals no other signs.

What tests would you arrange?

- FBC, U&Es.
- Blood cultures.
- MSU.
- CXR.

The Hb is 60 g/L, WCC 90×10^9/L and platelets are 30×10^9/L. Renal function is normal and the CXR shows minimal increased shadowing at the right base.

Remember

Don't wait until the next morning — the patient may succumb before then!

Is this an acute or chronic disorder?

A short history in an ill patient with severe anaemia and thrombocytopenia indicates an acute disorder.

You must ask what the white cells are, morphologically. If they are neutrophils (neutrophilia), this might reflect an underlying infection; this is unlikely with such a high WCC.

However, the technician looks at the blood film and tells you they look like blasts.

Kumar & Clark's Cases in Clinical Medicine

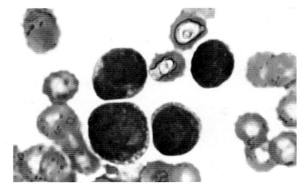

Figure 6.16 Bone marrow in acute myeloid leukaemia showing numerous large leukaemic blasts.

> **Remember**
>
> Blasts are primitive white cells present in bone marrow in small numbers. They are never seen in peripheral blood in health.

This suggests an **acute leukaemia** (Fig. 6.16). In a patient of this age, **acute myeloid leukaemia** is most likely (if he were a child, acute lymphoblastic leukaemia would be more likely).

Investigations

- Specific diagnostic tests (performed by Haematology department)
- Peripheral blood film examination (Are there Auer rods? If so, their presence confirms acute myeloid leukaemia, as are not all that common)
- Bone marrow aspirate and biopsy
- Cell marker analysis (determines pattern of antigens on white cells)
- Cytogenetic studies on marrow blasts: several karyotypic abnormalities are diagnostic
- Other tests, e.g. HLA typing

You should aim to perform only the initial treatment steps: IV fluids, empirical (blind) therapy for infection (send blood and urine cultures first), and then notification of Haematology staff as soon as possible.

Case history (3)

A 72-year-old former butcher is currently on the orthopaedic ward with collapse of one of his lumbar vertebrae. The orthopaedic trainee is concerned because some results have come back that she wishes to discuss with you.

The patient has mild anaemia with an elevated WCC (26×10^9/L, mainly neutrophils). The ESR is 120 mm/h. Blood film comment: red cell rouleaux.

There is mild renal impairment and hypercalcaemia (corrected calcium is 3.21 mmol/L).

The patient appears quite uncomfortable and has pain in the lower back pain, left rib cage, right humerus and right thigh. His general health was excellent until about 4 months ago, when he developed anorexia and mild weight loss. His wife, who is present, is concerned, as he is forgetful and confused at times (this has been much worse over the past 1–2 weeks).

What possible diagnoses are there?

Although not in extremis, this man is ill:

- An ESR of 120 mm/h suggests serious underlying pathology (an ESR of 120 could be due to serious infection, autoimmune disease, rheumatoid disease or malignancy).
- Red cell rouleaux, renal impairment and hypercalcaemia in a patient with bone disease suggest either a primary bone disorder (such as myeloma) or possible infiltration by malignancy, e.g. carcinoma.

If outside working hours, there is little else you can request. Your main objective is to treat the symptoms, e.g. rehydrate, start antibiotics if you think infection is present, and correct the elevated calcium level (see p. 427). Alert the Haematology team.

What to check as soon as possible

- Blood film.
- Immunoglobulin levels/serum protein electrophoresis/immunofixation.
- Repeat biochemistry to check renal function and calcium level.
- Send urine for Bence-Jones protein and plasma for free immunoglobulin light chains.
- Blood cultures if febrile.
- MSU.
- Arrange skeletal survey (plain radiology of skull, spine, pelvis, femora).

Results in this case

- Elevated total IgG with reduced IgA and IgM.
- Serum IgG M paraprotein (paraprotein is monoclonal immunoglobulin produced by the malignant clone of plasma cells).
- Bence-Jones protein present: kappa light chains.
- Widespread lytic lesions throughout skeleton.
- Subsequent bone marrow aspirate showed infiltration by abnormal plasma cells (Fig. 6.17).

   Diagnosis. Multiple myeloma.

The patient should be referred for specialist advice, i.e. treatment for his myeloma. He also needs bisphosphonate treatment for his bone disease and orthopaedic referral for possible kyphoplasty, which involves inflating a balloon in the affected vertebral body and filling this with methyl methacrylate cement in order to restore the vertebral shape.

Case history (4)

A 50-year-old bank manager is admitted with weight loss, sweats and splenomegaly.
Initial investigations show mild anaemia, WCC 200×10^9/L and platelets 600×10^9/L.

What further information do you require?

- White cells: are they blasts? No – there are neutrophils, eosinophils, basophils and early (i.e. immature) granulocytes (e.g. promyelocytes, myelocytes).
- How large is the spleen? Palpable to umbilicus (ultrasound = 24 cm).

Kumar & Clark's Cases in Clinical Medicine

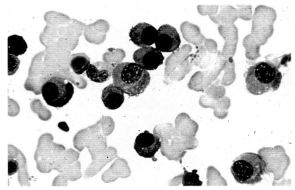

Figure 6.17 Bone marrow aspirate in myeloma showing large numbers of plasma cells.

Biochemical screen

- Normal, apart from elevated serum uric acid level.

Re-examine the patient yourself

Are there any other abnormal findings?
- There is no lymphadenopathy.
- Liver edge is palpable.
- Chest is clear.
- Fundi: nothing abnormal.

What is the underlying diagnosis?

There are several significant findings, i.e. very high WCC, splenomegaly with weight loss and sweats. Could the patient have an underlying infection/neoplasm producing these features (i.e. reactive process)? Yes, but it is much more suggestive of an underlying primary blood disorder such as **chronic myeloid leukaemia**, because the WCC is very high with the whole spectrum of granulocytic cells present (Fig. 6.18). If the blood picture were 'reactive', a neutrophilia would be more likely.

What single investigation will confirm the diagnosis?

Cytogenetic analysis of peripheral blood white cells or bone marrow white cells.

The Philadelphia chromosome will be present (translocation of DNA between chromosomes 9 and 22) in most cases (95%) of CML.

Remember

Philadelphia chromosome is present in some acute leukaemias but this patient does not have features of acute leukaemia; the bone marrow will confirm this.

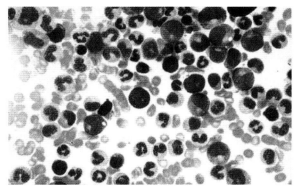

Figure 6.18 Blood film in chronic myeloid leukaemia. Note the large numbers of granulocytic cells, in particular neutrophils, at all stages of development.

Does he need urgent referral to the Haematology team?

Unless the patient is very unwell or has features of leucostasis (blood sludging in the lungs or brain due to a high WCC), there is no immediate need for urgent referral. You should, however, alert the Haematology staff, who should take over the patient's care the next day. Leucostasis can result in:

- Confusion
- Visual disturbance
- Cough and dyspnoea.

Features suggestive of acute leukaemia/high-grade lymphoma

- Acute onset.
- Unwell patient.
- Dramatic presentation.
- Extensive infection and/or bruising.
- Gum swelling.
- Fundal haemorrhage.
- Coagulopathy.
- Blasts/immature cells in peripheral blood.
- Auer rods (neutrophil granules join up to produce these rod-like structures, which are pathognomonic of acute myeloid leukaemia [AML]).

Features suggestive of chronic/low-grade haematological malignancy

- Less dramatic onset.
- Patient who is not particularly unwell.
- Previous infection (e.g. chest infection or herpes zoster).
- Absence of blasts in blood.
- Abnormal peripheral blood cells: lymphocytes with abnormal morphology or immature granulocytes. Generalised lymphadenopathy present for months.

Refer all patients suspected of having acute leukaemia to the Haematology team as soon as possible, for specialist management.

Remember

The WCC does not have to be high to diagnose acute (or chronic) leukaemia. In many cases acute leukaemia may present with normal or low WCC.

Not all patients with acute leukaemia are ill at presentation.

Is it lymphoma or leukaemia? (Fig. 6.19)

- Leukaemias generally involve bone marrow and blood. Lymph nodes and other organs might be involved.
- Lymphomas originate in lymphoid tissue (lymph nodes, spleen), sometimes spill over into blood and might involve marrow (especially low-grade lymphomas).
- High-grade lymphoma and acute lymphoblastic leukaemia are very similar.
- Low-grade lymphomas and chronic lymphoid leukaemias are similar.

Progress. This patient with CML was referred to the Haematologists, who treated him with imatinib. He achieved a complete haematological response.

ANAEMIA IN RHEUMATOID ARTHRITIS, CHRONIC KIDNEY DISEASE AND LIVER DISEASE

Anaemia in rheumatoid arthritis

Case history

A 53-year-old woman with rheumatoid arthritis was admitted for investigation of anaemia.

On examination, she has typical features of rheumatoid arthritis in her hands and arms. Her hands are grossly deformed and swollen, with redness over the MCPs. She has tender, subcutaneous nodules on her elbows. All these features are indicative of an acute flare-up of her condition.

Investigations showed an Hb of 92 g/L, MCV 84 fL, WBC 11.4×10^9/L and platelets 490×10^9/L. Serum vitamin B_{12}, folate and ferritin were checked and found to be normal.

There are several possible causes for this anaemia:

- Bleeding (e.g. due to NSAIDs): the patient denies obvious GI bleeding. If she had been bleeding chronically, her MCV would probably be reduced (iron deficiency). This woman's MCV is normal, making chronic blood loss unlikely.
- Poor diet: can induce folate deficiency, but we know her folate level is normal.
- Autoimmune causes: e.g. pernicious anaemia (she has rheumatoid arthritis and might possibly have pernicious anaemia, another associated autoimmune disease). However, her vitamin B_{12} level is normal.
- Felty's syndrome (see p. 111): rheumatoid arthritis, splenomegaly and neutropenia. This woman has no features of this disorder.
- Infiltrations, myelodysplasia: difficult to exclude these in the absence of additional information, e.g. bone marrow. In myelodysplasia and

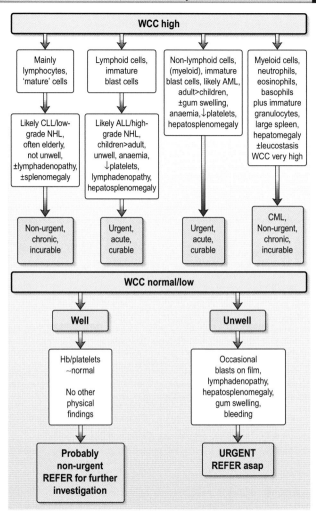

Figure 6.19 Summary of suspected haematological malignancy. ALL, acute lymphoblastic leukaemia; AML, acute myeloid leukaemia; CLL, chronic lymphocytic leukaemia; NHL, non-Hodgkin lymphoma.

marrow infiltration due to carcinoma in the presence of reduced Hb, it is likely (but not always the case) that the blood film would show morphological abnormalities such as 'tear-drop' red cells, nucleated red cells, hypogranular neutrophils or immature white cells. This woman's blood film simply showed RBC rouleaux.

- Renal impairment or liver disease: again, morphological abnormalities are usually present on the film, and the biochemical screen will assess liver and renal function.
- Drug-induced anaemia: several mechanisms, e.g. haemolysis. There are no features suggesting this. Remember the bone marrow suppressive effect of gold and azathioprine.

This woman's ESR was found to be >100 mm/h with a high CRP. Her rheumatoid disease was very active (flare-up), and 3 months before admission her Hb was 110 g/L. The drop in Hb has coincided with the flare-up: a common finding, especially in patients with rheumatoid arthritis.

A major diagnostic pitfall in the assessment of anaemia in patients with inflammatory disease is in the determination of iron status. Patients can be iron-deficient (confirmed by bone marrow aspirate stained for iron, the 'gold standard') yet have a normal serum ferritin, an acute-phase protein that rises to normal (or greater than normal) in patients with inflammation.

Assessment of iron status in patients with inflammatory disorders

- Ferritin: likely to be misleading for the reasons given above.
- Serum iron/total iron binding capacity (TIBC): there might be a reduction of both in chronic disease. These tests are seldom performed now because they are unreliable. Ferritin is the preferred assay.
- Bone marrow: will determine iron status, but is expensive, painful and to be avoided if possible.
- Serum transferrin receptor assay: the number of transferrin receptors on red cells rises in iron deficiency but remains normal in secondary anaemia. This test is replacing bone marrow aspirate in diagnosis of iron deficiency in patients such as this.

This woman had normal transferrin receptor levels, confirming anaemia of chronic disease. She failed treatment with sulfasalazine and methotrexate. She was therefore treated with etanercept SC, a fully humanised p75 TNF-α receptor IgG fusion protein, with a good response in her joints and the ESR. She is now attending the Rheumatology clinic for follow-up.

Anaemia in chronic kidney disease (CKD)

The kidney is the body's major site of erythropoietin (Epo) production. In renal disease, Epo levels fall, leading to chronic anaemia.

Additional factors in development of anaemia in CKD

- Reduced RBC lifespan.
- Iron deficiency (blood loss in dialysis tubing or GI tract).
- Folate loss due to dialysis.

What features should you look for?

- Low Hb.
- Normal MCV.

- Reticulocytes normal or reduced: low Epo reduces RBC production.
- Bizarre RBC shape on blood film: burr cells.

Management

Generally, Epo replacement given at dialysis improves the Hb in these patients ($50-100$ units/kg $\times 3$ per week IV). Alternatively, darbepoetin alfa can be given weekly or pegzerepoetin alfa monthly. The patient might also require additional iron and folic acid. The Hb should be kept within the range of $100-120$ g/L.

Anaemia in liver disease

Complex and multifactorial

Patients with chronic liver failure generally have moderate anaemia.

The red cells are often macrocytic and can have abnormal shapes — target cells and spur cells — owing to membrane abnormalities.

Vitamin B_{12} levels are normal or high; folate levels are often low, owing to poor dietary intake.

- Bleeding produces a hypochromic, microcytic picture.
- Alcohol causes macrocytosis, sometimes with leucopenia and thrombocytopenia due to bone marrow suppression.
- Hypersplenism results in pancytopenia.
- Cholestasis can often produce abnormal-shaped cells and also deficiency of vitamin K.
- Haemolysis accompanies acute liver failure and jaundice.
- Aplastic anaemia is present in up to 2% of patients with acute viral hepatitis.
- A raised serum ferritin with transferrin saturation ($> 60\%$) is seen in hereditary haemochromatosis.

ANAEMIA IN CANCER

Case history

A 55-year-old woman, who underwent a right mastectomy 10 years earlier, presents with a subcapsular fracture of the left humerus. This had followed minimal trauma sustained when she slipped on the floor in the supermarket. It was thought that she might have disseminated bony metastases.

The contributory information provided by the blood count is:

- Hb 86 g/L
- MCV 76 fL
- WCC 14.7×10^9/L
- Platelets 64×10^9/L
- Reticulocytes 2.0%
- Nucleated red cells
- Occasional myelocytes noted 4/100 WBCs
- Rouleaux +
- Platelets clumped + +

Information

ROULEAUX
The tendency of red cells on the blood film to stack up like a 'pile of coins' relates to an increase in plasma proteins, particularly fibrinogen, as part of the acute-phase response.

This patient has a microcytic anaemia with rouleaux formation on the blood film. The anaemia of chronic disorder is common in disseminated malignancy and many other inflammatory and infective illnesses.

Further investigations

- Blood:
  - Serum alkaline phosphatase 247 IU/L
  - CRP 80
  - Serum calcium 2.9 mmol/L.
- Imaging:
  - X-ray of shoulders showed humeral fracture.
  - Skeletal survey showed bony metastases in thoracic spine and pelvis.

  Diagnosis. Carcinoma of the breast with bony secondaries.

Anaemia of chronic disorder: pathophysiology

- Functional iron deficiency
- Reduced sensitivity to erythropoietin
- Reduced red cell lifespan.

This patient has a raised total WCC with nucleated red cells and immature granulocytes seen on the blood film. This is a **leucoerythroblastic picture;** such cells are normally confined to the bone marrow. Bone marrow infiltration by disseminated malignancy disrupts the normal mechanisms controlling release of haemopoietic cells into the blood.

Leucoerythroblastic anaemia

Causes include:
- Acute haemolysis
- Severe infection
- Severe hypoxia
- Bone marrow infiltration:
  - Carcinoma
  - Myeloma
  - Lymphoma
  - Tuberculosis
  - Myelofibrosis
  - Osteopetrosis.

Remember

Most blood count analysers can't distinguish nucleated RBCs (nRBCs) from white cells, and might give an inappropriately high WCC when nRBCs are present. Ask for the blood film to be reviewed.

The reticulocyte count is not increased and no red cell fragmentation is present on blood film review. Microangiopathic haemolytic anaemia (MAHA), which sometimes complicates disseminated breast, prostate or gastric carcinoma, is not likely to be a feature in this patient. MAHA results from mechanical disruption of red cells in small blood vessels and can be complicated by chronic DIC, with a coagulopathy, reduced fibrinogen concentration, elevated fibrin breakdown products and thrombocytopenia.

This patient has thrombocytopenia. The aetiology of thrombocytopenia in disseminated malignancy is complex and can be due to:
- Bone marrow infiltration
- Folate deficiency secondary to anorexia
- Cytotoxic chemotherapy
- DIC.

However, review of the blood film in this patient reveals that the thrombocytopenia is spurious — platelets are clumped on the blood film. Platelet clumping is a common phenomenon related to the EDTA anti-coagulant that blood is collected into.

Progress and management. This lady was treated symptomatically with NSAIDs and started on bisphosphonates. She was referred to the Oncology department for an MDT for discussion of further management.

INFECTION/SEPSIS

Bacterial sepsis

This results in a characteristic constellation of changes in the blood, which provide confirmatory evidence of sepsis and, in occasional patients with occult infection, may direct appropriate investigations.
- Neutrophil leucocytosis: increased numbers of neutrophils
- Immature granulocytes (= left-shift): occasional promyelocytes, myelocytes
- Toxic granulation: coarse neutrophil granulation
- Döhle bodies (white cells containing large RNA inclusions that are seen in, e.g., sepsis, malignancy, pregnancy).

Kumar & Clark's Cases in Clinical Medicine

Possible accompaniments of uncontrolled sepsis

- A falling white cell count/neutropenia.
- Granulocyte vacuolation.
- Bacteria visible on the stained blood film.
- Thrombocytopenia
- DIC.

Anaemia is common in bacterial sepsis and is usually related to the acute-phase response. Occasionally, haemolysis and red-cell fragmentation accompany DIC, and severe haemolysis might complicate *Clostridium welchii* septicaemia with spherocytosis on the blood film.

Malaria (see also case on p. 15)

This should be suspected in any individual with a fever who has recently visited/come from malarial parts of the world. Thrombocytopenia is a frequent accompaniment of malaria infection and haemolytic anaemia might develop, particularly if an individual also has G6PD deficiency.

Remember

If malaria is suspected:
- Ask for thick and thin blood film examination
- Repeat × 3–5 if the initial results are negative but clinical suspicion persists.
  If malaria is diagnosed:
- Ask for the species of *Plasmodium*
- If *P. falciparum*, ensure that you are given the parasite count. This indicates the severity of infection:
  - A high parasite count >5.0% indicates an increased risk of cerebral malaria.
  - Pre-schizont forms indicate an increased risk of cerebral malaria.

Some features of severe *falciparum* malaria

Remember

Treatment for severe malaria due to *P. falciparum* is a *medical emergency*. Give:
- Artesunate 2.4 mg/kg single bolus, and at 12 h and 24 h, and then daily, until oral medication can be tolerated.
- Quinine dihydrochloride 20 mg/kg IV over 4 h, then 10 mg/kg if artesunate unavailable.
  See your National Formulary for details, and p. 17 for other treatment.

- CNS: cerebral malaria (coma, convulsion).
- Renal:
  - Haemoglobinuria (blackwater fever)
  - Oliguria
  - Uraemia (acute tubular necrosis).
- Blood:
  - Severe anaemia (haemolysis and dyserythropoiesis)
  - DIC: haemorrhage.
- Respiratory: acute respiratory distress syndrome (see p. 373).
- Metabolic:
  - Hypoglycaemia (particularly in children)
  - Metabolic acidosis.

- Gastrointestinal/liver
  - Diarrhoea
  - Jaundice/splenic rupture.
- Other:
  - Shock: hypotension
  - Hyperpyrexia.

Beware

The parasite count in *falciparum* malaria may under-estimate the severity of the infection due to parasite sequestration. Always take a diagnosis of *falciparum* malaria seriously.

Viral infections

These produce a variety of specific and non-specific effects on the blood that might be helpful diagnostically.

Consider:
- Age of patient
- Length of history
- Clinical findings
- Morphology of lymphoid cells
- Monospot or Paul–Bunnell test
- Immunophenotyping

Non-specific effects

These are common to many viral illnesses:
- Mild neutropenia and thrombocytopenia
- Occasional reactive lymphoid cells on blood film.

Specific effects

- **Glandular fever** is produced by Epstein–Barr virus infection (see p. 18). Similar features are seen in CMV infection and also in toxoplasmosis. The reactive lymphocytosis must be distinguished from a malignant lymphoid proliferation.
- **Erythrovirus B19** causes Fifth's disease and specifically infects erythroid progenitor cells, resulting in transient erythroid hypoplasia and failure of red cell production. This is of no consequence in otherwise healthy individuals, but in those with chronic haemolytic anaemia it causes a sudden fall in the Hb concentration, with absent reticulocytes. Urgent blood transfusion can be life-saving.

Remember

Erythrovirus B19 is infective and chronic haemolytic anaemias can be inherited, e.g. sickle-cell disease. Ask about other family members with haemolysis: 'Are they well?'

- **HIV infection** results in anaemia, thrombocytopenia and neutropenia in most patients. The severity of the cytopenia is related to the stage of the disease and is reflected by ineffective haemopoiesis with dysplastic changes in bone marrow precursor cells. It can be exacerbated by intercurrent infection and therapy.

Further reading

Microcytic and macrocytic anaemia

British Committee for Standards in Haematology. Guidelines for the diagnosis and treatment of cobalamin and folate disorders. *British Journal of Haematology*. 2014; **166**: 496—513.

Camaschella C. Iron deficiency anaemia. *New England Journal of Medicine*. 2015; **372**: 1832—1843.

Sickle-cell disease

Piel FB, Steinberg MH, Rees DC. Sickle cell disease. *New England Journal of Medicine*. 2017; **376**: 1561—1573.

Elevated white blood cell count

Stock W, Hoffman R. White blood cells 1: non-malignant disorders. *Lancet*. 2000; **355**: 1351—1357.

Platelet disorders

Imbach P, Crowther M. Thrombopoietin receptor agonists for primary immune thrombocytopenia. *New England Journal of Medicine*. 2011; **365**: 734—741.

Provan D, Newland A. Fifty years of idiopathic thrombocytopenic purpura (ITP): management of refractory ITP in adults. *British Journal of Haematology*. 2002; **118**: 933—944.

Blood transfusion

Murphy MF, Roberts DJ, eds. *Practical Blood Transfusion*. 5th edn. Oxford: Wiley—Blackwell; 2017.

British Society for Haematology (BSH). Guidelines. www.transfusion-guidelines.org.

Haematological oncology

Devereaux S, Cuthill K. Chronic lymphocytic leukaemia. *Medicine*. 2017; **455**: 292—295.

Longo DL. Imatinib changed everything. *New England Journal of Medicine*. 2017; **376**: 982—983.

BLACKOUTS

This implies either altered consciousness, with or without falling, or sometimes a visual disturbance.

Case history

An 86-year-old woman is brought into A&E with a 'blackout'. She had been found on the floor but had regained consciousness on the way to hospital.

On examination, pulse and BP were normal and there was no abnormality found on neurological examination.

What should you ascertain from the history?

- Any previous episodes.
- What the patient was doing at the time (e.g. micturition, change in posture, coughing).
- Symptoms preceding blackout:
  - Chest pain or palpitations, suggesting cardiac cause.
  - Aura, suggesting epilepsy.
- Witness history: any witness(es) to give a description of the blackout.
  Differential diagnosis. Common causes include neurological or cardiovascular events.

Epilepsy in the elderly

- Focal fits or a focal origin of generalised seizures are common in the elderly (accounting for 80% of fits in this age group).
- Post-ictal confusion, headache and focal signs (Todd's paresis) are common.
- 35–50% of fits in the elderly are caused by vascular disease.
- 20% of patients with stroke have seizures within the first year.
- Elderly persons are more susceptible to pharmacological causes of fits, e.g. neuroleptics, tricyclics, and to alcohol withdrawal.
- An EEG can be useful but a normal or non-diagnostic EEG does not rule out epilepsy.
- Don't forget hypoglycaemia as a cause of fits.
- Anti-convulsant drugs should be started after the first fit if a vascular or structural cause is suspected.
- Pallor suggests a cardiac cause.
- Tonic–clonic contractions or incontinence suggest epilepsy.
- Was there a history of head turning or tight neckwear? This suggests carotid sinus syndrome.
- Was there a period of drowsiness after the blackout? This suggests epilepsy but might also occur in cardiac causes.

Remember

Epilepsy might be secondary to reduced cardiac output.

Investigations

- FBC, U&Es, glucose, TFTs, Ca^{2+}
- ECG
- 24-h tape if ECG abnormal or history suggestive of cardiac cause
- EEG and/or CT scan if history suggests epilepsy
- Specialist intervention: carotid sinus massage — undertaken if carotid sinus syndrome suspected (**Note:** contraindications for massage include presence of carotid bruit and history of carotid territory neurological events)

Cardiovascular causes of blackouts

- Arrhythmias (brady- or tachy-) can be difficult to diagnose and sometimes require repeated 24-h tapes or 2–3-week 'event recorders' (see p. 264).
- Myocardial infarction can be pain-free in older people.
- Aortic stenosis typically causes exertional syncope, also shortness of breath on exertion and angina.
- Hypertrophic cardiomyopathy is diagnosed on echocardiogram.
- Postural hypotension.
- Carotid sinus syndrome is an under-diagnosed cause of unexplained blackouts. It is caused by an exaggerated response of baroreceptors in the carotid sinus and requires specialist investigation by carotid sinus massage with close observation. There are three variants. The **cardio-inhibitory variant** is diagnosed by >3-s asystole on massage. The **vasopressor variant** is diagnosed by a 50-mmHg drop in BP or systolic BP drop to <90 mmHg. Third, up to one-third of cases are mixed.
- Vasovagal syncope occasionally presents for the first time in older people. Consider if there is a long history of 'funny turns'.

Treatment

In this patient an ECG, CXR and blood tests were normal. It was thought that the blackout could be due to an **arrhythmia** so a 24-h tape ECG was performed. This showed episodes of tachycardia and bradycardia, with two episodes of sinus arrest, compatible with the **sick sinus syndrome.**

Progress. This patient was fitted with a pacemaker/DDD and has had no further attacks.

FALLS IN THE ELDERLY

Case history

A 79-year-old man was brought into A&E following a fall. He was taking atenolol 100 mg daily, aspirin 75 mg daily and bendroflumethiazide 2.5 mg daily.

On examination, he was well. His pulse was normal but BP low at 90/50; he had no abnormal neurological signs. He had symptomatic **postural hypotension** on standing up.

What questions should you ask?

- What was he doing when he fell, e.g. was there a postural element?
- What does he remember about the fall?
- Did he lose consciousness?
- What happened immediately before the fall?
- Were there any preceding symptoms?

- Was there a witness?
- Were there any physical hazards, e.g. wet floor, carpet edge?
- Had he fallen before?

These features can help distinguish pathological causes (intrinsic) from those with a major external factor (extrinsic), although in practice most falls are multi-factorial. Falls or 'collapse' can be seen as a final common pathway for many frequently encountered diseases in the elderly.

Examination after falls

Full physical examination, especially:
- Cardiovascular:
  - BP including postural changes after 1–3 min
  - Evidence of heart failure or rhythm disturbance
  - Murmurs.
- Musculoskeletal:
  - Arthritis: acute or chronic, and evidence of joint instability
  - Muscle wasting, especially quadriceps.
- Neurological:
  - Focal signs; don't forget cerebellar/brainstem
  - Hearing or visual impairment
  - Gait: observation of the patient standing from sitting (with arms folded) and walking (with turns) provides a good assessment of risk for falling.
- Frailty: the Fried Frailty score assesses:
  - Slowness in walking
  - Exhaustion
  - Weakness (decreased hand grip strength)
  - Physical inactivity (low energy expenditure)
  - Weight loss (body mass index [BMI] <18.5 or >5% weight loss in the last year).
    Score of 3 or more defines frailty.

Orthostatic hypotension

This is defined as a >20-mmHg drop in systolic BP on standing or during head-up tilt:
- Common in elderly: occurs in up to 30% of healthy older people and it is not clear why some develop symptoms.
- 'Physiological' changes in elderly: decreased baroreceptor sensitivity increases risk of postural hypotension.
- 'Pathological' changes: e.g. sepsis with vasodilatation; poor left ventricular function; neurological disease affecting reflex pathways.
- Pharmacological causes: beta-blockers, vasodilators, anti-parkinsonian drugs, sedatives, neuroleptics, diuretics.

Investigation of falls

- BP and heart rate measurement with patient lying flat, standing upright or at 45 degrees on tilt table after 1, 3 and 5 min.
- FBC for evidence of infection, anaemia.
- U&Es, creatinine for evidence of dehydration, renal impairment (eGFR is calculated).
- Blood glucose for hypo-/hyperglycaemia.
- TFTs for subclinical hypothyroidism.
- CXR for infection, tumour.

- ECG for ischaemia, arrhythmias, silent MI.
- Heart beat monitoring (beat-to-beat variation) for autonomic neuropathy.
- MSU and Stix testing for infection.

Management of falls

- Review medications and withdraw exacerbating drugs if possible.
- Treat medical factors, e.g. sepsis.
- Assessment and reduction of osteoporosis risk.
- Advice to patients (see later).
- Drug treatment occasionally used in patients with persistent disabling symptoms:
  1. Fludrocortisone 100−200 µg at night. Watch for fluid retention and hypokalaemia.
  2. If still symptomatic, add sympathomimetic agent, e.g. ephedrine 15 mg × 3 daily. This can be increased to 45 mg × 3 (side-effects: hypertension, tachycardia, tremor).

Progress. In this patient with postural hypotension, the atenolol was stopped and a careful watch was kept on his BP (he had his own BP machine) over the following few weeks. He should stay on aspirin and bendroflumethiazide. His BP stabilised at 115/80 and therefore no further medication was required.

Advice for patients with postural hypotension

- Get out of bed in stages.
- Pause between positional changes.
- Wear leg support tights during the day; take them off at night.
- Raise head of bed.
- Avoid alcohol.

DELIRIUM

Delirium (see p. 485) is also known as 'toxic confusional state'. It is the commonest psychosis seen in the general medical setting. It is 'brain failure' with impairment of attention and abnormalities of perception and mood.

Case history

A 76-year-old female is admitted to the MAU with a 3-day history of confusion associated with hallucinations.

On examination, she has signs of consolidation at the left lung base. Her temperature and WCC, however, were within normal limits.

Delirium in the elderly

An elderly person presenting with acute confusion associated with disorientation and agitation ± hallucinations is a common medical emergency. In a hospital setting the elderly develop delirium while receiving treatment for other medical or surgical problems, the reported incidence varying from 10 to 60%.

As a condition (syndrome), it is associated with increased morbidity and mortality.

> **Box 7.1** Delirium: diagnostic criteria (derived from DSM-5)
>
> - Disturbance of consciousness:
>   - Clarity of awareness of environment
>   - Ability to focus, sustain or shift attention
> - Change in cognition:
>   - Memory deficit, disorientation
>   - Language disturbance, perceptual disturbance
> - Disturbance develops over a short period (hours or days)
> - Fluctuation over course of day

Diagnosis

Information

The Diagnostic and Statistical Manual (DSM) is published by the American Psychiatric Association and provides clear descriptions of diagnostic categories. Text revision (DSM-5) Washington, DC: American Psychiatric Association, 2013.

Use DSM-5 criteria or the Confusional Assessment Method (CAM), which is based on the DSM criteria (Box 7.1).

Confusional assessment method (CAM) criteria

Need points 1 and 2:
1. **Acute onset +fluctuating course:** this history is usually obtained from the family/carer or from the nurse caring for a patient who is already in hospital.
2. **Inattention:** is the patient easily distractible or does he/she have difficulty keeping track of what is being said?
   ... and either 3 or 4:
3. **Disorganised thinking:** is the patient incoherent? Is the conversation irrelevant?
4. **Altered level of consciousness:** the patient might be hyperactive, hypoactive/lethargic or semi-conscious.

Remember

- One in four patients with delirium is hypoactive.
- Although history/observations can confirm the presence of CAM features, it is also useful to assess the patient's cognitive functioning using serial mental test scores, e.g. Abbreviated Mental Test (AMT; Box 7.2). Other tests using questions on orientation (e.g. time, place, date), registration (naming objects), attention and calculation (simple arithmetic), recall (previously mentioned objects) and language (understanding commands) can be used.

What should you do when delirium is suspected/diagnosed?

- Identify the cause by taking a medical history, and performing a physical examination and appropriate investigations.
- Manage the delirium.

Box 7.2 Abbreviated Mental Test (AMT)

Total score 10 (1 point for each item)

- Age
- Time (to nearest hour)
- Address for recall
- Year
- Where do you live (town or road)?
- Recognition of two persons
- Date of birth (day and month)
- Year of the start of the First World War
- Name of present leader of the country
- Count backwards 20 to 1

Medical history. Illness in old age can present in a non-specific or atypical way. It is therefore necessary to go through a systematic enquiry to detect symptoms of physical illness, particularly those relating to chest infection and urinary tract infection (UTI). The family/carer or doctor should also be questioned about recent changes to drug therapy.

Physical examination. Full physical examination, including neurological examination, is essential, as any physical illness in older people can lead to delirium.

Investigations

- FBC
- U&Es
- Liver biochemistry
- Calcium
- Phosphate
- TFTs
- CXR
- ECG, MSU
- Other investigations as indicated by clinical findings

Causes

For causes, remember the mnemonic **delirium** and think of common conditions:

D drugs: side-effects, toxicity of drugs, e.g. hypotensives, sedatives

E electrolyte/endocrine disturbance, e.g. hyponatraemia, hypernatraemia, hypothyroidism

L lack of drugs: withdrawal of drugs

I infections, e.g. pneumonia, cellulitis

R reduced sensory input, e.g. visual impairment

I intracranial: transient ischaemic attack (TIA), epilepsy

U urinary retention/faecal impaction

M myocardial: ischaemia/infarct, arrhythmias, chronic heart failure (CHF).

Remember

The presentation of illness in the elderly can be altered, e.g. not all patients with pneumonia will have a raised temperature or raised WCC.

Risk factors for delirium

- Dementia.
- Severe physical illness.
- Raised urea/creatinine.
- Visual impairment.
- More than three prescribed drugs.

How would you manage a patient with delirium?

- Treat cause(s) of delirium. Review present drug therapy.
- Environmental measures and general support: fluids/nutrition; bladder/bowel care + environment (nurse in quiet, dimly lit room if possible), providing reassurance and reorientation.
- Pharmacological management: only appropriate if general supportive measures are not adequate to reduce patient's distress and if there is danger to patient. Drugs of choice:
  1. Lorazepam up to 2 mg IV or IM up to 4-hourly
  2. Haloperidol 0.5 mg IV or IM, repeating if necessary after 30 min
  3. Olanzapine 5 mg is also used.

Progress. The cause of this patient's delirium was pneumonia. She didn't mount a raised white count or have a temperature. Her delirium resolved on treatment with antibiotics.

DEMENTIA

Definition. Dementia is defined by the Royal College of Physicians as global impairment of higher cortical functions, including memory:

- The capacity to solve problems of day-to-day living.
- The performance of learned perceptuomotor skills.
- The correct use of social skills.
- The control of emotional reactions in the absence of gross clouding of consciousness.

Case history

An 89-year-old man with a 6-month history of deteriorating short-term memory and increasing confusion is referred to A&E because of self-neglect. He has become even more confused over the previous 24 h. He was diagnosed as having **dementia** and referred to the Care of the Elderly team.

Remember

You should distinguish delirium from dementia, but remember that delirium can and does occur commonly in patients with dementia, as in this case.

- Dementia is often irreversible and progressive, and has a number of causes.
- Assessment: this is performed using the 10-point AMT (see Box 7.2) or Clock-drawing test (Fig. 7.1).
- Although screening tests are useful in demonstrating the presence of deficits in cognition, they can't be used for making the diagnosis of dementia or identifying the underlying cause. This requires imaging

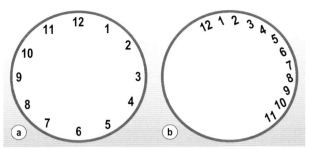

Figure 7.1 Clock drawing test. (a) Normal. (b) Abnormal — inappropriate spread.

(CT or MRI scan) and, in some patients, assessment by a clinical psychologist and/or a psychiatrist. A history of progressive decline in memory or cognition over 6 months is significant.

Investigations

INITIAL INVESTIGATIONS FOR DEMENTIA

- FBC and film
- U&Es
- Random blood glucose
- Liver biochemistry
- TFTs
- Vitamin B_{12} and folate
- Syphilis serology
- CXR
- ECG
- CT/MRI scan of brain or PET scan

Causes

The common causes of dementia include Alzheimer's disease (AD), vascular dementia, Lewy body dementia and Creutzfeldt–Jakob disease, but other conditions can produce a dementia-like syndrome (Box 7.3).

Management

- AD: although there is no cure, research on acetylcholine esterase inhibitors has shown that in selected patients with mild to moderate AD the decline can be slowed down. The National Institute for Health and Care Excellence (NICE) has produced guidance on use of donepezil, rivastigmine, memantine and galantamine in patients with mild to moderate AD by specialists. Other agents/drugs that have some benefit in patients with AD include vitamin E and *Ginkgo biloba* extract.
- Vascular dementia: treat the risk factors, such as hypertension. Aspirin also has a role in preventing further strokes. *Ginkgo biloba* (120–240 mg daily) can also help.

> **Box 7.3** Examples of treatable causes of dementia-like syndrome (see also p. 492)
>
> - Hypothyroidism
> - Vitamin B_{12} deficiency
> - Folate deficiency
> - Recurrent hypoglycaemia
> - Alcohol excess
> - Depression ('pseudodementia')
> - Subdural haematoma
> - Normal pressure hydrocephalus

- As dementia progresses, the management focus changes to care provision for patients plus support for carers.
- Lewy body dementia: avoid anti-psychotics, as they can increase confusion. Some of these patients respond to acetylcholine esterase inhibitors.

Remember

Acetylcholine esterase inhibitors for AD are initiated only by a specialist (psychiatrist, neurologist or geriatrician):

- Donepezil 5–10 mg daily
- Rivastigmine 3–12 mg daily
- Galantamine 8–24 mg daily
- Memantine 5–20 mg daily.

Progress and management. This patient's previous history of hypertension and two small strokes suggested vascular dementia. The diagnosis was confirmed by an MRI. The Care of the Elderly team arranged for full support in the community and he was continued on his treatment for hypertension. He is being assessed regularly to see if pharmacological treatment for his dementia is required.

Remember

In all types of dementia, it might be necessary to use pharmacological agents to control agitation and other behavioural disturbances, but it is important to remember that patients with Lewy body dementia are very susceptible to the side-effects of anti-psychotic drugs.

DEPRESSION

Depression is common in old age (see also p. 145). Community studies have revealed a prevalence of 11.3% for depressive symptoms and 3% for depression in the UK. Studies of elderly hospital inpatients have shown that up to 33% have depression. It is common in the elderly with chronic physical illnesses such as stroke, and it can also be the presentation of an occult physical illness such as hypothyroidism, hypercalcaemia or carcinoma of the lung. Physical illness is the biggest risk factor for depression in old age.

Remember

Whereas the clinical features of depression in old age can be the same as in younger patients, somatic complaints, delusions and decline in cognition ('pseudodementia') are more frequently noted in the elderly.

Case history

A senior nurse noted that an 83-year-old man with a cerebrovascular accident (CVA) is eating poorly and is losing weight. On direct questioning, the patient admits to being depressed and feels he has no future.

Examination showed no abnormality, apart from slight residual neurological signs from his CVA.

Assessment

- Geriatric Depression Scale (Table 7.1), shorter version, is a reliable and valid screening instrument of depression in the elderly. A score <5 indicates probable depression.
- Physical examination and investigations to detect/exclude physical causes of depression, such as hypothyroidism, hypercalcaemia, malignancy. In a patient with a normal physical examination, the recommendation is that FBC, U&Es, liver biochemistry, vitamin B_{12}, Ca^{2+}, TFTs and CXR are performed.

  In this patient, these blood tests and the CXR showed no abnormality.

Remember

Always ask the patient about suicidal thoughts/intent.

Management

Significantly depressed patients can be treated successfully with drugs. Drugs commonly used for treating depression in older people include:

- Citalopram: a selective serotonin reuptake inhibitor (SSRI), 8–32 mg daily.
- Mirtazapine: a pre-synaptic alpha-2 antagonist is particularly useful in patients with poor appetite, 15 mg daily, increased according to response to 45 mg daily.
- Venlafaxine: a serotonin and noradrenaline reuptake inhibitor, 75–150 mg daily.

  Severely depressed patients with or without suicidal ideation need urgent referral to a psychiatrist for further assessment.

  Progress and treatment. Management of this patient consisted of multidisciplinary support in the community with short-term use of venlafaxine 75 mg daily to help his depression.

NON-SPECIFIC PRESENTATION OF ILLNESS IN THE ELDERLY

Many illnesses in the elderly population can present in a non-specific manner. Taking a detailed and informative history can be very difficult because underlying memory loss due to dementia can be exacerbated by an acute medical problem (delirium). Information regarding the previous medical,

Table 7.1 Geriatric Depression Scale

CHOOSE THE BEST ANSWER FOR HOW YOU HAVE FELT OVER THE PAST WEEK:

1.	Are you basically satisfied with your life?	Yes/No
2.	Have you dropped many of your activities and interests?	Yes/No
3.	Do you feel that your life is empty?	Yes/No
4.	Do you often get bored?	Yes/No
5.	Are you in good spirits most of the time?	Yes/No
6.	Are you afraid that something bad is going to happen to you?	Yes/No
7.	Do you feel happy most of the time?	Yes/No
8.	Do you often feel helpless?	Yes/No
9.	Do you prefer to stay at home, rather than going out and doing new things?	Yes/No
10.	Do you feel you have more problems with memory than most?	Yes/No
11.	Do you think it is wonderful to be alive now?	Yes/No
12.	Do you feel pretty worthless the way you are now?	Yes/No
13.	Do you feel full of energy?	Yes/No
14.	Do you feel that your situation is hopeless?	Yes/No
15.	Do you think that most people are better off than you are?	Yes/No

The following answers count as 1 point:

A total score >5 indicates probable depression

1.	No
2.	Yes
3.	Yes
4.	Yes
5.	No
6.	Yes
7.	No
8.	Yes
9.	Yes
10.	Yes
11.	No
12.	Yes
13.	No

(Continued)

Table 7.1 Geriatric Depression Scale—cont'd		
CHOOSE THE BEST ANSWER FOR HOW YOU HAVE FELT OVER THE PAST WEEK:		
14.	Yes	
15.	Yes	

From Sheikh JI, Yesavage JA. Geriatric Depression Scale (GDS). *Clinical Gerontologist* 1986; **5:** 165–173.

mental, functional and social conditions is needed to make an accurate assessment of the patient's current state.

History obtained from the patient should be augmented by information from the patient's doctor, district nurse, carers, relations and neighbours, if necessary, particularly if the patient is confused.

These problems are highlighted in the following case. NEWS (see Figs 1.1 and 1.2) is a simple physiological scoring system that can be used at the bedside in a MAU. It identifies patients at risk of deterioration and who may require more specialised care.

Case history (1)

Mr S. is 85 years old and lives alone in a bungalow. His neighbours noticed that he had failed to collect the milk from the front door for 2 days. They called the family doctor, who found Mr S. sitting in a chair with grossly swollen feet. In his letter referring the patient to hospital the doctor confirmed that Mr S. had been on salbutamol and ipratropium inhalers for 5 years. However, he had not visited the surgery for some time.

On arrival in hospital, Mr S. was very confused and unable to give a detailed history. His AMT score (see Box 7.2) was 3 out of 10.

On examination, he had a low-grade temperature of 37.6°C and appeared breathless on minimal exertion, with central cyanosis and had signs of congestive heart failure: high JVP, an enlarged liver, and leg swelling up to the groin.

A CXR showed signs of left **heart failure** and there was left basal shadowing suggestive of **left lower lobe pneumonia** (Fig. 7.2).

It was not clear how long he had been confused or how mobile he had been before these problems.

His next of kin was a younger brother who lived far away. He was contacted by telephone and confirmed that the patient was not married and had been able to go out to the local shops (a quarter of a mile away) until 3 weeks ago. He also commented that the patient had been mildly confused and needed some help in running his own affairs for several years, but was self-caring and didn't need help at home.

Treatment. Mr S. was started on antibiotics — amoxicillin 500 mg × 3 daily — bendroflumethiazide 2.5 mg daily and enalapril 2.5 mg × 2 daily for his pneumonia and heart failure. He was also found to be hypothyroid and was started on levothyroxine 25 μg initially. His general condition gradually improved and his AMT rose to 7 out of 10.

Progress. With the help of the physiotherapist, Mr S. was able to get back on his feet using a Zimmer frame. A home visit was successful and he returned to his bungalow with daily home-care support and follow-up in the day hospital, with adjustment of his medication, to maintain his mobility.

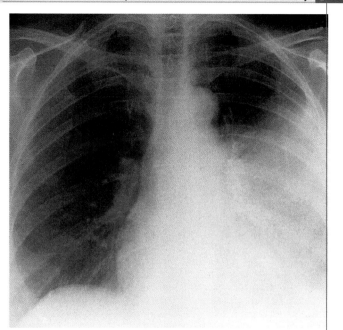

Figure 7.2 CXR showing lobar pneumonia. (From Feather A, Randall D, Waterhouse M, eds. *Kumar and Clark's Clinical Medicine*, 10th edn. Elsevier, 2021; Fig. 28.28.)

Remember

All elderly persons presenting to hospital with non-specific complaints should have full physical examinations and investigations that include FBC, U&Es, liver biochemistry, Ca^{2+}, phosphate, TFTs, ECG, MSU and CXR, plus any other investigations as indicated by the findings on examination.

Case history (2)

A 79-year-old man was admitted after having an unexplained fall. He was mildly confused but on direct questioning denied any symptoms.

On examination, he had a tachycardia of 100 bpm, normal heart sounds and a clear chest. An ECG revealed raised ST segment in leads II, III and AVF, i.e. an acute inferior myocardial infarct (STEMI). He had a raised serum troponin.

- Any illness in old age can present with any of the so-called 'giants' of geriatric medicine, i.e. confusion, falls/instability and incontinence.
- In addition, some illnesses present atypically. Examples of this include:
  - 'Silent' MI
  - Pneumonia without pyrexia or rise in WCC

• 'Silent' peptic ulcer perforation, i.e. peptic ulcers might perforate with little or no pain but the patient becomes non-specifically unwell, anorexic and bed-bound.

Diagnosis. This patient has had a 'silent' myocardial infarction.

Management. Aspirin 300 mg chewed with clopidogrel 300 mg oral gel were given. He was assessed urgently by the Cardiac team, who felt that, despite his age, he should be treated urgently with percutaneous coronary intervention (PCI). He responded well, with a fall in the ST segment to normal, without any complications of treatment.

Progress. The patient was discharged, given post-MI drug treatment and was followed up by the cardiac rehabilitation nurse.

Drug therapy and assessment post acute coronary syndrome (ACS)

Extensive clinical trial evidence has been gathered in post-MI patients, demonstrating that a range of pharmaceuticals is advantageous in reducing mortality over the following years. Therefore, after MI, most patients should be taking most of the following medications:

- Aspirin 75 mg daily
- An adenosine diphosphate (ADP)-receptor blocker
- An oral beta-blocker to maintain heart rate <60 bpm
- Angiotensin-converting enzyme (ACE) inhibitors or angiotensin receptor blockers, particularly if left ventricular ejection fraction (LVEF) is <40%
- High-intensity statins with target low-density lipoprotein (LDL) cholesterol <1.8 mmol/L
- An aldosterone antagonist, if there is clinical evidence of heart failure and LVEF is <40%; the serum creatinine is <221 μmol/L (men) or <177 μmol/L (women); and the serum potassium is <5.0 mEq/L.

Remember

Older patients often do well with active treatment of STEMI (fibrinolysis or PCI). There is no evidence to support not giving therapy to elderly patients.

APPROPRIATE ASSESSMENT SCALES

The Royal College of Physicians has produced a list of useful assessment scales/tools for the day-to-day management of the elderly. The following scales are recommended:

- **Barthel Index:** for activities of daily living (ADL) (Table 7.2)
- **Mini-Mental State Examination (MMSE):** cognitive screening test for dementia and delirium
- **Geriatric Depression Scale:** screening instrument test for depression (see Table 7.1)
- **Waterlow Score:** for risk quantification for pressure ulcers (Table 7.3)
- **Philadelphia Geriatric Center Morale Scale:** for quality of life (Table 7.4); provides a multidimensional approach to assessing the psychological state of older people, i.e. well-being/life satisfaction/quality of life.

Other scales, e.g. Braden, Walsall and Maelor, are also available.

The Barthel Index should be used as a record of what a patient does (not as a record of what the patient could do). The main aim is to establish the degree of dependence on any help, physical or verbal. A need for supervision means that

Table 7.2 Barthel Index	
Item	**Categories**
Bowels	0 = incontinent (or needs to be given an enema)
	1 = occasional accident (once per week)
	2 = continent
Bladder	0 = incontinent/catheterised, unable to manage
	1 = occasional accident (max. once every 24 h)
	2 = continent (for over 7 days)
Grooming	0 = needs help with personal care
	1 = independent face/hair/teeth/shaving (implements provided)
Toilet use	0 = dependent
	1 = needs some help but can do something alone
	2 = independent (on and off, dressing, wiping)
Feeding	0 = unable
	1 = needs help cutting, spreading butter, etc.
	2 = independent (food provided in reach)
Transfer	0 = unable − no sitting balance
	1 = major help (one or two people, physical), can sit
	2 = minor help (verbal or physical)
	3 = independent
Mobility	0 = immobile
	1 = wheelchair independent (includes corners)
	2 = walks with help of one (verbal/physical)
	3 = independent (may use any aid, e.g. stick)
Dressing	0 = dependent
	1 = needs help, does about half unaided
	2 = independent, includes buttons, zips, shoes
Stairs	0 = unable
	1 = needs help (verbal, physical), carrying aid
	2 = independent
Bathing	0 = dependent
	1 = independent (may use shower)

the patient is not independent. Performance over the preceding 24–48 h is used when completing the Barthel Index but longer periods of assessment might be more relevant. A patient's performance should be established using the best available evidence. Ask the patient or carer but also observe what the

Table 7.3 Waterlow pressure ulcer risk assessment

Build/weight for height		Visual skin type		Continence		Mobility		Sex/Age		Appetite	
Average	0	Healthy	0	Complete	0	Fully mobile	0	Male	1	Average	0
Above average	2	Tissue paper	1	Occasionally incontinent	1	Restricted/difficult	1	Female	2	Poor	1
		Dry	1					14–18	1	Anorectic	2
Below average	3	Oedematous	1	Catheter/incontinent of faeces	2	Restless, fidgety	2	50–64	2		
		Clammy	1					65–75	3		
		Discoloured	2			Apathetic	3	75–80	4		
		Broken/spot	3	Doubly incontinent	3	Inert/traction	3	81 +	5		

Special risk factors		Assessment value	
1. Poor nutrition, e.g. terminal cachexia	8	At risk	10
2. Sensory deprivation, e.g. diabetes, paraplegia, cerebrovascular event	6	High risk	15
3. High-dose anti-inflammatory or steroid in use	3	Very high risk	20
4. Smoking 10 + per day	1		
5. Orthopaedic surgery/fracture below waist	3		

The Waterlow assessment is mainly used in acute hospital settings in order to highlight patients at risk of pressure sores who will require special nursing care, including aids, and to prevent the development of pressure sores.

Table 7.4 Philadelphia Geriatric Center Morale Scale

	High morale response	Low morale response
Do little things bother you more this year?	No	Yes
Do you sometimes worry so much that you can't sleep?	No	Yes
Are you afraid of a lot of things?	No	Yes
Do you get mad more than you used to?	No	Yes
Do you take things hard?	No	Yes
Do you get upset easily?	No	Yes
Do things keep getting worse as you get older?	No	Yes
Do you have as much pep as you had last year?	No	Yes
Do you feel that as you get older you are less useful?	No	Yes
As you get older, are things . . . than you thought?	Better	Worse or same
Are you as happy now as you were when you were younger?	No	Yes
How much do you feel lonely?	Not much	A lot
Do you see enough of your friends and relatives?	Yes	No
Do you sometimes feel that life isn't worth living?	No	Yes
Do you have a lot to be sad about?	No	Yes
Is life hard much of the time?	No	Yes
How satisfied are you with your life today?	Satisfied	Not satisfied

References: Lawton MP. The Philadelphia Geriatric Center Morale Scale: a revision. *Journal of Gerontology* 1975; **30:** 85–89; Royal College of Physicians. *Report of A Joint Workshop with the Royal College of Physicians and the British Geriatrics Society Standardised Assessment Scales for Elderly People.* London: RCP, 1992.

patient can do. The use of aids to be independent is allowed. Direct testing is not needed. Unconscious patients score '0' throughout.

STROKE

This is the sudden onset of focal neurological symptoms caused by interruption of the vascular supply to the brain (ischaemic stroke) or intra-cerebral haemorrhage (haemorrhagic stroke).

Case history

A 78-year-old man presents with a reduced conscious level, GCS of 12, weakness of the right arm and leg, and inability to speak. His daughter thinks that he has had a stroke. She also says that her father has been well and is still working 2 days a week.

Information

Each year in England about 100 000 (1.6—2 per 1000) people have a first stroke. Stroke is the most common cause of severe disability in adult life. There are 64 000 deaths attributed to first or recurrent strokes, which makes it the third commonest cause of death in the UK.

Paramedics and members of the public are encouraged to make the diagnosis of stroke on a history and simple examination (FAST test):

- Face — sudden weakness of the face
- Arm — sudden weakness of one or both arms
- Speech — difficulty speaking/slurred speech
- Time — the sooner the treatment can be started, the better.

! Stroke is a medical emergency and prompt treatment can improve prognosis.

Questions you need to address

- Is it a stroke?
- What type of stroke?
- What part of the brain is affected?
- What is the prognosis?
- Are there complications to treat or prevent?

Pathology

- 80—90% of strokes are ischaemic, i.e. due to thrombosis or embolism.
- 10—20% are the result of primary cerebral haemorrhage or aneurysm rupture.

Common sources of emboli

- Carotid artery and aortic arch atheroma.
- Intra-cardiac sources, e.g. left atrium in atrial fibrillation (AF), left ventricle mural thrombus, left-sided heart valves.
- Vertebral artery atheroma or dissection.

Uncommon causes of thrombotic stroke

- Giant cell arteritis.
- Other vasculitides.
- Haematological disorders, e.g. polycythaemia vera, hyperviscosity syndrome.

Typical signs of a stroke

The typical signs of a stroke are listed in Table 7.5.

Features of a stroke involving the brainstem

- Hemiplegia/quadriplegia.
- Ataxia/vertigo/tinnitus.
- Dysphagia.

Table 7.5 Clinical deficits associated with different vascular territories of the brain

Anatomical location	Common neurological deficits
Left middle cerebral artery	Right-sided weakness involving face and arm > leg with expressive, receptive or mixed dysphasia
Right middle cerebral artery	Left-sided weakness, face and arm > leg, visual and/or sensory neglect or inattention of left side, denial of disability (anosognosia)
Lateral medulla (posterior inferior cerebellar artery and/or parent vertebral artery)	Ipsilateral Horner's syndrome, Xth nerve palsy (due to infarction of nucleus ambiguus), facial sensory loss (trigeminal nerve), limb ataxia with contralateral spinothalamic sensory loss Typically, patients are vertiginous and unable to feed by mouth due (mainly) to failure of laryngeal closure during swallowing and ineffective coughing Cervical radiculopathies may occur due to involvement of radicular branches of the vertebral artery
Posterior cerebral artery	Homonymous hemianopia with variable additional deficits due to involvement of parietal and/or temporal lobe
Internal capsule	Motor, sensory or sensorimotor loss, involving face, arm and leg to a roughly similar extent There may be profound dysarthria due to involvement of corticobulbar fibres but the patient should not be dysphasic or have other cortical type deficits such as dyslexia or dysgraphia
Bilateral paramedian thalamus (30% of population have a single common arterial stem	Coma or disturbed vigilance at presentation, ophthalmoplegia (internal

(Continued)

Kumar & Clark's Cases in Clinical Medicine

Table 7.5 Clinical deficits associated with different vascular territories of the brain—cont'd

Anatomical location	Common neurological deficits
supplying medial aspect of both thalami)	and/or external), ataxia and memory impairment Some patients require ventilation
Carotid artery dissection	Ipsilateral Horner's syndrome due to compression of the sympathetic plexus around the carotid artery; the same process can also affect the lower cranial nerves (Xth and XIIth most obvious clinically) in the carotid sheath, or the VIth nerve in the cavernous sinus If ipsilateral cerebral infarction follows (due to hypoperfusion or embolisation), the clinical picture can mimic a brainstem event; in this way, carotid artery dissection can mimic vertebral artery dissection

- Dysarthria.
- Gaze paresis.
- Temperature control disturbance.
- Altered respiratory pattern.

Is your diagnosis of a stroke correct?

Most strokes are easily diagnosed clinically but errors do occur. Not all acute neurological impairments are due to stroke and other conditions can be misdiagnosed as stroke.

Unusual symptoms and signs should make you question the diagnosis, e.g.:
- Papilloedema
- Persistent headache
- Fluctuating signs
- Unexplained fever
- History of trauma to head or neck.

Examples of misdiagnosis

- Todd's paresis secondary to epileptic fit.
- Space-occupying lesions:
  - Primary tumours, metastases
  - Subdural haematoma
  - Cerebral abscess.
- Venous sinus thrombosis.
- Carotid or vertebral artery dissection.

- Infections:
  - Meningitis
  - Encephalitis.
- Metabolic disturbance:
  - Hypo-/hyperglycaemia
  - Hypo-/hypernatraemia
  - Chronic kidney disease.
- Intoxication/overdose:
  - Alcohol
  - Drugs, e.g. sedatives, tricyclics. (**Note:** focal neurological signs are common with tricyclic overdose.)
- Hypotension:
  - Hypovolaemia
  - Cardiac dysrhythmia
  - Cardiogenic shock.
- Old neurological deficits, e.g. previous stroke.

Stroke management (Fig. 7.3)

Clinical problems associated with a stroke (see Table 7.5)
Neurological deficit
Early management of a stroke

- Thrombolytic treatment with IV alteplase (tPA) (see p. 450): needs to be given in <4.5 h (ideally 90 min) of onset of stroke, once haemorrhage has been excluded on scanning. Tenecteplase is an alternative agent. Endovascular thrombectomy is performed after thrombolytic treatment in many units.

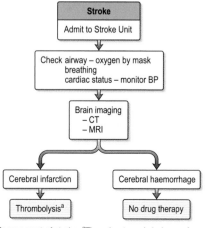

Figure 7.3 Management of stroke. [a]Thrombectomy is being performed after thrombolysis in many units. (From Kumar P, Clark M, eds. *Medical Management & Therapeutics*. Edinburgh: Saunders/Elsevier; 2011; Fig. 20.20.)

Kumar & Clark's Cases in Clinical Medicine

- Aspirin: 300 mg and clopidrogel 75 mg after CT scanning (to rule out haemorrhage), if fibrinolysis is not being used.
- Hydration and/or feeding: early nasogastric (NG) or percutaneous endoscopic gastrostomy (PEG) feeding improves outcome in stroke patients who have unsafe swallowing (see later).
- Treatment of hyperglycaemia with insulin regimen initially.
- Paracetamol for pyrexia: if present.
- Prevention of complications:
  - Chest infection: attention to swallowing and chest physiotherapy.
  - DVT. TED stockings have been shown not to be helpful. Prophylactic low-molecular-weight (LMW) heparin (if haemorrhage has been ruled out) should be used early.
  - Pressure ulcers.
  - Contractures.
- Rapid treatment of infection (most commonly chest and urinary tract).
- Hypertension: BP often rises in acute stroke but usually settles. Lowering of BP is only necessary in the early stage for severe hypertension. Persistently raised BP requires treatment for its secondary prevention benefits (see below).
- Support and interventions for the patient and family: stroke is a major life event and both the patient and family need information and support.

  Dysphagia and aspiration. These can occur in up to 50% of patients at presentation. The ability to swallow should be tested by asking the patient to swallow a teaspoon of water and *not* by putting a spatula in the throat. Some patients need further assessment by a Speech and Language Therapist (SALT) and investigation by videofluoroscopy.

  If the patient's conscious level is impaired, don't assess the swallow until it improves.

  Skin condition
- Are there any pressure ulcers?
- Are there any areas of skin at risk?

  Bladder function
- Incontinence can result from the neurological problem or from immobility.
- Catheterisation is required only if the patient is incontinent and there is a risk of pressure ulcers.

Remember

The specific symptoms and signs detected will depend on site of the lesion. Some 75% of strokes occur in middle cerebral artery territory; 15% are in the vertebrobasilar territory (see Table 7.5).

How would you investigate and treat this patient?

A CT scan (MRI not available) was performed approximately 3 h after the onset of the stroke. This showed a middle cerebral artery thrombus.

The National Stroke Guidelines state that fibrinolytic therapy should be commenced; fibrinolytic therapy is indicated in patients with a cerebral infarct due to a thrombus which occurred less than 4.5 hours ago (see p. 157). Therapy should be given as soon as possible, however, to allow the damaged brain to recover. A CT scan in the first 24 h after an infarct might appear normal; if so, it will need to be repeated if MRI can't be performed. Haemorrhage can usually be seen. An MRI scan shows an infarct early in the diagnosis.

Investigations

- FBCs
- U&Es
- Random blood glucose
- ESR
- ECG
- CXR
- CT or MRI scan of brain

Major risk factors for stroke

- Smoking.
- Hypertension.
- Peripheral vascular disease.
- Diabetes.
- AF.
- Hypercholesterolaemia.
- Previous stroke.
- Coronary artery disease.

Remember

POOR PROGNOSTIC SIGNS IN STROKE
- Reduced conscious level on admission
- Gaze paresis
- Early and persisting urinary incontinence
- Sensory inattention
- Pre-existing disability
- Previous cognitive impairment

Further management — rehabilitation

- Physiotherapy to maximise functional recovery and prevent contractures.
- Occupational therapy for functional assessment, aids and adaptations.
- SALT for assessment and management of speech and swallowing problems.
- Continuing medical review.
  Post-stroke care and rehabilitation in Stroke Units have been shown to reduce mortality and early disability.

Secondary prevention after stroke

- Hypertension: if persisting at 28 days after stroke, this should be treated according to British Hypertension Society Guidelines (see p. 299).
- Anti-platelet agents: aspirin 75–150 mg daily and clopidogrel 75 mg daily should be started. Dipyridamole MR 200 mg is used if clopidogrel 75 mg daily is contraindicated or not tolerated.
- Anti-coagulation: given in patients with ischaemic stroke who make a reasonable recovery and have AF, mitral valve disease or a prosthetic heart valve, or are within 3 months of MI.

- Carotid endarterectomy: if carotid stenosis of 70—90% is present in patients who are not severely disabled by their stroke. Early investigation and surgery should be performed within 1 week.
- Statins: for those with cholesterol >3.5 mmol/L.
- Smoking cessation: refer to anti-smoking clinic.

Progress. This 78-year-old man improved a few hours after the fibrolytic therapy. Two days later he was able to stand with help. With physiotherapy and speech therapy he became fully ambulant in 6 days and his speech was improving. At assessment, 3 months later, he was living an independent life.

HEART DISEASE IN THE ELDERLY

Case history

A 78-year-old man with long-standing atrial fibrillation was admitted with tiredness and breathlessness. He also complained of indigestion and recent falls.

Examination revealed a radial pulse of 96, apical rate 110 irregular, a raised JVP, swollen ankles and crackles up to both lung mid-zones.

He was taking digoxin 125 μg daily and aspirin 75 mg daily.

What investigations would you do?

- FBC
- U&Es.
- Liver biochemistry.
- TFTs.
- Troponins.
- ECG.
- CXR.

Investigations revealed AF with no R wave progression on his ECG, suggesting a possible **acute myocardial infarct.**

His CXR showed pulmonary oedema (Fig. 7.4a). The FBC showed an Hb of 98 g/L with an MCV of 70 fL, suggesting an iron deficiency anaemia, possibly related to his aspirin intake.

Learning points

- Cardiac failure in the elderly may present with non-specific symptoms such as tiredness and falls.
- Aspirin, even at low dose, can be associated with occult GI blood loss.
- Always check compliance in older people, especially if the patient thinks that the medication is not effective.
- Benefits have been shown for anti-coagulation of elderly patients in AF up to age 85, but contraindications (e.g. falls or GI haemorrhage) are more common in this population. In this case the microcytic anaemia (see p. 71) would need to be investigated before starting anti-coagulants.
- Risks of anti-coagulation in the over-85s are high and no study has shown a benefit in this age group.
- ACE inhibitors should be used in hypertension in the elderly, starting with a low dose, and renal function closely monitored due to increased risk of renal impairment (see p. 223).

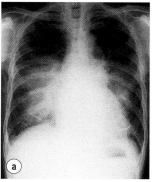 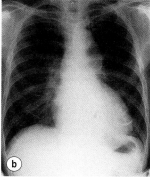

(a)　(b)

Figure 7.4 A pair of chest X-rays taken from a patient before (a) and after (b) treatment of acute pulmonary oedema. The CXR taken when the oedema was present demonstrates hilar haziness, Kerley B lines, upper lobe venous engorgement and fluid in the right horizontal interlobar fissure. These abnormalities are resolved on the film taken after successful treatment.

Acute MI

The management principles of heart disease in the elderly are the same as those in young people, with a few exceptions.

Age alone is not a contraindication to thrombolysis/PCI in acute MI; in fact, the greatest benefits are seen in older patients. However, other co-morbidities causing contraindications are more common in older people.

Acute MI may present silently (with no pain) more commonly in the elderly.

Treatment

This patient was given diuretic therapy with furosemide 40 mg orally daily. This helped his breathlessness and his ankles became less swollen. His CXR improved (Fig. 7.4b). As his presentation was over a few days, he was not given fibrinolytic therapy. He was started on an ACE inhibitor with enalapril 2.5 mg.

Endoscopy was performed and he was found to have gastric and duodenal erosions due to his aspirin intake. The aspirin was stopped. Colonoscopy showed no lesion.

Progress. Three weeks later he was feeling much better. He was given iron therapy and started on anti-coagulation with apixaban.

TRANSIENT ISCHAEMIC ATTACK (TIA)

This is a transient episode of neurological dysfunction caused by focal brain, spinal cord or retinal ischaemia without acute infarction. The arbitrary time of <24 h is no longer used; the criteria depend on having no demonstrable lesion on imaging.

Case history

A 68-year-old man presents to A&E with weakness of the right arm and leg, expressive dysphasia and a facial palsy. While he is being examined, his symptoms and signs start to improve and have resolved by the time he returns from the X-ray department. A diagnosis of a TIA is made.

What points do you need to ascertain in the history?

- Previous similar episodes, especially recently.
- Previous episodes of amaurosis fugax (sudden transient loss of vision in one eye).
- History of palpitations, hypertension, diabetes, high cholesterol or stroke.
- Smoking history.
- Current and previous medication.
- Functional status: mental and physical.

What are the major aspects of the examination?

- The neurological examination.
- BP.
- Pulse rate and rhythm.
- Presence of cardiac murmurs, carotid bruits.
- Papilloedema, visual field deficit, signs of retinal emboli.

Investigations

- FBC
- ESR
- U&Es
- Blood sugar
- Cholesterol
- ECG/24-h tape in selected patients
- CXR
- CT head
- Echocardiogram in patients with suspected valvular disease or mural thrombus
- Carotid duplex ultrasonography in patients with carotid territory TIAs

Should you admit this patient?

Updated National Stroke guidelines for the UK recommend that a patient with a TIA should be admitted to hospital if he/she can't be assessed and investigated in a neurovascular clinic within 7 days of TIA.

Other reasons for admission:

- Doubt over diagnosis, e.g. need to exclude space-occupying lesion
- Multiple TIAs in a short time: these patients should also be fast-tracked to carotid endarterectomy
- Identification of pathology requiring immediate intervention, e.g. cardiac arrhythmia
- Background disability with poor social circumstances.

How would you manage a case of TIA?

- Aspirin 75–150 mg per day and clopidogrel 75 mg.
- Anti-coagulation with apixaban in patients with AF.
- Statins for those with hypercholesterolaemia (cholesterol >3.5 mmol/L).

- Treatment of risk factors, e.g. hypertension.
- Smoking cessation.
- Advice not to drive for 1 month following the event.

Further management — carotid endarterectomy

Carotid endarterectomy is recommended for patients with TIAs and minor strokes who have 70—90% stenosis of the relevant carotid artery and who are otherwise fit, with no major persisting disability.

Investigation and treatment should be performed within 1 week. MR angiography is required prior to surgery. Carotid endarterectomy has a 1—2% perioperative stroke risk in the most experienced hands but reduces the incidence of stroke by 75% over the next 2—3 years.

The **ABCD^2 score** can help to stratify stroke risk in the first 2 days (Table 7.6).

Note: asymptomatic carotid stenosis is associated with a lower stroke risk but benefit from surgery is not proven.

Prognosis after untreated TIA over 4 years

- 25% dead.
- 25% stroke.
- 10% MI.

Progress. This man had a carotid endarterectomy performed 6 days after his admission to hospital. He made a good recovery; at 6-month review

Table 7.6 ABCD^2 score in the stratification of stroke risk

Parameter	Score
Age >60 years	1
BP >140 mmHg systolic and/or diastolic >90 mmHg	1
Clinical features	
Unilateral weakness	2
Isolated speech disturbance	1
Other	0
Duration of symptoms (min)	
>60	2
10—59	1
<10	0
Diabetes	1
A score of <4 is associated with a minimal risk whereas >6 is high-risk for a stroke within 7 days of a TIA	

(From Feather A, Randall D, Waterhouse M, eds. *Kumar and Clark's Clinical Medicine*, 10th edn. Edinburgh: Elsevier, 2020; Box 26.33.)

he was still taking treatment for stroke prevention and had started on an exercise programme.

HYPOTHERMIA

Information

Hypothermia is defined as core body temperature of <35°C. It is associated with many clinical conditions and in most patients aetiology is multifactorial.

Case history

An 89-year-old female is found lying on the floor by her carer. On arrival at the A&E department, she is noted to be confused and has a rectal temperature of 34°C.

Aetiological factors

- Exposure to cold.
- Impaired thermoregulation.
- Impaired shivering thermogenesis.
- Low metabolic heat production.
- Impaired temperature perception.
- Drugs, e.g. phenothiazines, hypnotics, alcohol.
- Hypothyroidism.
- Intercurrent illness.

Clinical features

These vary with the degree of hypothermia. Whereas those with a core temperature of 33–34°C can be confused and have slow cerebration, those with a temperature of 30°C are more likely to be drowsy and have muscular stiffness.

Some patients with hypothermia have features such as slow relaxing reflexes, which are suggestive of hypothyroidism.

The ECG can show changes such as sinus bradycardia, slow AF, prolonged PR interval, and 'J' waves (commonly seen in leads V_3-V_4) (Fig. 7.5).

Complications of hypothermia include pancreatitis, oliguria, cardiac arrhythmias (particularly during rewarming) and aspiration pneumonia.

Investigations

- FBC
- U&Es
- Glucose

Figure 7.5 ECG showing J waves.

- Amylase
- Liver biochemistry
- Calcium
- Arterial blood gases
- ECG
- CXR
- TFTs

This patient was found to be grossly hypothyroid with a TSH of 14.3 mU/L and a T_4 of 4 pmol/L.

How would you manage this patient?

She was managed as follows:
- Nursing with space blanket in a warm room (allowing temperature to rise by 0.5°C/h)
- Oxygen: remember that patients with COPD might require 24% oxygen
- IV fluids (through blood warmer)
- Triiodothyronine 5–10 µg slowly IV 12-hourly for her severe hypothyroidism.

A severely hypothermic patient will require admission to ITU for positive pressure ventilation, CVP line and ECG monitoring.

Progress. This woman made a slow but steady recovery and was discharged home on levothyroxine 125 µg daily with a follow-up appointment.

PRESSURE ULCERS

Pressure ulcers are common. Ill elderly people are most at risk of developing pressure ulcers. The reported prevalence rates vary widely – on average 5–10% of this group.

Case history

A 78-year-old woman with a right hemiplegia from a previous stroke was brought to A&E, having fallen at home. She had been on the floor for at least 24 h because she was unable to get up.

On examination, she was conscious and aware of her surroundings. There were no specific abnormalities on physical examination, apart from evidence of a right hemiparesis. When examining her, you notice a dusky area over the right hip overlying the greater trochanter.

Risk factors for developing pressure ulcers

- Low/excessive body weight.
- Poor nutritional state.
- Motor deficit/immobility.
- Sensory deficit.
- Presence of intercurrent illness.
- Incontinence: bladder/bowel.
- Use of certain medication, e.g. long-term prednisolone, sedatives and analgesics, which reduce sensation and hence stimulation to move.

Other patients at special risk

- Those undergoing surgery, particularly orthopaedic.
- Those with neurological disease.

- Those with spinal cord injury, including cord compression.
- Those receiving palliative care.

Why do pressure ulcers occur?

Pressure greater than the mean capillary pressure (25–32 mmHg) will occlude blood vessels and lead to anoxia of the skin. Hard surfaces can generate pressures of >100 mmHg; damage to the skin therefore results from the pressure applied and the length of time exposed to the pressure. In addition to pressure, shearing force is another significant factor.

Pressure ulcers can be graded into superficial (grades 1 and 2) and deep (grades 3 and 4).

Clinical assessment

Document pressure ulcers fully:
- Site, size and grade of pressure ulcer
- Condition of the surrounding skin
- Presence/absence of infection.

Photography is a good method of recording pressure ulcers and monitoring change.

Perform a general examination of the patient with special regard to:
- Nutritional state, including body weight
- Full neurological examination
- Abdominal examination, especially bladder and bowel.

How would you investigate?

Investigations will be directed by the physical examination, but special attention should be paid to those in the Investigations box.

Investigations

- FBC: presence of anaemia will delay wound healing
- Albumin: marker of nutrition; low albumin will delay wound healing
- Blood sugar: hyperglycaemia delays healing
- Wound swabs: for culture and sensitivity
- Blood cultures: if concern about septicaemia
- X-ray of the underlying bone: to rule out osteomyelitis if the wound is deep, overlies a bony prominence and has been present for some time

How would you manage pressure ulcers?

Prevention is definitely better than cure and all at-risk patients require immediate assessment.

Remember

- Pressure ulcers can develop in 1–2 h.
- Beware of leaving patients on hard A&E trolleys or X-ray tables for too long.

- Relief of pressure with appropriate support mattress and/or cushion for chair:
  - Low-risk patients: a soft overlay to the mattress may be adequate
  - High-risk patients: an alternating pressure support system, e.g. special pressure-relieving mattresses.
- Appropriate dressings for wounds. **Note:** dry dressings should not be used on moist wounds. Examples of dressings include:

- Hydrocolloid for superficial granulating wounds
- Alginates for exuding or bleeding wounds.
- Treatment of infection (cellulitis or associated septicaemia), when present, with appropriate systemic antibiotics.
- General management of the patient:
  - Pain relief
  - Treatment of medical conditions, including anaemia
  - Review of drug treatment: NSAIDs and steroids delay wound healing
  - Review of nutrition: including use of supplements, such as vitamin C and zinc
  - Management of incontinence.
- Severe pressure ulcers often require surgical debridement and skin grafting by plastic surgeons, when non-infected.

Most hospitals have tissue viability specialist nurses to advise on prevention and treatment of pressure ulcers. For quantification of risk, these nurses can use the Waterlow score or Norton Scale (see p. 152).

Progress. This patient was admitted to the MAU and the tissue viability nurse was contacted to assess her pressure areas. Despite immediate treatment, she developed a pressure ulcer over her right hip.

URINARY TRACT INFECTION AND INCONTINENCE

Case history

An 80-year-old woman with mild dementia presented with 24 h of increasing confusion and drowsiness. She had a 3-day history of urinary incontinence and diarrhoea. She was taking co-dydramol for arthritis.

    Examination revealed a woman with confusion, with no knowledge of her surroundings or time of day. Her GCS score was 12. Examination of her abdomen was normal but rectal examination showed constipation with faecal impaction and overflow diarrhoea. A urine sample was offensive, and positive to Stix testing for nitrites, leucocytes, blood and protein.

Particular points to note in the history

- UTI in the elderly can present with non-specific symptoms such as confusion, drowsiness or falls.
- Recurrent UTIs should be investigated (>3 in a woman, >1 in a man) with renal tract ultrasound, including assessment of post-micturition bladder volume.
- New urge incontinence may be precipitated by infection, leading to an unstable bladder.
- Infection can be precipitated by obstruction: most commonly caused by constipation or prostatic hypertrophy.
- Drug history for precipitating causes: drugs causing constipation, diuretics, sedatives.

Examination

Examination of this patient included:
- Full physical examination for coexisting causes of confusion, e.g. chest infection
- Rectal examination, to assess for constipation/overflow (prostatic enlargement in men)

Kumar & Clark's Cases in Clinical Medicine

- Neurological examination, to exclude neurological causes of urinary retention and constipation.

- Stix testing positive for both leucocytes and nitrites is highly specific and sensitive for infection; blood and protein Stix are much less useful. **Note:** bacteriuria without symptoms (urgency, frequency, dysuria or systemic symptoms) is common in hospitalised/institutionalised older people and should not be treated, even if bacterial count is $>10^5$
- In—out catheterisation can be useful for obtaining specimens or assessing residual volumes. However, catheterisation should not be used as a treatment for incontinence
- FBC
- Blood cultures
- U&Es
- Creatinine (eGFR)
- AXR for evidence of constipation
- Further assessment of incontinence if it doesn't settle on treatment of infection

How would you treat this patient?

- Treat infection with oral antibiotics:
  - Trimethoprim 200 mg × 2 for 3—5 days is a good first-line treatment. Use parenteral antibiotics only if the patient is very ill or vomiting.
- Treat constipation: enemas and laxatives (see p. 36). Stop co-dydramol. Repeat residual volumes after constipation is treated, as this patient's constipation was likely to be due to the codeine in co-dydramol. The latter was replaced by paracetamol.

Progress. This patient's confusion and drowsiness improved with successful treatment of her UTI. Her faecal impaction was relieved by the enemas, but she is still inclined to constipation and this is treated symptomatically with Macrogol.

ARTERITIS

An 82-year-old widower was admitted with left-sided temporal headache of 3 days' duration. He is known to have type 2 diabetes (on insulin), visual impairment due to macular degeneration, hypertension and an old left hemiparesis. He lives alone in a house and has one son who lives far away.

Medical assessment

On examination, the patient had signs of an old left hemiparesis and a peripheral neuropathy (probably due to long-standing diabetes) and visual impairment. His BP was 150/80 on losartan therapy. In addition, it was noted that the left temporal artery was pulsatile but tender.

Investigations revealed a significantly elevated ESR (>100 mm in 1 h).

A clinical diagnosis of **temporal arteritis** (see p. 197) was made. A temporal artery biopsy showed:

- Cellular infiltrate of CD4 and T lymphocytes
- Macrophages in the vessel wall
- Granulomatous inflammation of the intima and media
- Breaking up of the internal elastic lamina

- Giant cells, lymphocytes and plasma cells in the internal elastic lamina.
  His response to steroids was very good, although he remained tired and slightly frailer than previously.

How would you organise his discharge?

The patient needs a multidisciplinary assessment before discharge to ensure his safety. His son should also be contacted, with the patient's permission.

General points for discharge planning

Discharge planning of an elderly person should start as early as possible after admission. Once the person's medical problems have been accurately diagnosed and treated, his/her potential for returning home should be assessed by an MDT of professionals, taking into account the elderly person's views.

Remember

A competent adult has a right to decide whether he/she wishes to go home, even if this decision is against the advice offered by member(s) of the MDT.

The MDT review includes:
- Assessment by a physiotherapist to assess the patient's mobility, transfers and ability to climb stairs
- Assessment by an occupational therapist to assess independence and safety in ADL, kitchen assessment and/or a home visit
- Social work assessment that will take into account the assessments of other professionals to quantify his/her needs for care on discharge
- Assessment by a SALT, a dietitian or a psychologist in some cases
- Referral to a district nurse, e.g. for treatment of leg ulcers, monitoring of diabetic control, monitoring of medication
- Discussion with GP about on-going medical care.

Following discharge, it might be possible to continue further rehabilitation or monitoring of medical or nursing care in a day-hospital setting.

Progress. This patient was keen to go home, even though he was still frail. He required full support at his house, with community nurses managing his insulin therapy. His headaches disappeared on steroid therapy, which was reduced, making his diabetes easier to manage. He continues to improve.

ACUTE HOT JOINT

Case history

An 80-year-old man presents with a hot, painful, swollen knee joint. He takes a thiazide diuretic for hypertension and has recently had a chest infection treated by his GP.

What are the possible causes?

- Acute gout (see p. 194).
- Acute pseudo-gout (pyrophosphate arthropathy) (see p. 194).
- Septic arthritis (see p. 195).

- Acute flare-up of chronic arthritis, e.g. rheumatoid arthritis (RA; see p. 182).
- Traumatic haemarthrosis with fracture of patella or tibial plateau.
- Ruptured Baker's cyst in osteoarthritis (OA; see p. 178).

Particular points you should elicit in the history

- Trauma or injury: entry for infection.
- Drug history: particularly diuretic.
- Known arthritis or previous episodes, e.g. of gout.
- History of intercurrent illness.

What should you look for on examination?

- Temperature, pulse: systemic signs of infection/inflammation.
- Joint colour, temperature and tenderness.
- Evidence of trauma.
- Other joint disease, including evidence of RA or OA.

Joint fluid should be sent for culture, cell count and examination under polarised light. Urate crystals are distinguished by being negatively birefringent. Calcium pyrophosphate consists of weakly positively birefringent rhomboidal crystals.

Investigations

- X-ray joint
- Tap joint under sterile conditions: fluid for culture, crystal detection and cell count
- Blood cultures
- FBC for WCC and ESR
- Serum uric acid
- Rheumatoid factor, ACPA and autoantibody screen if appropriate

How would you manage this patient?

This patient's serum uric acid is in the high range: 700 μmol/L, which is compatible with gout.

His joint aspiration showed a cloudy, viscous fluid containing 4020 μWCC/mm^3 and negative birefringent, needle-shaped crystals.

Diagnosis. Gout.

Treatment

There are three acute options:

- An NSAID: e.g. ibuprofen 400 mg $\times$ 3 daily or diclofenac with misoprostol one tablet $\times$ 3 daily. (Misoprostol is a cytoprotective agent to the gastric mucosa.)
- Colchicine (rarely used only because it causes diarrhoea): 1 mg initially, 0.5 mg every 2 h until attack subsides or 0.5 mg $\times$ 2 daily for 5 days if symptoms are not severe.
- Intra-articular corticosteroids: injection with methylprednisolone 40 mg with 1 mL of 1% lidocaine.

Allopurinol *should not* be used acutely. *Prophylactically*, it is started at least 4 weeks after the acute attack has settled, to prevent further attacks of gout.

Progress. This man's knee became less painful and the swelling settled after 1 week's NSAID therapy. His thiazide diuretic was stopped and replaced with losartan. He has had no further attacks of gout.

PARKINSON'S DISEASE

Case history

An 80-year-old man with a history of hypertension presents with a fall. He has had numerous falls recently and, on questioning, said he had slowed down generally.

You immediately notice a tremor in his left arm, lack of facial expression and a monotonous voice. The diagnosis is **Parkinson's disease** (PD).

Features of PD

- Akinesia/bradykinesia:
  - Poor initiation of movement
  - Slowing of repetitive movements
  - Fatigue.
- Rigidity:
  - Lead pipe *and/or*
  - Cogwheel (if tremor is present).
- Tremor: 70% of patients present with tremor, usually unilateral:
  - Rest tremor
  - 3–7 Hz
  - Absent in 30% at presentation.
- Postural instability is usually a late feature of idiopathic PD.
- Response to levodopa (L-dopa) suggests idiopathic PD.

Remember

- The disease is often asymmetrical at presentation.
- Depression is a common association, often missed.

Clinical diagnosis of PD

PD is a clinical diagnosis; there are no diagnostic tests. Diagnosis requires two cardinal features, including:
- Akinesia/bradykinesia of the upper body
- Asymmetrical onset with resting tremor
- Clear response to L-dopa.

What is the differential diagnosis of PD?

- Essential tremor:
  - Isolated tremor, can affect the head (Yes/Yes or No/No pattern)
  - Becomes more prominent with increasing age
  - Autosomal dominant inheritance
  - Responds to alcohol, beta-blockers.
- Arteriosclerotic parkinsonism:
  - History of cerebrovascular disease and hypertension common
  - Wide-based, short-stepped gait: *marche à petit pas*
  - Upper part of body not affected
  - Limited/transient response to L-dopa.
- Drug-induced parkinsonism:
  - Anti-psychotic drugs, especially depot preparations
  - Metoclopramide: acute.
- Rarer causes of parkinsonism:

• Multiple system atrophy, Shy–Drager parkinsonism: autonomic failure and dementia
• Steele–Richardson–Olszewski parkinsonism: loss of voluntary conjugate deviation of gaze, and pseudobulbar dysarthria.

WHEN TO QUESTION A DIAGNOSIS OF PD
• Poor response to L-dopa
• Early instability
• Pyramidal or cerebellar signs
• Early autonomic failure, e.g. postural hypotension, incontinence
• Dementia early in course of disease
• Voluntary downward gaze palsy

How would you manage this patient?

• This patient was started on L-dopa as first-line treatment (e.g. co-beneldopa 62.5 mg × 2 daily), as it is useful in the elderly. Dose requires titration, depending on improvement and side-effects of medication, e.g. postural hypotension, nausea, hallucinations.
• Synthetic dopamine agonists (ropinirole, pramipexole) are less effective but might be useful in early disease. Hallucinations and somnolence are common side-effects but are tolerated by approximately 46% of very elderly patients. They may need to be used with domperidone to avoid GI side-effects. Other dopamine agonists have ergot side-effects and are poorly tolerated by the elderly.
• The monoamine oxidase inhibitor (MAOI-B) selegiline should be avoided in patients with postural hypotension or hallucinations.
• Catechol-O-methyl transferase (COMT) inhibitors (e.g. tolcapone, entacapone) are used as adjuncts to L-dopa.
• Apomorphine SC infusion is used in specialist centres.

The frequency of this patient's falls improved with PD therapy, but nevertheless, exercise and balance training was started. He was referred to an MDT to assess the need for walking aids and changes in the home environment.

Progress. The patient was commenced on co-beneldopa 62.5 mg × 2 daily and was able to return home with community support.

DRUGS AS A CAUSE OF ILLNESS, ADMISSION TO HOSPITAL AND DELAYED DISCHARGE

Individuals over the age of 65 make up approximately 18% of the population but represent 25–30% of drug expenditure. Approximately 87% of the elderly take one prescribed medication and one-third of this group take three or more drugs.

Age-associated increases in the incidence of adverse reactions have been well described for certain groups of drugs, e.g. benzodiazepines.

The most frequently used classes are cardiovascular drugs, analgesics, GI preparations and sedatives (Table 7.7).

Case history (1)

A 75-year-old woman was admitted to the MAU with a severe cough and purulent sputum. She was known to have COPD and this was thought to be an infective exacerbation.

Table 7.7 Drugs that are more likely to produce adverse effects in the elderly

Drug	Adverse effects
Benzodiazepines	Sedation, drowsiness, confusion, ataxia
NSAIDs	Gastric erosions, fluid retention, renal impairment and drug interaction, e.g. diuretics
Opiates	Sedation, confusion, constipation
Anti-muscarinic	Urinary retention, glaucoma
Anti-arrhythmics	Confusion, urinary retention, thyroid problems
Anti-psychotics	Confusion, sedation, tardive dyskinesia, malignant hyperthermia
Diuretics	Dehydration, hyponatraemia, hypo- or hyperkalaemia, postural hypotension, renal impairment, gout
Antibiotics	Renal failure, diarrhoea, auditory complications

On examination, she was tachypnoeic but not cyanosed. Examination of her chest showed diffuse wheeze with some basal crackles. Her oxygen saturation was 92%.

She was started on amoxicillin 500 mg × 3 daily and erythromycin 500 mg × 4 daily, in addition to nebulised salbutamol and ipratropium, with a good response.

A few days later she developed watery diarrhoea, which was bad enough to require IV fluids. Her stool analysis was positive for *Clostridium difficile* toxin (see p. 261). She was prescribed a 10-day course of metronidazole 400 mg × 3 daily. Apart from transient nausea, she made a good recovery from her diarrhoea and was able to go home after 6 days.

Case history (2)

A 71-year-old woman was admitted with malaise, fatigue, weight loss and a general feeling of being unwell.

On examination, she looked anxious, underweight and tremulous with a tachycardia.

In the past, she had suffered from atrial fibrillation and was taking amiodarone 200 mg once daily.

Investigations revealed thyrotoxicosis (thought to be due to amiodarone) with undetectable TSH <0.05 mU/L and very high free T_3 (10 pmol/L and T_4 35 pmol/L).

The amiodarone was stopped and her Cardiologist contacted about alternative therapy for her AF (see p. 261). She was started on anti-thyroid therapy (carbimazole 10 mg × 3 daily) and steroids (prednisolone 40 mg once daily). Her response was slow and she remained an inpatient for 2 weeks before her condition was brought under control. She was seen in the Endocrine clinic for dose adjustment of her carbimazole.

Case history (3)

A 79-year-old woman with a background of type 2 diabetes and ischaemic heart disease was admitted to the MAU with uncontrolled diabetes and progressive shortness of breath. She was taking gliclazide 160 mg × 2 daily and co-amilofruse (5 mg amiloride, 40 mg furosemide) one tablet in the morning. A few weeks prior to admission, she complained of back pain and her doctor prescribed diclofenac 50 mg × 3 a day (an NSAID).

On examination, she was in acute left ventricular failure with a tachycardia, raised venous pressure, gallop rhythm and basal crackles. She was treated acutely with oxygen, IV furosemide 50 mg and buccal glyceryl trinitrate 2 mg repeated every 20 min. There was no evidence of an acute ischaemic episode or chest infection.

Progress. The NSAID was stopped. The dose of furosemide was doubled to 80 mg daily with 2.5 mg of amiloride. Her symptoms settled gradually over the next few days and her furosemide was then reduced without recurrence of her left ventricular failure. Her diabetes is well controlled on gliclazide with an HbA_{1c} of 6.5% (48 mmol/mol).

Remember

NSAIDs cause fluid retention, and can precipitate heart failure in susceptible individuals (e.g. patients with diabetes, hypertension or renal failure).

DO NOT ATTEMPT RESUSCITATION (DNAR) DECISION-MAKING

Case history (1)

A fit, elderly, 72-year-old man presents with an acute myocardial infarct. If he has a cardiac arrest, would you resuscitate him?

Case history (2)

A 75-year-old woman presents with hypercalcaemia secondary to disseminated lung carcinoma. You treat her hypercalcaemia aggressively. A nurse asks whether the patient should be recorded for resuscitation or not.

What would you say?

Cardiopulmonary resuscitation (CPR) is an everyday practice in most hospitals. Despite success in selected patients, there is a consensus that CPR might be inappropriate (e.g. in terminal illness) or ineffective (e.g. very severe pneumonia) in some. Age alone is not a contraindication to CPR.

All decisions should be made by senior medical staff after discussion with the patient (if competent), other members of the team and family/carers (if the patient lacks mental capacity).

What principles might guide you to decide to withhold CPR?

- Likely effectiveness of CPR: only 6–15% of patients who undergo CPR leave hospital alive. A number of factors predict a poor outcome from CPR attempts. These include:

- Pneumonia
- Chronic kidney disease
- Anaemia (<90 g/L)
- A high level of dependency, including housebound lifestyle
- More than two acute medical conditions.
- Patient's wishes: these can be ascertained in advance, or from advance directives and living wills. Mentally competent patients who express their wishes about treatment, including CPR, must have those wishes respected. The guidance also recommends that a patient can refuse to accept a DNAR order made by a clinician and that, under the Human Rights Act, doctors must respect this decision and record the change. If a patient is not mentally competent to decide whether to accept CPR, the doctor must consult family/carers and/or the family doctor to ascertain what the patient's wishes would have been. The doctor then uses this information to 'act in the patient's best interest'. **Note:** there is no provision in law in England and Wales for relatives to make medical decisions, including CPR, on behalf of an adult.
- Quality of life: this is the most difficult aspect to address. It includes quality of life as it is now and also as it would be after a CPR attempt, which might be worse. Difficulties arise because it involves professionals making value judgements about other people's lives.

Remember

- If no DNAR decision is documented, the patient is for resuscitation.
- Any DNAR decision made should be communicated to all members of the healthcare team involved with the patient.
- DNAR decisions should be reviewed if appropriate (i.e. not necessarily in terminal illness).

Case 1. This man should be resuscitated. Many patients recover from an MI, even if elderly.

Case 2. This woman should have a DNAR note in her clinical records, as she is suffering from disseminated cancer.

Further reading

General

https://www.bgs.org.uk British Geriatrics Society.

Falls in the elderly

Rodriguez-Mañas L, Fried LP. Frailty in the clinical scenario. *Lancet* 2015; **385**: 67.

Delirium

Folstein MF, Folstein SE, McHugh PR. Mini-mental state: a practical method for grading cognitive state of patients for the clinician. *Journal of Psychiatric Research* 1975; **12**: 189–198.

Marcantonio ER. Delirium in hospitalized older adults. *New England Journal of Medicine* 2017; **377**: 1456–1466.

http://hospitalelderlifeprogram.org HELP website.

Dementia

National Institute for Health and Care Excellence. Dementia: assessment, management and support for people living with dementia and their carers. *NICE Guideline* 2018; **97**. www.nice.org.uk.

Scheptens P. Alzheimer's disease. *Lancet* 2016; **388**: 505–517.

http://en.wikipedia.org/wiki/Mini%E2%80%93mental_state_examination Mini-Mental State Examination.

Depression

Carvalho AF, Firth J, Vieta E. Bipolar disorder. *New England Journal of Medicine* 2020; **383**: 58–66.

Stroke

Baird AE. Paving the way for improved treatment of acute stroke with tenecteplase. *New England Journal of Medicine* 2018; **378**: 1635–1636.

Hughes T. Stroke on the acute medical take. *Clinical Medicine* 2011; **10**: 68–72.

Langhorne P, Bernhardt J, Kwakkel G. Stroke care 2. *Lancet* 2011; **377**: 1693–1702.

Rothwell PM, Algra A, Amarenco P. Stroke care 1. *Lancet* 2011; **377**: 1681–1692.

https://www.rcplondon.ac.uk/stroke Royal College of Physicians stroke programme.

Hypothermia

Morrison G. Management of acute hypothermia. *Medicine* 2017; **45**: 135–138.

Pressure ulcers

National Institute for Health and Care Excellence. Nutrition support for adults. *Clinical Guideline* 2006; **32**. www.nice.org.uk.

Reddy M, Gill SS, Rochon PA. Preventing pressure ulcers; a systematic review. *Journal of the American Medical Association* 2006; **296**: 974–984.

Urinary tract infection

Elements of provisional discharge plan. *Clinical Medicine* 2011; 80.

Acute hot joint

Malay SR, Anders HJ. Crystallopathies. *New England Journal of Medicine* 2016; **374**: 2465–2476.

Parkinson's disease

Bressman S, Saunders-Pullman R. When to start levodopa therapy for Parkinson's disease. *New England Journal of Medicine* 2019; **380**: 389–390.

Kalia LV, Lang AE. Parkinson's disease. *Lancet* 2015; **386**: 896–912.

DNAR decision-making

https://www.resus.org.uk Resuscitation Council (UK).

OSTEOARTHRITIS (OA)

Case history

A 75-year-old woman attends the A&E department with pain in the left groin. The pain has been present for several months but she has not sought medical advice until now. The pain is now so severe that she is unable to walk more than a few yards and it is keeping her awake at night. She lives alone and is unable either to manage her pain or to cope alone at home.

On examination, movements at the left hip were decreased compared to the right and movement was painful, compatible with OA of the hip.

The medical doctor in A&E has arranged for a pelvic X-ray, which shows OA of the left hip. You are asked to see her for possible admission.

Describe the main radiological features of OA of the hip

The X-ray shows joint space narrowing, periarticular sclerosis, cyst formation and osteophytes. These are the four classic features of OA (Fig. 8.1).

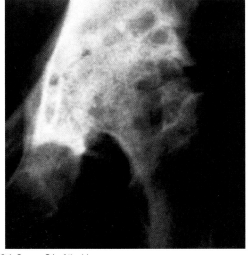

Figure 8.1 Severe OA of the hip.

How would you assess this patient?

The long-standing history suggests a gradual onset of the pain. A short history or systemic symptoms might have indicated joint sepsis or a pathological fracture.

The main site of the pain — especially in the left groin radiating into the left thigh/knee — indicates that the hip is the source of the pain. Beware referred pain either from the lumbar spine (common) or the knee (less common).

A full musculoskeletal examination is needed. The GALS (gait, arms, leg, spine) is a useful screen (see Further reading) (Fig. 8.2).

Diagnostic clues

Look for Heberden's (distal interphalangeal [DIP] joints)/Bouchard's (proximal) nodes, 'square' hands, painful thumb and carpometacarpal joints, which indicate primary nodal OA. Fig. 8.3 shows the distributions of generalised OA and pyrophosphate arthropathy.

Examine

- Other joints for evidence of inflammatory arthritis, e.g. psoriatic arthritis, rheumatoid arthritis (RA).
- Lumbar spine for referred pain.
- Hips:
  - Ask patient to walk to assess gait.
  - Measure leg lengths.

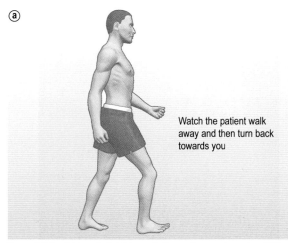

(a)

Watch the patient walk away and then turn back towards you

Figure 8.2 (a–d) Musculoskeletal examination: gait, arms, leg, spine. MCP, metacarpophalangeal; MT, metatarsal.

(b)

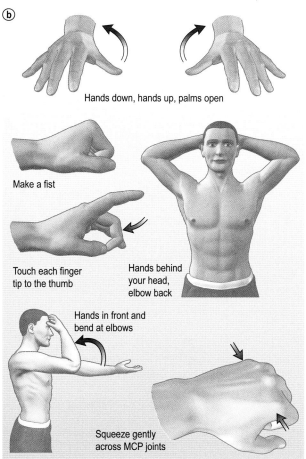

Hands down, hands up, palms open

Make a fist

Touch each finger tip to the thumb

Hands behind your head, elbow back

Hands in front and bend at elbows

Squeeze gently across MCP joints

Figure 8.2, cont'd

(c)

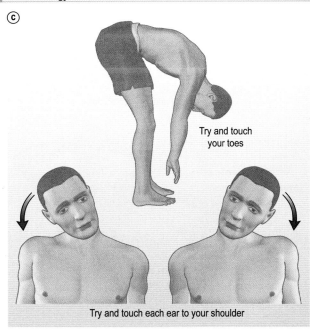

Try and touch
your toes

Try and touch each ear to your shoulder

(d)

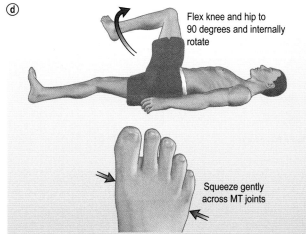

Flex knee and hip to
90 degrees and internally
rotate

Squeeze gently
across MT joints

Figure 8.2, cont'd

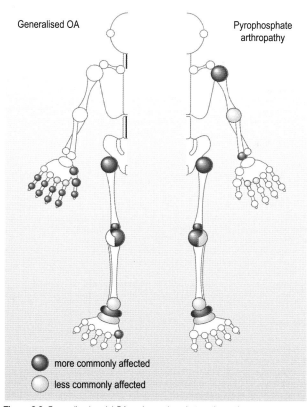

Generalised OA

Pyrophosphate arthropathy

● more commonly affected

○ less commonly affected

Figure 8.3 Generalised nodal OA and pyrophosphate arthropathy.

- Assess range of all movements fully and compare with right hip. Examine from behind to look for pelvic tilt and perform Trendelenburg's test.

What points would you consider when deciding if admission is appropriate?

Full general medical examination is essential because co-morbid conditions in this age group are common. For example, in a patient with significant disability, consider the possibilities of pneumonia, cardiac disease or urinary tract infection. The patient's nutrition might be poor, raising the possibility of osteomalacia – a well-described problem in the elderly.

A full assessment of the patient's ability to cope is essential and you should ask her about her ability to wash, dress and feed herself. This disability assessment will weigh strongly when discussing admission to hospital.

Initial treatment

- Admit because:
  - The patient lives alone.
  - She needs pain control.
  - She is considerably disabled.
- Give analgesia: paracetamol is no longer used, as trials have shown little or no effect on pain in OA. A short course of an NSAID, e.g. diclofenac, usually helps the pain. There is a high risk of GI toxicity with long-term NSAID use in her age group. A gastro-cytoprotective agent, e.g. lansoprazole, should be co-prescribed. Opiates should be avoided unless other analgesia has not worked because of sedation/confusion and constipation.

Investigations

- FBC
- CRP or ESR
  N.B. If she had been febrile, blood cultures would have had to be taken.

Later management

Refer to a Rheumatologist or Medicine for the Elderly consultant. In the mean time, organise:

- Physiotherapy:
  - Mobilise hip, joint protection exercises.
  - Assess walking aids, e.g. stick, Zimmer frame.
  - Hydrotherapy.
- Occupational therapy and social work assessments.
  There should be detailed planning before discharge, including liaison with her doctor and a home visit.

Indications for surgery

Referral to orthopaedics for surgery:

- Severe pain, especially at night
- Poor mobility.
  Progress. The general health of the patient was good and hip surgery is a very effective treatment. She therefore underwent a total hip replacement (THR). The postoperative recovery was excellent and she was able to walk without pain.

RHEUMATOID ARTHRITIS (RA)

Case history

A 26-year-old woman presents at A&E with sudden onset of severe, widespread joint pain and swelling affecting her hands, wrists and feet symmetrically. She has lost half a stone in weight and feels systemically unwell.

On examination, you find that she has hot joints with a symmetrical synovitis, joint restriction of the wrists, metacarpophalangeal (MCP) and proximal interphalangeal (PIP) joints, and painful metatarsophalangeal (MTP) joints. You suspect this is an acute onset of RA.

What other conditions could give a similar clinical picture?

- Systemic lupus erythematosus (SLE).
- Erythrovirus B_{19} infection.
- Post-streptococcal arthritis.

- Psoriatic arthritis.
- Primary Sjögren's syndrome.
- Some systemic vasculitides.

In the first two differential diagnoses there are often other features. In SLE, photosensitive rashes, hair loss, serositis and oral ulceration are seen. Erythrovirus B_{19} nearly always presents with flu-like symptoms and a widespread rash.

Post-streptococcal arthritis may be preceded by a sore throat but is rare. Psoriatic arthritis is usually asymmetrical but can occasionally present with a symmetrical pattern. Psoriatic nail changes and other evidence of psoriasis are usually present, although these might develop after the onset of arthritis.

Sjögren's syndrome can be associated with intermittent parotid swelling and sicca symptoms: dry eyes (keratoconjuctivitis sicca) and dry mouth (xerostomia).

How would you manage this patient?

Remember

RA is a multisystem disease, so look carefully for pulmonary, cardiac or neurological involvement, although these are less common at presentation.

A full history and general medical examination are essential. Specific points are as follows:
- Look for nodules or vasculitis: uncommon at first presentation.
- Perform a full musculoskeletal examination, noting the symmetry of the joint involvement.
- Look for persistent inflammatory symmetrical arthritis (PISA). The most common cause of this is RA.

The most commonly involved joints at onset in RA are the wrists, MCP, PIP and MTP joints.

Admission is necessary to manage a patient who is very unwell systemically and to exclude other pathology.

Investigations

- FBC/ESR, biochemistry including globulin level, CRP (the finding of a high ESR but normal CRP is characteristic of SLE)
- Anti-nuclear antibodies (ANA)/rheumatoid factor (RhF)
- Anti-citrullinated peptide antibodies (ACPA) are positive early in the disease
- X-ray hands and feet for erosions, periarticular osteopenia (Fig. 8.4) (MRI if necessary)
- ASO titre if sore throat
- Blood cultures if febrile
- Erythrovirus B_{19} titres if the ANA/RhF are negative

Initial management

- A short period of bed rest and ice packs: if only a few joints are involved.
- NSAIDs: ibuprofen is the safest; other NSAIDs have a higher risk of GI toxicity, although this patient is young.
- Disease-modifying anti-rheumatic drugs (DMARDs): these should be given at the earliest opportunity because RA is a systemic disease

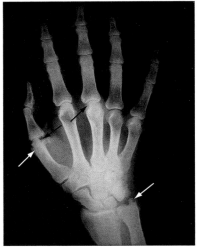

Figure 8.4 X-ray of early RA showing typical erosions at the thumb and middle MCP joints, and at the ulnar styloid (arrows).

that leads rapidly to joint damage and disability. It is no longer acceptable to treat RA with NSAIDs alone. There is accumulating evidence to show that early DMARD use delays joint damage and functional disability.

Initial DMARDs commonly used include sulfasalazine, methotrexate or azathioprine. Others, such as IM gold and D-penicillamine, are less commonly used but still effective. Hydroxychloroquine and auranofin are the least effective but can be used in combination regimens. Combination therapies are showing good results.

Anti-TNF-α agents, e.g. infliximab and etanercept, are effective when initial DMARD therapy has failed. Infectious complications, such as tuberculosis, are a concern with these agents.

Late manifestations of RA

Changes in the hand are shown in Fig. 8.5. Other joints, such as knees and hips, become involved later in the disease course.

All drugs need careful explanation to the patient and close monitoring for toxicity.

Prednisolone is not used in young patients but IM methylprednisolone 40–120 mg gives excellent short-term benefit.

The addition of prednisolone 7.5 mg to existing DMARD therapy might retard the progression of erosions, but studies in this area remain controversial and this is not recommended for general use at present.

Diagnosis. This patient had a high ESR of 60 mm/h and a CRP of 90 mg/L, indicating active disease. Her ACPA and RhF were positive in the

Ulnar deviation

Boutonnière deformity

Swan-neck deformity

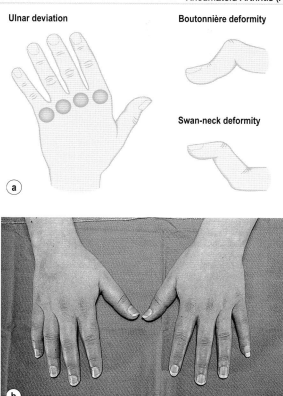

(a)

(b)

Figure 8.5 (a–b) RA: late manifestations.

serum, typical of RA. The X-rays of her hands showed soft tissue swelling only. An MRI was therefore performed and showed early erosions, confirming the diagnosis.

Progress. This patient was admitted and treated symptomatically with analgesics. She was started on prednisolone and methotrexate. The pain and swelling improved and she was discharged, still with some residual problems. She was given a follow-up appointment for clinic in 2 weeks' time.

Targeted synthetic DMARDs (ts DMARD) are now available. Baricitinib (a Janus kinase inhibitor) with methotrexate has kept this patient in long-term remission. Belimumab and anifrolumab, inhibitors of the interferon pathway, are also available.

SYSTEMIC LUPUS ERYTHEMATOSUS (SLE) AND VASCULITIS

Case history

A 28-year-old woman is referred to you by her doctor. Six weeks ago, she delivered her first baby and the pregnancy and delivery were uneventful. Two weeks after delivery she developed a widespread polyarthritis affecting her hands, feet and knees, and a photosensitive rash on her face. In the last week or two, she has become extremely unwell with weight loss and painful lesions on her hands and feet.

On examination, she is clearly unwell, with a facial rash and severe oral ulceration. Examination of her hands and feet shows extensive digital infarcts with necrotic ulceration on the palms, finger pulps and soles of the feet. There are splinter haemorrhages and nail-fold infarcts.

Discuss the differential diagnosis, investigation and management

The differential diagnosis includes an inflammatory autoimmune rheumatic disease such as SLE, which has developed after delivery of her baby. The lesions on her hands (Fig. 8.6) and feet are strongly suggestive of vasculitis, which is a serious prognostic factor that requires immediate therapy.

Investigations (Table 8.1) are performed to look for the possibility of major organ involvement, which might be vasculitic. Her urine must be tested immediately for blood and protein, and sent for urine cytology to look for fragmented red cells and/or casts. The presence of an 'active' urine sediment with fragmented or dysmorphic red cells and granular casts has a >90% specificity for glomerulonephritis.

Remember

The major risk of vasculitis is organ involvement including renal, cerebral and pulmonary disease, which can be life-threatening.

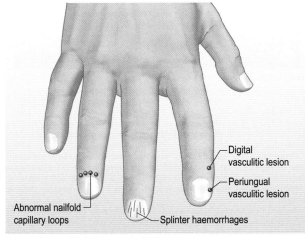

Digital
vasculitic lesion

Periungual
vasculitic lesion

Abnormal nailfold
capillary loops

Splinter haemorrhages

Figure 8.6 Vasculitic lesions seen in the fingers.

Table 8.1 Investigations for SLE and vasculitis

Investigation	Typical finding
FBC	Immune cytopenias, especially neutropenia and thrombocytopenia, are common in SLE
	There may be anaemia of chronic disease or haemolytic anaemia – check Coombs' test
ESR and CRP	The pattern of a high ESR but normal CRP is characteristic of SLE
Renal function	U&Es, 24-h urine protein/eGFR
Liver biochemistry	Hypoalbuminaemia is common
Lupus serology	
ANA	Present in 95% of SLE patients
dsDNA	Specific marker for SLE; a negative dsDNA, however, does not exclude SLE
Extractable nuclear antigen (ENA)	Ro/La photosensitivity/Sjögren's
	RNP/Sm often seen in severe SLE
Complement	Low values indicate activation of complement or, rarely, congenital deficiency
Anti-neutrophil cytoplasmic antibody (ANCA)	A marker of vasculitis: a systemic vasculitis is an alternative to SLE

Diagnosis. The patient was found to be anaemic with an Hb of 50 g/L, a raised ESR of 80 mm/h, normal CRP, a raised ANA and anti-dsDNA auto-antibodies. A diagnosis of **systemic lupus erythematosus** was reached.

Once the diagnosis of lupus and vasculitis is established on clinical and serological grounds, therapy is with prednisolone and IV pulse methylpred-nisolone 500 mg on alternate days for three doses.

Immunosuppressive therapy is commonly used to treat vasculitis. One commonly adopted approach is IV 500 mg cyclophosphamide therapy given 2-weekly or monthly. The patient should be carefully counselled about the risks and benefits of cyclophosphamide; these include adverse effects, such as cytopenias, haemorrhagic cystitis and infections, including herpes zoster and infertility. If the patient is breastfeeding, she should stop because cyclophosphamide and other immunosuppressives such as azathio-prine are excreted in breast milk.

Remember

Specialist advice from a Rheumatologist or Immunologist should be sought.

Progress. On treatment with steroids (see earlier) her symptoms settled and a decision was taken to delay immunosuppressive therapy until after she had stopped breastfeeding.

Kumar & Clark's Cases in Clinical Medicine

ACUTE AUTOIMMUNE RHEUMATIC DISEASE

Case history

A 33-year-old woman of African origin is admitted through A&E, complaining of breathlessness and swollen legs. Two years ago she was admitted with a psychotic illness that had features of schizophrenia and improved with anti-psychotic medication.

In the last 6 months she has developed a symmetrical small joint inflammatory arthritis, mouth ulcers and photosensitive facial rashes. Over the last 2 weeks she has become breathless and her legs have become severely swollen.

On examination, she is anaemic and has a pulse rate of 120/min with pulsus paradoxus. Her BP is 90/60. She has bilateral pleural effusions, a raised JVP with a sharp rise and y descent (Friedreich's sign) and pitting oedema to her waist. There is synovitis of the small joints of her fingers and she has florid splinter haemorrhages. Her urine showed heavy proteinuria.

What is the likely diagnosis?

Diagnosis is likely to be **SLE complicated by the nephrotic syndrome**. In addition, she may have cardiac tamponade from a pericardial effusion.

SLE is nine times more common in females than in males, and is found more often in people of African and Far Eastern ancestry; it is often more severe in these ethnic groups.

This patient has many characteristic features of SLE: inflammatory polyarthritis, mouth ulcers, photosensitive rashes, psychotic illness, serositis with pleural and probably pericardial effusions, and renal disease with nephrotic syndrome (Fig. 8.7). The high JVP might indicate early tamponade.

How would you manage this patient?

The most urgent priority is to establish whether this patient has cardiac tamponade. The low BP and the presence of pulsus paradoxus, tachycardia and raised JVP, with increased distension during inspiration and cardiomegaly on CXR, are strong pointers to this. An echocardiogram is performed urgently, which shows an echo-free region between the myocardium and the intense echo of the parietal pericardium. This confirms the effusion and the clinical signs confirm tamponade.

The overwhelming majority of patients with lupus who have cardiac tamponade associated with a pericardial effusion respond to high-dose oral corticosteroids and do not need pericardiocentesis. This should be performed, however, if the patient deteriorates despite corticosteroid therapy or if sepsis is present. A normal CRP makes infection less likely.

The next priority is to determine the extent and severity of the renal disease. Serum creatinine, eGFR, albumin and 24-h urine protein are essential. If there is an 'active' (see p. 29) urine sediment, e.g. fragmented red cells and granular casts, indicating glomerulonephritis, renal biopsy is required.

Investigations

- FBC with reticulocyte count, Coombs' (direct anti-globulin test) if positive: the anaemia is haemolytic
- U&Es (eGFR): renal impairment may be present
- Biochemistry: serum albumin will be low
- 24-h urine protein should be started
- Urine cytology for fragmented red cells and granular casts: a useful marker of glomerulonephritis

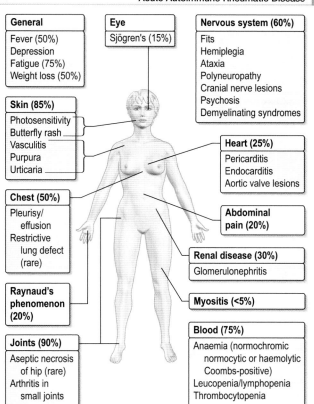

Figure 8.7 Clinical features of SLE.

- CXR: to document pleural effusions and cardiomegaly (Fig. 8.8)
- Echocardiogram: to document pericardial effusion and possible valve lesions
- ECG
- Blood gases
- Blood cultures/urine cultures: to exclude sepsis, especially endocarditis, prior to corticosteroid and immunosuppressive therapy
- Full autoantibody screen: ANA, DNA, ENA, RhF, ACPA, anti-cardiolipin antibodies, lupus anti-coagulant, ANCA (Table 8.2)
- Complement studies
- A diagnostic renal biopsy may be required later

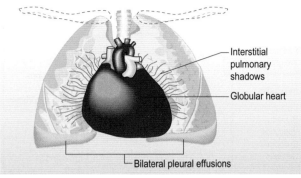

Figure 8.8 Diagram of a CXR showing pleural effusions and cardiomegaly.

Table 8.2 Antinuclear autoantibodies and disease associations		
Antibody	**Disease**	**Prevalence**
ds-DNA	SLE	70%
Anti-histone	Drug-induced lupus	–
Anti-centromeric	Limited scleroderma	70%
Anti-Ro (SS-A)	SLE	40–60%
	Primary Sjögren's	60–90%
Anti-La (SS-B)	SLE	15%
	Primary Sjögren's	35–85%
Anti-Sm	SLE	10–25% (Caucasian)
		30–50% (Black African)
Anti-UI-RNP	SLE	30%
	Overlap syndrome	
Anti-Jo-1 (anti-synthetase)	Polymyositis	30%
	Dermatomyositis	
Anti-topoisomerase-1 (Scl-70)	Diffuse cutaneous SSc	30%

RNP, ribonucleoprotein; Ro, La, first two letters of name of patients; Sm, Smith, patient's name; SS-A, SS-B, Sjögren's syndrome A and B; SSc, systemic scleroderma. (From Feather A, Randall D, Waterhouse M, eds. *Kumar and Clark's Clinical Medicine*, 10th edn. Elsevier, 2021; Box 18.38.)

Other points

A normal protein diet is necessary with salt restriction and diuretic therapy using a thiazide, e.g. bendroflumethiazide 5 mg daily.

- Thrombosis prophylaxis: this patient is at high risk of deep vein thrombosis (DVT)/pulmonary embolus (PE). TED stockings and prophylactic low-molecular-weight heparin should be given.
- Is the anaemia haemolytic? If so, it should respond to corticosteroids.
- Angiotensin-converting enzyme (ACE) inhibition: when the BP has normalised as a result of treatment of the tamponade, start an ACE inhibitor. This is especially useful in proteinuric patients.
- If renal biopsy confirms proliferative glomerulonephritis: the treatment of choice is corticosteroid therapy and intermittent IV cyclophosphamide, followed by azathioprine.
- This patient's lipid profile might well be deranged, especially in the nephrotic syndrome: this will need to be assessed and managed actively. Measurement of serum lipids is performed and the patient started on a statin immediately if hypercholesterolaemia is present.
- Prophylaxis against corticosteroid-induced osteoporosis: a baseline dual energy X-ray absorptiometry (DXA) scan should be performed and calcium supplementation should be started.

Long-term prognosis

The majority of patients with SLE have a good prognosis, although clearly this woman has a serious disease with life-threatening complications. Mortality in SLE occurs at two peak periods: those patients who die from overwhelming disease, thrombosis or sepsis, and those who die prematurely from accelerated atherosclerosis. Prognosis has been considerably improved by earlier recognition and effective therapy.

Progress. This patient had several problems. Her cardiac effusion gradually responded to high-dose oral steroids and her BP improved. She had a haemolytic anaemia of 95 g/L. She was discharged on steroids and an ACE inhibitor after an inpatient stay of 2 weeks. She later had a renal biopsy, which confirmed a proliferative glomerulonephritis, and was seen by the Nephrologists for treatment. A DXA scan did not show osteoporosis.

THROMBOSIS AND THE ANTI-PHOSPHOLIPID SYNDROME

Case history

A 25-year-old woman presents with a 2-day history of left leg swelling, and on the day of admission she notices breathlessness and chest pains that are worse on deep inspiration.

In her past medical history you find that she has had three miscarriages and one successful pregnancy. This pregnancy was complicated by hypertension and intra-uterine growth retardation, with a premature delivery at 31 weeks. On further questioning, you note that she has had oral ulceration, with rashes that are worse in the sunlight, and has also been having headaches.

Drug history: she is on the oral contraceptive pill.

On examination, she has extensive splinter haemorrhages on most fingers. Her pulse is 100 and BP 110/70, but she is not cyanosed. Her heart sounds are normal but there is a soft murmur of mitral regurgitation. She also has a soft left pleural rub.

> **Abdominal examination and neurological examination** are normal. The left calf is swollen and the calf circumference is 3 cm greater than on the right. You note extensive livedo reticularis on her arms, thighs and knees.

What is the differential diagnosis and what investigations are required?

This young woman (who is on the oral contraceptive pill) is deemed to have a DVT and a PE until it is proved otherwise.

An FBC revealed thrombocytopenia, which is commonly seen in the antiphospholipid syndrome.

Investigations

- ECG: look for the classic (but seldom seen) S1, Q3, T3 pattern of PE (Fig. 8.9)
- CXR: likely to be normal. However, it is useful to exclude other causes of pleuritic chest pain, including infective causes
- Ultrasound scan of the leg veins: to document the extent of the left calf thrombosis
- A $\dot{V}/\dot{Q}$ scan: to show the extent of the pulmonary emboli: still useful
- Plasma D-dimers: if these are undetectable, the diagnosis of PE and DVT is excluded
- Multidetector CT with contrast: good specificity 96% and sensitivity 85% for medium-sized pulmonary emboli
  Choose the imaging techniques according to local availability.

An echocardiogram and blood cultures in women are essential because the differential diagnosis includes Libman—Sacks endocarditis and infective endocarditis.

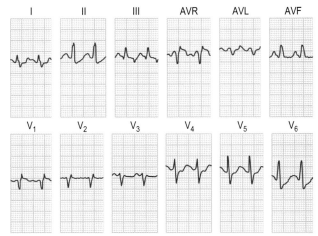

Figure 8.9 Acute pulmonary embolism shown on a 12-lead ECG. There is an S wave in lead I, a Q wave in lead III and an inverted T wave in lead III (the S1, Q3, T3 pattern). There is sinus tachycardia (160 bpm) and an incomplete right bundle branch block pattern (an R wave in AVR and V_1 and an S wave in V_6).

Differential diagnosis

In this case, this includes the anti-phospholipid syndrome with a DVT and pulmonary emboli, along with an increased risk of thrombosis from the oral contraceptive pill. The history is rather suggestive of SLE, and this should be investigated further with autoantibodies to ANA, DNA and ENA and complement studies. The features favouring a diagnosis of the anti-phospholipid syndrome in this case would include the three previous miscarriages and one pregnancy complicated by intra-uterine growth retardation and premature delivery. There is accumulating evidence in the literature to suggest that intra-uterine growth retardation is due to recurrent placental thrombosis and this is often manifested by reduced umbilical artery flow patterns on Doppler studies, with an increased resistance index, notching or even reversed flow in the umbilical vessels.

Information

- The anti-phospholipid syndrome is due to the presence of antibodies that bind phospholipids, leading to both venous and arterial occlusion.
- The syndrome is most commonly seen in SLE but can occur in isolation: primary anti-phospholipid syndrome.

The anti-phospholipid syndrome

Anti-cardiolipin antibodies and the lupus anti-coagulant should be measured. Both of these are anti-phospholipid antibodies and both tests should be requested because a small percentage of patients have either one or the other antibody but not both. A thrombophilia screen can exclude other factors, including the factor V Leiden mutation. Patients with the anti-phospholipid syndrome also have reduced protein C and S levels, which are associated with the lupus anticoagulant.

Libman—Sacks endocarditis

Splinter haemorrhages and a mitral murmur indicate Libman—Sacks endocarditis, which is a feature of the anti-phospholipid syndrome and SLE. These patients have mucinous degeneration of the mitral valve leaflets, and occasionally thrombus (which might embolise) is seen on the damaged valves. Similarly, the damaged valves might become secondarily infected, leading to infective endocarditis. The splinter haemorrhages could represent micro-emboli and are a feature of both the anti-phospholipid syndrome and infective endocarditis.

How would you manage this patient?

This woman should be admitted and commenced on heparin. This can be given intravenously as a continuous infusion but many hospitals use once-daily low-molecular-weight heparin. Warfarin should be commenced and the eventual target INR should be 2.5. Rivaroxaban is being used instead of warfarin in some centres.

Progress. The diagnosis of the anti-phospholipid syndrome was confirmed and therapy with life-long warfarin at the target INR was started. These patients are often resistant to warfarin and occasionally require high doses, e.g. 15—20 mg warfarin daily.

In terms of the mitral valve disease, the patient needed counselling about appropriate antibiotic therapy for any infection. Prophylactic antibiotics are not required. Infective endocarditis was excluded and she was monitored regularly because a small percentage of these patients require mitral valve replacement.

CRYSTAL ARTHRITIS

Two main types of crystal account for the majority of crystal-induced arthritis. They are sodium urate (gout) and calcium pyrophosphate (pseudo-gout), and are distinguished by their different shapes and refringence properties under polarised light with a red filter. Rarely, crystals of calcium apatite or cholesterol cause acute synovitis.

Case history

A 73-year-old woman was admitted a week ago to the Stroke Unit, having had a right hemiparesis. She has developed a hot, swollen right knee. You have been asked to see the patient for your advice on whether this might be a septic arthritis.

On further questioning, you discover that the patient has attended the hypertension clinic for many years and has been taking bendroflumethiazide. She has also complained of knee pain intermittently over the last 5 years but the joint has never previously swelled up. She is making a reasonable recovery from her stroke and there is no other relevant history.

Clinically, there is no evidence of tophi. The knee is hot and movement is restricted due to a large tense effusion. She is afebrile.

How would you manage this patient?

The X-ray showed chondrocalcinosis (Fig. 8.10) and patello-femoral and tibio-femoral OA. The serum uric acid was elevated (520 μmol/L); she is taking a thiazide diuretic. The differential diagnosis thus includes gout or pseudo-gout, of which pseudo-gout is probably more likely in this clinical context. The uric acid level, although high, is usually >600 μmol/L with gout.

Investigations

- FBC
- ESR
- U&Es
- Bone and liver biochemistry
- Serum urate
- X-ray of the knee
- Blood cultures
- Aspiration of the joint using a sterile technique; fluid should be sent for cells, crystals and culture

Pseudo-gout

This patient has the typical presentation of pseudo-gout: an acute onset of a swollen joint in an elderly patient who has been admitted for other reasons, usually a stroke, MI or chest infection.

Calcium pyrophosphate is the most common crystal associated with pseudo-gout (Fig. 8.11). The crystals are diagnosed on synovial fluid analysis using polarised light microscopy. They are rhomboidal and positively birefringent, and can be idiopathic or associated with OA. A number of metabolic conditions are also associated with calcium pyrophosphate deposition; these include hypothyroidism, hyperparathyroidism, acromegaly, Wilson's disease, haemochromatosis, hypophosphatasia and hypomagnesaemia.

The differential diagnosis of gout is also confirmed on crystal examination. These urate crystals are negatively birefringent needle-shaped crystals.

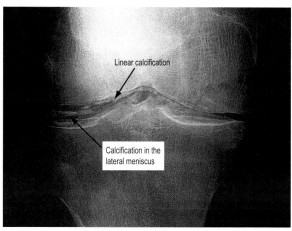

Figure 8.10 Chondrocalcinosis of the knee. Note the linear calcification in the hyaline cartilage and calcification of the lateral meniscus (plus mild secondary OA).

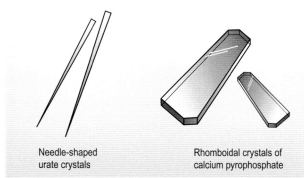

Figure 8.11 Urate and calcium pyrophosphate crystals.

Management

Septic arthritis, although unlikely, should be excluded and, providing joint aspiration and synovial fluid culture and blood cultures are all negative, the knee should be aspirated to dryness and injected with a steroid such as 40 mg of methylprednisolone. Risk factors should be minimised and, in particular, the thiazide diuretic (which can precipitate gout) should be switched to an alternative anti-hypertensive medication. Intensive physiotherapy is necessary, with particular attention to quadriceps exercises and maintenance of mobility and hydration in the patient.

Progress. She was started on diclofenac 50 mg × 3 daily and was able to be gradually mobilised with the help of physiotherapy. Her speech improved over the first 2 weeks but she was left severely disabled by her right-sided weakness. She was eventually transferred to long-term care.

POLYMYALGIA RHEUMATICA/CRANIAL ARTERITIS

Polymyalgia rheumatica (PMR) and giant cell (cranial) arteritis (GCA) are systemic vasculitides affecting people over 50 years of age. Both are associated with the finding of a giant cell arteritis on temporal artery biopsy.

Case history

A 73-year-old woman presents to A&E, feeling non-specifically unwell. On further questioning, she has a headache and joint aches, particularly of her shoulders and hips, in addition to widespread aches and pains. She has marked joint stiffness, particularly of the shoulders and hips, lasting for several hours each morning, and occasionally all day. The headache is predominantly right-sided and the patient says that it is painful when she brushes her hair. In addition, she has pains in the left jaw on talking or eating.

On examination, the scalp is tender and it is difficult to palpate the temporal arteries. The rest of the examination is normal. Her shoulders and hips ache at the extremes of the range of movement but are otherwise normal.

Differential diagnosis and management

The most likely diagnosis in a patient over 50 years is temporal arteritis with PMR and there is therefore a significant risk of blindness from arteritis of the ophthalmic artery. A differential diagnosis includes malignancy of any cause and myeloma, which can, rarely, mimic PMR. The ESR is nearly always significantly elevated but approximately 1–5% of patients with PMR have a normal ESR.

Investigations

The following are essential:
- FBC
- ESR or CRP
- U&Es
- Liver biochemistry
- Temporal artery biopsy

This patient should be commenced on 60 mg of prednisolone immediately and a temporal artery biopsy should be arranged within the next 24 h. The clinical diagnosis is **giant cell arteritis.**

> **Box 8.1** Histological features of cranial arteritis
> - Intimal hypertrophy
> - Inflammation of the intima and sub-intima
> - Breaking up of the internal elastic lamina
> - Giant cells, lymphocytes and plasma cells in the internal elastic lamina

The histological features of GCA are shown in Box 8.1.

The response to steroids is usually dramatic in these patients and a response is often seen within 24–48 h. The steroid therapy can then be reduced reasonably quickly, over a few months, to 15–20 mg daily; if this is not possible, a steroid-sparing agent such as azathioprine should be added to achieve this. The addition of low-dose aspirin may reduce the risk of blindness. This patient is also at high risk of osteoporosis and subsequent vertebral fractures, and calcium and vitamin D supplementation should be co-prescribed routinely. A baseline DXA should be requested. If there is already osteoporosis, bisphosphonates should be given.

Progress. This patient's headache quickly disappeared on steroid therapy and in 6 months she was well on prednisolone 10 mg daily with a normal ESR. Her steroids will be continued for at least 1 year, with regular checks of her ESR.

Patients who fail to respond to steroids

Such patients should be investigated in detail for an underlying malignancy, especially multiple myeloma. Occasionally, other conditions such as severe hypothyroidism might also present with similar joint aches but the clinical picture of temporal arteritis with a good response to steroids is usually characteristic enough to establish the diagnosis.

ACUTE BACK PAIN

This is usually due to acute lumbar disc prolapse. The central disc gel may extrude into a fissure in the surrounding fibrous zone and cause acute pain and muscle spasm, which in turn leads to a forward and sideways tilt when standing.

Case history

A 36-year-old publican presents to A&E, having just lifted a barrel of beer. He experienced severe buttock and back pain. The pain radiated down the left leg to the sole of the foot with associated paraesthesiae. On further questioning, he finds that it is extremely painful to move his back and that the pain is worse on coughing or sneezing. The pain is also worse in the leg than in the back. He says that he has not passed any urine for 6 h.

On examination, he is found to be in severe pain and is lying flat on the examination couch. He finds it too painful to stand up but the hips, knees and other joints are all normal on examination. Straight-leg raising on the right is 40 degrees but on the left is only 10 degrees, with a strongly positive sciatic stretch test. The femoral nerve stretch test is also strongly positive on the left and neurological examination reveals an absent left ankle jerk and sacral anaesthesia.

Discuss your further investigations, diagnosis and management

The history and clinical examination are almost diagnostic for a large L5/S1 disc protrusion with compromise of the cauda equina, which can lead to urinary retention. This is therefore a neurosurgical emergency.

The most urgent investigation is imaging (MRI) of the lumbar spine and pelvis (Fig. 8.12). The patient should be catheterised and analgesia should be given. This includes IM non-steroidals, such as IM diclofenac, or opiate analgesics, including morphine if needed. The patient should be referred immediately to a neurosurgeon or orthopaedic surgeon with an interest in acute spinal problems for urgent decompressive surgery with a laminectomy and discectomy. Any delay in diagnosis or decompression might lead to a permanent neurological deficit.

In patients without sacral anaesthesia or neurological deficit, the evidence-based advice is not to recommend bed rest but to mobilise the patient as soon as possible using adequate analgesia. Rapid access to physiotherapy can improve outcome, and procedures such as sacral or lumbar epidurals might be necessary to relieve pain while recovery occurs.

Progress. This patient required urgent surgery, as the MRI showed a large L5/S1 disc protrusion. He made a good recovery and had no permanent neurological deficit.

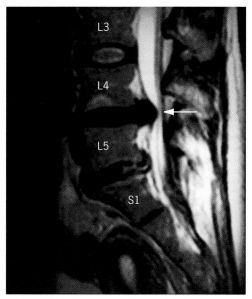

Figure 8.12 MRI of the lumbar spine showing a central disc prolapse at the L4/L5 level (arrow). The signal from the L4/L5 and L5/S1 discs indicates dehydration, whereas the appearance of the L3/L4 signal is normal.

SEVERE BACK PAIN/OSTEOPOROSIS

Osteoporosis is characterised by reduced bone density and micro-architectural deterioration of bone tissue, leading to increased bone fragility and the susceptibility to fracture.

Case history

A 71-year-old woman presents with severe thoracic spinal pain, which came on suddenly 6 h previously. The pain is severe and radiates around the thoracic spine and front of the chest; it is worse on coughing or sneezing. In the past medical history she has had rheumatoid arthritis for the last 25 years and is currently taking 7.5 mg of prednisolone daily. Her RA has been in remission for 5 years on this therapy and she is on no other medication. Disease-modifying drugs used in the past either have induced toxicity or have been ineffective.

On examination, there is evidence of quiescent RA with classic rheumatoid deformities, nodules and synovial thickening, but no active synovitis. On examination of the thoracic spine there is a marked kyphosis and she is exquisitely tender over T8. The thoracic spine is markedly restricted on rotation, reproducing her pain radiating around the chest to the anterior aspect of the chest.

What investigations would you do?

Investigations

- FBC
- ESR
- Renal function
- Bone and liver biochemistry
- CRP
- X-ray chest and thoracic spine

Discuss your differential diagnosis and management

The most likely diagnosis is steroid-associated osteoporosis with an acute vertebral fracture. The differential diagnosis should include myeloma and other malignancies because these can also present with vertebral fractures.

Imaging should include a CXR and specific views of the dorsal spine, which are likely to show one or more vertebral crush fractures. Crush fractures have a fairly characteristic appearance and on the AP view of the thoracic spine all the pedicles should be visible. Should any pedicles be missing, this should immediately raise the suspicion of metastatic malignancy as a cause of the vertebral fracture.

Later, a myeloma screen, including protein immunofixation, serum light chain assay and urine for Bence Jones protein, should be done.

A DXA scan is performed to establish the degree of osteoporosis (Fig. 8.13). This gives an accurate index of bone mineral density in relation to the normal range for an age-, sex- and race-matched population. The World Health Organisation definition of osteopenia is a T score of −1.5 to 2.5. The definition of osteoporosis is a T score of greater than −2.5 standard deviations below the mean, and established or severe osteoporosis is a T score of greater than −2.5 with an established fracture.

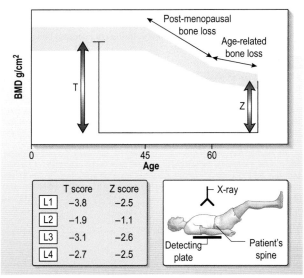

Figure 8.13 DXA scan. Graph showing bone mineral density (BMD; vertical axis) against age. T score is the number of standard deviations by which the patient's BMD differs from the population average for a healthy young adult. Z score is as the T score but BMD deviations from the population average for the patient's age.

Initial management

In the acute setting of a recent vertebral fracture, give strong analgesia, e.g. meptazinol 200 mg every 3–6 h IM or IV if necessary. A single IV infusion of a bisphosphonate (pamidronate 60–90 mg) gives some pain relief. Salmon calcitonin is not now used as first-line therapy.

Progress. This woman's pain proved difficult to control and kyphoplasty was performed. This involves injecting methyl methacrylate through a needle placed directly into the damaged vertebra. This allowed mobilisation with physiotherapy help.

Later management

This patient should commence specific therapy for osteoporosis.

Therapies include cyclical etidronate with calcium or weekly alendronate or risedronate. These therapies are well tolerated in this age group but alendronate and risedronate are associated with a small but significant risk of oesophagitis. All the bisphosphonate drugs are poorly absorbed and should be taken at least 2 h before a meal with a full glass of water; particularly with alendronate, the patient should not lie down for at least 2 h after taking the medication to reduce the risk of oesophagitis. Strontium ranelate is used in post-menopausal osteoporosis. These medications increase bone mineral density over a 3- to 5-year period and also reduce fracture risk.

Hormone replacement therapy (HRT) is not usually used in women of this age because of the adverse effects, which include breast tenderness and a return of menses. Raloxifene, a selective oestrogen-receptor modulator (SERM), has been shown to increase bone mineral density. The main adverse effects of raloxifene include a risk of thrombosis and possible endometrial/uterine malignancy. There is evidence that raloxifene protects against the risk of breast cancer.

Other factors used in the treatment of osteoporosis include stopping smoking, keeping alcohol intake to a moderate level and encouraging active weight-bearing exercise. Attention to diet is necessary, particularly in this age group, and a broad, varied diet containing a reasonable calcium intake should be advised; if necessary, a specific dietitian referral would be helpful. These patients should be monitored with DXA scan to check on progress.

Progress. This woman had not been given prophylactic bisphosphonate therapy, which is usually necessary in addition to calcium for patients on long-term steroids; nor did she have regular DXA scans to assess the development of osteoporosis.

Her prednisolone 7.5 mg daily was gradually tapered and stopped, and her RA remained in remission, with some analgesia and an NSAID being required. She has continued on alendronate calcium and has regular DXA scans.

OSTEOMYELITIS

Case history

A 56-year-old Asian woman presents with a 2-month history of upper back pain and weight loss. She has just arrived home after visiting relatives in Bangladesh for the last year.

There is no relevant past history and she is taking no medication.

On examination, she is in pain and looks thin. Her pulse is 110/min and regular; her temperature is 38°C. Cardiovascular, respiratory and abdominal examinations are all normal and neurological examinations, including power, tone and reflexes, are within normal limits. There are no sensory signs.

All her joints are normal but she is tender over the thoracic spine, which is exquisitely painful on rotation of the thoracic spine.

Investigations

- Hb 106 g/L, MCV 83
- ESR 102 mm/h, CRP 94
- U&Es normal
- Biochemistry: serum Ca 2.3 mmol/L; phosphate 1.2 mmol/L; serum alkaline phosphatase 103 IU/L

A thoracic spine X-ray was normal. A CXR showed no evidence of TB.

What is the differential diagnosis?

The differential diagnosis is **spinal tuberculous osteomyelitis** (Pott's disease), despite the normal CXR. A differential diagnosis would include *Staphylococcus aureus* discitis, although this tends to affect the lumbar spine, whereas tuberculous spinal disease characteristically affects the thoracic spine or the thoraco-lumbar junction.

The most useful investigation is an MRI scan of the thoracic spine. This showed destruction of the T4 vertebral body with evidence of discitis at T4/ T5. A paravertebral abscess accompanied the bone destruction. These findings are typical of thoracic spine tuberculosis. There was no evidence of cord compression and so a neurosurgical opinion was not required. Aspiration of the vertebral abscess was carried out to culture the tubercle bacillus and to obtain the sensitivities. She was commenced on isoniazid, pyrazinamide, rifampicin and ethambutol, to be given for 9 months (reducing drugs when sensitivities are known; see p. 345). Other risk factors should always be considered, such as immunosuppression and HIV disease.

As vertebral collapse was not present, the prognosis is usually excellent in these patients if the organism is fully sensitive to therapy and compliance with therapy is maintained.

Progress. This patient made an excellent recovery and was left with no sequelae from her spinal abscess.

SEPTIC ARTHRITIS

Septic arthritis is due to haematogenous spread from skin or a respiratory tract infection. It is also seen after surgery or sometimes following trauma to the joint.

Case history

A 21-year-old man presents with pain and swelling of his right knee. On further questioning, he had no other symptoms. He had no relevant past medical history. Specifically, he has had no diarrhoea, urethritis, rashes or oral ulceration, and has had no problems with inflammation of his eyes. His sexual history revealed many sexual contacts, including oral/ anal sex with other men.

How would you investigate and manage this patient?

The most common diagnosis in a young man with a monoarthritis is a reactive arthritis associated either with diarrhoea or with urethritis, usually chlamydial in origin (Fig. 8.14). However, clinical questioning here has excluded any associated features that would point to reactive arthritis (a triad of urethritis, arthritis and conjunctivitis, formerly known as Reiter's disease), and septic arthritis should be considered as the most likely diagnosis, raising the possibility of HIV disease.

This patient's results were as follows:
- FBC normal
- ESR 74 mm/h
- Biochemistry, including a serum uric acid 420 μmol/L

The joint should be X-rayed and a series of blood cultures performed following admission to the MAU.

The joint should be aspirated using a sterile technique, and the fluid sent for microscopy, culture and crystals.

Information

KNEE ASPIRATION
- Explain procedure and obtain consent
- Strict aseptic technique
- 2% lidocaine as local anaesthetic
- Medial or lateral approach 0.5–1 cm below the patella

- Use a white needle to ensure that even viscous or purulent fluid can be aspirated easily
- Caution in patients on warfarin
- Don't inject steroids if fluid is purulent

The most common organism is *Staphylococcus aureus*, which is seen in 40–70% of patients. Gram-negative organisms are the next most common, but a careful search for gonorrhoea should be conducted and the patient should be referred to the genitourinary medicine clinic for urethral swabs and other tests.

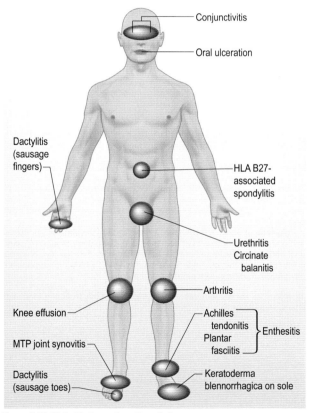

Figure 8.14 Clinical features of reactive arthritis.

Table 8.3 Examination of synovial fluid

Characteristics of synovial fluid	Diagnosis	WCC/mm³
Clear, yellow and viscous	Osteoarthritis	<3000
Translucent and thin	Rheumatoid arthritis	3000–40 000
Very cloudy	Seronegative arthritis	
	Reactive arthritis	
	Crystal arthritis	
	Sepsis	750 000

Polarised light microscopy with a red filter needs to be undertaken by an expert:
- Gout: negatively birefringent, needle-shaped crystals of sodium urate
- Pyrophosphate arthropathy (pseudo-gout): rhomboidal, weakly positively birefringent crystals of calcium pyrophosphate

Gram staining is essential if septic arthritis is suspected and may identify the organism immediately. Joint fluid should be cultured and antibiotic sensitivities requested

The fluid can be examined directly in a clear syringe or sterile pot. The characteristics of synovial fluid show a trend from clear to purulent, which roughly indicates the type of arthritis

This man is at risk for HIV and an HIV test is performed. Should HIV be proven, microbiology assessment of the synovial fluid is crucial, particularly for atypical organisms such as *Mycobacterium avium intracellulare* and other forms of TB.

Progress. A septic arthritis due to *Staph. aureus* infection was confirmed on blood and synovial fluid culture (Table 8.3). The patient required 6 weeks of IV antibiotics: flucloxacillin plus oral fusidic acid. Arthroscopic drainage and washout of the joint was performed at 48 h, which minimised joint damage. He made a good recovery.

Further reading

Osteoarthritis
Doherty M, Dacre J, Dieppe P, et al. The GALS locomotor screen. *Annals of Rheumatological Disease* 1992; **51**: 1165.

Rheumatoid arthritis
Fleischmann R. Interleukin-6 inhibitors for rheumatoid arthritis. *Lancet* 2017; **389**: 1168–1170.

Fleischmann R, van Adelsberg J, Lin Y, et al. Sarilumab and non-biologic disease-modifying antirheumatic drugs in patients with active rheumatoid arthritis and inadequate response or intolerance to tumor necrosis factor inhibitors. *Arthritis Rheumatology* 2017; **69**: 277–290.

Acute autoimmune rheumatic disease

Salmon JE, Niewold TB. A successful trial for lupus. *New England Journal of Medicine* 2020; **382**: 287–288.

Tsokos GC. Systemic lupus erythematosus. *New England Journal of Medicine* 2011; **378**: 1949–1961.

Thrombosis and the anti-phospholipid syndrome

Garcia D, Erkan D. Diagnosis and management of antiphospholipid syndrome. *New England Journal of Medicine* 2018; **378**: 2010–2021.

Hughes GRV. Hughes' syndrome: the anti-phospholipid syndrome. *Journal of the Royal College of Physicians of London* 1998; **32**: 260–264.

Crystal arthritis

Mulay SR, Anders HJ. Crystallopathies. *New England Journal of Medicine* 2016; **374**: 2465–2476.

Axial spondyloarthritis

Taurog JD, Chhabra A, Colbert RA. Ankylosing spondylitis and axial spondyloarthritis. *New England Journal of Medicine* 2016; **374**: 2563–2574.

Psoriatic arthritis

Ritchlin CT, Colbert RA, Gladman DD. Psoriatic arthritis. *New England Journal of Medicine* 2017; **376**: 957–970.

Kidney and Urinary Tract Disease

Presentation of kidney and urinary tract disease

- Patients' complaints directly related to the urinary tract or urine output, e.g. frequency, dysuria, burning micturition, urgency, colic, polyuria, nocturia, haematuria, oliguria and anuria.
- Discovery of abnormal laboratory findings during routine investigations, e.g. proteinuria, haematuria, elevated plasma creatinine, electrolyte and acid–base disturbances.
- Symptoms and signs of renal disease (e.g. uraemia, anaemia, anuria, hypertension and oedema) in the absence of prior renal disease.
- Discovery of renal and urinary tract disease as part of involvement in systemic disease, e.g.:
  - Metabolic disease (e.g. diabetes mellitus): the most common cause of end-stage renal disease (ESRD) in the Western world
  - Autoimmune rheumatic diseases (e.g. systemic lupus erythematosus [SLE], vasculitis, systemic sclerosis, rheumatoid arthritis)
  - Infectious diseases (e.g. Gram-negative sepsis, infective endocarditis, mycobacterial, protozoal, viral)
  - Cardiovascular diseases (e.g. hypertension, heart failure)
  - Blood dyscrasia (e.g. multiple myeloma, amyloidosis, lymphoma, haemolytic uraemic syndrome/thrombotic thrombocytopenic purpura, HUS/TTP).

Information

- Decline in GFR: is this due to pre-renal, post-renal or intra-renal disease?
- Intrinsic renal disease: divide into glomerular or non-glomerular disorders (e.g. tubular, interstitial or vascular).
- Differentiate between primary renal diseases and renal disorders secondary to systemic disease.
- Identify preventable or reversible diseases.

FLUID BALANCE AND ELECTROLYTES: ASSESSING FLUID STATUS

Clinical assessment

Take a quick history, particularly of fluid and electrolyte intake (oral or IV) and output (renal, GI tract or skin), and then examine the patient (Fig. 9.1, Table 9.1).

Case history (1)

A 43-year-old man is brought to A&E with a 4-day history of severe abdominal pain and watery diarrhoea up to 10 times daily. He has felt so bad that he has hardly drunk or eaten anything over the last few days. He has lost 5 kg in weight.

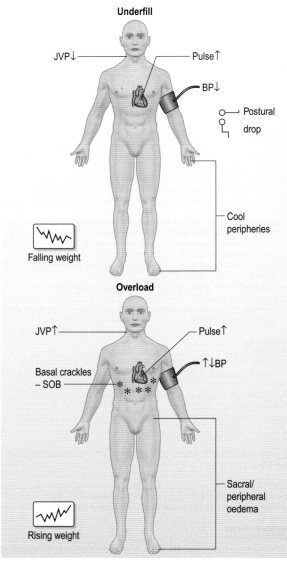

Figure 9.1 Examining the patient: underfill and overload. SOB, short of breath.

Table 9.1 Tools to assess fluid status

Useful	Not so useful
Clinical examinations	
BP (especially postural or post-exercise drop) Oedema JVP Peripheral perfusion Pulse Basal crackles	Skin turgor Eye turgor Mucous membranes
Charts	
Serial weight (on same machine)	Fluid balance (input/output)
Additional tools	
CVP line − use dynamically CXR Pulmonary artery flow catheter	CVP − absolute Urine Na^+ Osmolality

He is normally fit and well, and he wonders whether he has some form of severe gastroenteritis.

On examination, he is dehydrated with dry tongue. Abdominal examination reveals some generalised tenderness.

Fig. 9.1(a) shows the other signs of hypovolaemia.

Investigations:

- Serum Na 123 mmol/L
- Serum K 2.1 mmol/L
- Chloride 86 mmol/L
- Urea 35 mmol/L
- Creatinine 120 μmol/L
- Hb 154 g/L
- Packed cell volume (PCV) 0.58.

Diagnosis

Dehydration, secondary to GI fluid loss plus pre-renal failure.

Management

Volume replacement can often be achieved with oral rehydration solutions, but because of hypotension this man was given IV 0.9% saline initially over 1 h, followed by 1 L of 0.9% saline plus 20 mmol K^+ 4-hourly for 24 h. He quickly improved and clinically appeared euvolaemic (normal venous pressure, pulse and BP) by the next day. (*N.B.* Stool cultures grew *Campylobacter*, which is a common cause of severe gastroenteritis.)

Remember

- Examine the patient again!
- Then again later (today)!!

- And again (tomorrow)!!!
  Laboratory tests are no substitute for clinical assessment.

Case history (2)

A 24-year-old man is involved in an RTA, receiving injuries to his chest and abdomen.

On admission to the Trauma Unit he is shocked, with a tachycardia of 120 bpm, BP 90/55 and cold, clammy peripheries. His GCS score is 12.

Examination of his chest reveals a right haemothorax. Abdominal examination shows a tender, rigid abdomen with no bowel sounds, suggestive of peritonitis.

Management

Airways, circulation and breathing were quickly assessed and ventilation started with a very tight-fitting facial mask.

IV access was achieved with a large-bore intravenous cannula and 0.9% saline started. A urinary catheter was inserted.

An emergency CT scan confirmed the haemothorax and an intercostal tube drain was inserted.

Abdominal CT confirmed free fluid in the abdomen and an abnormal small intestine, suggestive of ischaemia. Liver, spleen and other organs seemed normal.

A CVP line was inserted to assess fluid balance. Fluid challenge (Box 9.1, Fig. 9.2) indicated hypovolaemia, and blood transfusion (2 units) was started with repeated checks on his fluid status.

A laparotomy was performed and 20 cm of small bowel resected.

Postoperatively, his vital signs were stable but he had not passed urine despite IV furosemide and adequate fluid replacement. His urea and creatinine have risen, indicating acute kidney injury (AKI) due to acute tubular necrosis.

Further management is provided by the Renal Unit with the aim of controlling fluid and electrolyte balance, and treating sepsis until the kidneys spontaneously recover. After 10 days' management, including haemofiltration (necessary for uncontrolled hyperkalaemia), he started to pass urine and eventually made a good recovery.

Box 9.1 Fluid challenge

Use CVP dynamically (see Fig. 9.2). Take reading

↓

Give IV bolus (100 mL 0.9% saline) fluid challenge

↓

Repeat reading

CVP ↑ — full

CVP ↓ — not full

There is no absolute value

Do this yourself! If done correctly, it gives accurate information

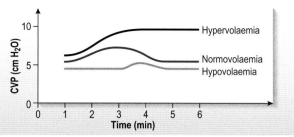

Figure 9.2 Fluid challenge.

FLUID BALANCE AND ELECTROLYTES: SODIUM PROBLEMS

What are you actually measuring when you measure the serum sodium? A ratio of:

- Extracellular Na^+ in mmol
- Extracellular water in litres.

Using this concept, you can describe how serum Na^+ becomes abnormally low (hyponatraemia) or high (hypernatraemia) (Table 9.2).

How do I work out why?

The key is to determine the extracellular water. Examine the patient (see Fig. 9.1).

Hyponatraemia

This is defined as sodium <135 mmol/L.

Case history

The Gynaecology trainee is worried about a 53-year-old woman who had a transabdominal hysterectomy 3 days ago. Her serum Na^+ has fallen to 123 mmol/L. The trainee asks whether the woman should be given some 1.8% (twice normal) saline. The polite answer is 'No'!

Remember

Wherever sodium goes, water is sure to follow, and vice versa.

Management

- Fluid assessment
- Examine fluid charts.

On examination, there were no features of fluid depletion, which excludes true Na^+ depletion.

You then discover that she had been receiving 5% glucose by IV infusion since surgery 3 days ago. This is probably the most common cause of hyponatraemia in a surgical patient. Other causes are listed in Box 9.2.

Table 9.2 Hyponatraemia and hypernatraemia

Ratio (Na⁺ : water)	Extracellular water
Hyponatraemia	
Water ↑	→ or ↓
Water ↑ > Na⁺ ↑	↓↓
Na⁺ ↓	↓
Hypernatraemia	
Water ↓	→ or ↓
Water ↓ > Na⁺ ↓	↓↓
Na⁺ ↑	↑

Note: In the table, Na⁺ is written as Na^+.

Box 9.2 Other causes of hyponatraemia

- Diuretic therapy: loop diuretics in particular cause large renal losses of salt and water, and metabolic alkalosis
- Severe heart failure, advanced liver cirrhosis or nephrotic syndrome: hyponatraemia with increased total body sodium and even greater excess of water, resulting in ascites and oedema. Plasma osmolality is low. Increased water orally continues in the face of salt restriction, diuretic therapy or both, and will aggravate the ascites and oedema
- Syndrome of inappropriate anti-diuretic hormone (SIADH) production (see p. 436)
- Pseudohyponatraemia: e.g. hyperlipidaemic states where sodium is confined to the aqueous phase or monoclonal gammopathies, hyperglycaemia (10 mmol rise reduces sodium by approximately 2 mmol)

Action

- Stop IV fluids, restrict oral fluids to 1 L daily and allow food as requested by the patient.
  Forty-eight hours later, her serum sodium is 132 mmol/L.

Hypernatraemia

Case history

A 47-year-old man is in the Neurosurgical Unit, having had a pituitary tumour removed by trans-sphenoidal surgery. He has made a normal postoperative recovery but on review, prior to discharge, he complains of excess thirst and nocturia.

Review of the fluid balance charts show that he is drinking nearly 5 L a day, with a urinary output of 3.5 L.

Recent blood tests show a serum Na^+ of 153 mmol/L.

You diagnose cranial diabetes insipidus, which you know occurs transiently for a few days or weeks after pituitary surgery.

Hypernatraemia is defined as sodium >145 mmol/L.

- Iatrogenic: IV infusion of hypertonic sodium bicarbonate, hyper-alimentation by IV route or nasogastric tube, sodium chloride tablets, sea water drowning or mineralocorticoid excess; total body sodium is elevated in these conditions. Signs are of hypervolaemia.
- Impaired thirst/unconscious patient: total body sodium is low because of both sodium and water deficit but water losses are greater than the losses of sodium. Signs are of hypovolaemia.
- Osmotic diuresis, e.g. diabetic ketoacidosis, radiocontrast, mannitol: total body sodium is low because of both sodium and water deficit, but water losses are greater than sodium losses. Urine is not maximally concentrated despite the hyperosmolar state, in contrast to GI losses of sodium and water where urine is maximally concentrated. Signs are of hypovolaemia.
- Water loss, e.g. diabetes insipidus: normal total body sodium. Signs are of euvolaemia.

Remember

True Na^+ overload is invariably iatrogenic and gives a clinical picture of fluid overload.

Treatment

- Reassure the patient.
- Avoid rapid correction (Fig. 9.3). Serum Na^+ should not fall by >1 mmol every 2 h, i.e. 10 mmol/24 h.
- Initially give IV 0.45% saline. This is followed by 5% glucose with 20 mmol/L K^+ with frequent monitoring of volume status and serum Na^+ level. This stays in the extracellular compartment (see assessing fluid status, p. 207).

Key points

- Examine the patient: know where their water is.
- Correction should be slow.
- Hyponatraemia is a more common problem in clinical practice than hypernatraemia.
- Hypernatraemia is generally found in ITU patients.

PATIENT STOPPED PASSING URINE

Information

- Oliguria: urine output <500 mL/day
- Anuria: urine output <50 mL/day

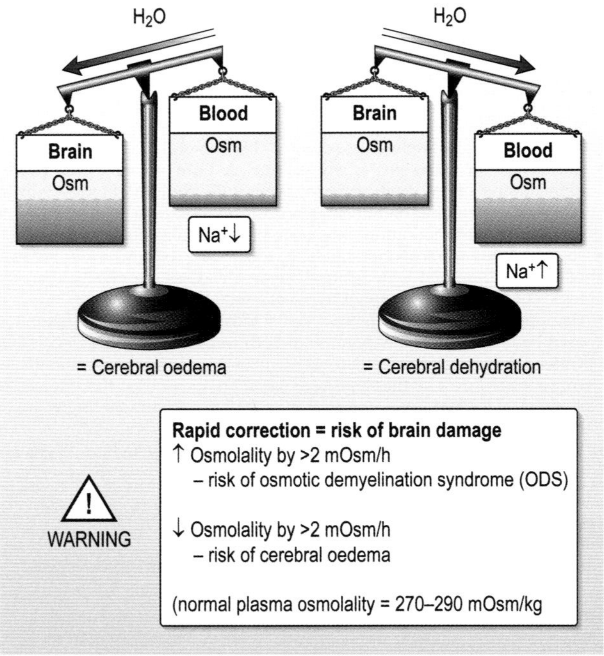

Figure 9.3 Effect on the brain of changes in sodium concentration.

Case history

The surgical registrar calls you at 10 p.m. to say that she has a 62-year-old man who is 2 days post laparotomy and who isn't passing urine.

What should you do?

- Do: see the patient.
- Don't: simply give telephone advice.

Take a detailed history of the type of surgical procedure. Ask about GI bleeding, dehydration or other fluid losses, nephrotoxic drugs, drugs associated with hypersensitivity reaction causing tubulo-interstitial nephritis (e.g. penicillins, NSAIDs, cephalosporins), evidence of previous renal insufficiency, and any radiological procedure with contrast enhancement. Anuria usually means obstructive uropathy or vasculitides rather than acute tubulo-nephritis (ATN); evidence of these conditions should be sought.

On examination, the patient has a tachycardia of 110 bpm with a low BP of 90/50.

Examination of his abdomen shows a healing laparotomy scar, no tenderness and no evidence of a palpable bladder.

Common causes of poor urinary output

- Urine retention: always catheterise.
- Dehydration: assess fluid status (see Fig. 9.1). Look at fluid balance charts.
- Shock: Table 9.3.
- Drugs: look at medicines chart.

Results in this man

- No urine from catheter.
- Your clinical assessment – hypovolaemic.
- Fluid charts incorrectly filled in but patient seems to have received 2 L of fluid (IV and oral) over the last 48 h.

Initial management

This man is fluid-depleted and needs fluid replacement (Table 9.4):
- Add 0.9% saline IV (20 mmol/K^+) to each litre.
- Write up initial regimen: modulate according to patient age/size and severity of fluid depletion.
- Reassess fluid status regularly.
- When in doubt, use a CVP line.

Aim

To establish a diuresis of at least 100 mL/h. In most cases, failure to achieve this is because of inadequate fluid replacement.

Other actions

- Check U&Es.
- Stop potentially nephrotoxic drugs.

Table 9.3 Shock – failure of organ perfusion				
	BP	**Peripheral perfusion**	**CVP**	**Brief action**
Hypovolaemia	↓	↓	↓	Look for overt/covert loss and replace with appropriate fluid, e.g. saline or blood
Cardiogenic	↓	↓	→ ↑	Myocardial infarction might need inotropes
Sepsis	↓	→ ↓	→ ↓	Look for source, give antimicrobials ± inotropes if hypotensive

Kumar & Clark's Cases in Clinical Medicine

Table 9.4 Fluid replacement

IV fluid	Na$^+$ (mmol/L)	K$^+$ (mmol/L)	HCO$_3$ or equivalent (mmol/L)	Cl$^-$ (mmol/L)	Ca^{2+} (mmol/L)	Indication (see below)
Normal plasma values	**142**	**4.5**	**26**	**103**	**2.5**	
1. Sodium chloride 0.9%	150	–	–	150	–	1
2. Sodium chloride 0.18% + glucose 4%	30	–	–	30	–	2
3. Glucose 5% + potassium chloride 0.3%	–	40	–	40	–	3
4. Sodium bicarbonate 1.26%	150	–	150	–	–	4
5. Compound sodium lactate (Hartmann's)	131	5	29	111	2	5
6. Plasma-Lyte 148	140	5		98		

1. Volume expansion in hypovolaemic patients. Rarely to maintain fluid balance when there are large losses of sodium. The sodium (150 mmol) is greater than plasma and hypernatraemia can result. It is often necessary to add KCl 20–40 mmol/L.

2. Maintenance of fluid balance in normovolaemic, normonatraemic patients.

3. To replace water. Can be given with or without potassium chloride. May be alternated with 0.9% saline as an alternative to (2).

(Continued)

Table 9.4 Fluid replacement—cont'd

IV fluid	Na⁺ (mmol/L)	K⁺ (mmol/L)	HCO₃ or equivalent (mmol/L)	Cl⁻ (mmol/L)	Ca²⁺ (mmol/L)	Indication (see below)

4. For volume expansion in hypovolaemic, acidotic patients alternating with (1). Occasionally for maintenance of fluid balance combined with (2) in salt-wasting, acidotic patients.

5. Used for maintenance of fluid balance after surgery. The potassium content may be dangerous in renal failure but occasionally useful in the diuretic phase of acute tubular necrosis where hypokalaemia occurs.

6. (6) For fluid replacement with glucose and electrolytes. Used for head injury, intra-operative fluid replacement, fracture and infection.

Modified from Kumar P, Clark M, eds. *Kumar and Clark's Clinical Medicine*, 9th edn. Edinburgh: Elsevier, 2017.

- Stop anti-hypertensive drugs.
- Ask nurses to record daily weights and to make careful note of fluid intake and urine output on the fluid chart.

Still no urine?

- Are you certain that the patient is adequately fluid-replete?
- Check that the urine catheter is not blocked or misplaced.
- Give a loop diuretic, e.g. furosemide.
- The patient might now have established AKI. Refer to a Nephrologist.
  Fortunately, this man responded to fluid replacement and produced urine, initially 50 mL/h.

Key points

- Don't miss urine retention.
- Recognise shock.
- Assess fluid status regularly.
- Most cases will need fluid replacement, and failure to achieve this can result in established renal failure.

ACUTE HEART FAILURE

Acute heart failure occurs when cardiac function falls, causing elevated cardiac filling pressure. This causes severe breathlessness with fluid accumulating in the interstitial and alveolar spaces of the lung (pulmonary oedema).

Case history

A 65-year-old, 50-kg woman, who smokes 20 cigarettes per day and has a past history of intermittent claudication, presented to A&E with acute shortness of breath. She is on no medication.

On examination, she was centrally and peripherally cyanosed, and peripherally cold and clammy, with a raised JVP, gallop rhythm and bilateral coarse crackles up to both mid-zones. She had absent foot pulses and bilateral femoral bruits. Her BP at presentation was 195/98.

Her ECG showed hypertensive changes (with left ventricular hypertrophy) and a CXR showed bilateral perihilar shadowing. Initially, her biochemistry was:

- Na: 142 mmol/L
- K: 3.1 mmol/L
- Urea: 12 mmol/L
- Creatinine: 115 μmol/L; eGFR 44 mL/min per 1.73 m².

Diagnosis
Flash pulmonary oedema.

Treatment
She responded well to oxygen, IV morphine 10 mg, IV furosemide 50 mg and a vasodilator (captopril 12.5 mg) but 4 days later her biochemistry was:

- Na: 142 mmol/L
- K: 6.0 mmol/L
- Urea: 54 mmol/L
- Creatinine: 500 μmol/L (Fig. 9.4); eGFR 8 mL/min/1.73 m².

What has gone wrong?

It is very likely that she has developed acute kidney injury (AKI). This is because she has underlying renovascular disease.

Diagnostic criteria for AKI

The definition of AKI used in clinical and epidemiological studies is based on specific criteria that have been sequentially developed. The Kidney Disease: Improving Global Outcomes (KDIGO) definition and staging system is the most recent and preferred (Table 9.5). Others include the RIFLE criteria (risk, injury, failure, loss of kidney function and end-stage kidney disease; Table 9.6) and a subsequent modification proposed by the Acute Kidney Injury Network (AKIN) and others.

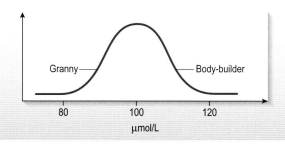

Figure 9.4 Interpreting serum creatinine. The serum creatinine in the healthy population is normally distributed according to muscle bulk. Only large, well-muscled men will usually have a creatinine >110 if their renal function is normal. Therefore, for small people, creatinine does not enter the 'abnormal' range until half their renal function has been lost.

Stage	Serum creatinine concentration (SCr)	Urine output criteria
Table 9.5 KDIGO classification of acute kidney injury			
1	SCr 1.5–1.9 times baseline OR ≥26.5 μmol/L (0.3 mg/dL) increase	<0.5 mL/kg per h for 6–12 h
2	SCr 2–2.9 times baseline	<0.5 mL/kg per h for 6–12 h
3	SCr 3 times baseline OR Initiation of renal replacement therapy OR In patients <18 years, decrease in eGFR to <35 mL/min per 1.73 m²	Anuria for ≥12 h

SCr, serum creatinine.

Table 9.6 RIFLE criteria for acute kidney injury[a]

Grade	GFR criteria	UO criteria
Risk	SCr × 1.5 or GFR decrease >25% (within 48 h)	<0.5 mL/kg per h × 6 h
Injury	SCr × 2 or GFR decrease >50%	<0.5 mL/kg per h × 12 h
Failure	SCr × 3, GFR decrease >75%, SCr >350 μmol/L with an acute rise >40 μmol/L	<0.3 mL/kg per h × 24 h
Loss	Persistent AKI >4 weeks	
ESKD	Persistent ESKD >3 months	

ESKD, end-stage kidney disease; UO, urinary output; SCr, serum creatinine.
[a]There is a consensus definition that merges RIFLE criteria and the Acute Kidney Injury Network definition (Kidney Disease: Improving Global Outcomes [KDIGO] group 2012).
From Bellomo R, Kellum JA, Ronco C. Acute kidney injury. *Lancet* 2012; **380:** 756–766.

The KDIGO criteria differ from the RIFLE classification in that the former utilise only changes in serum creatinine and urine output for staging, not changes in GFR; the exception is made for children under the age of 18 years, for whom an acute decrease in eGFR to <35 mL/min per $1.73m^2$ is included in the criteria for stage 3 AKI.

Clinical suspicion of renovascular disease

- Most patients will have disseminated atheroma with missing pulses and/or bruits and a history of smoking.
- Abdominal/renal bruits are rare (although they have a very strong association with renal artery stenosis, RAS).
- 'Flash pulmonary oedema' (without an obvious precipitant) is a good predictor of renovascular disease.
- There is a brittle response to volume loading or off-loading (Fig. 9.5). *Note:* this patient's renal function was abnormal at presentation.
   Angiotensin-converting enzyme (ACE) inhibitors can cause acute kidney injury in patients with renovascular disease (Fig. 9.6).

How should patients like this be managed?

The key to successful management is very careful fluid control.

Managing acute heart failure (AHF) in the presence of suspected renovascular disease

- Treat the pulmonary oedema: it is a dangerous and very distressing condition.
- Avoid ACE inhibitors (ACEIs)/A II blockers: use other vasodilators (this patient was given captopril!).
- Avoid rapid volume off-loading: titrate the diuretic dose against renal function.
- Insert a CVP line and use it properly (see Fig. 9.1).

NORMAL

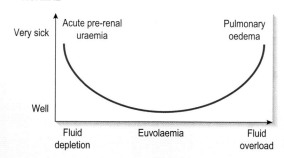

RENOVASCULAR DISEASE

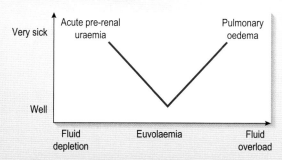

Patients with renovascular disease (who also often have
a stiff, non-compliant left ventricle) will develop acute kidney
injury or LVF rapidly in the face of mild depletion or overload

Figure 9.5 Fluid status in normal and renovascular disease. LVF, left ventricular
failure.

- Examine (and weigh) the patient regularly: use low-dose dopamine
  (can be given via peripheral line at 2.5 mg/kg per min) for its
  natriuretic effect if no response to initial therapy.

Renal imaging investigations

- Ultrasound: unequal renal size (>2 cm difference) is a good predictor
  of renovascular disease but its absence does not exclude RAS. Duplex
  ultrasound is used to demonstrate renal artery perfusion.
- Isotope renography: unequal function, slow transit and altered
  dynamics with captopril are all suggestive of renovascular disease. In
  experienced hands and with good renal function, its sensitivity and

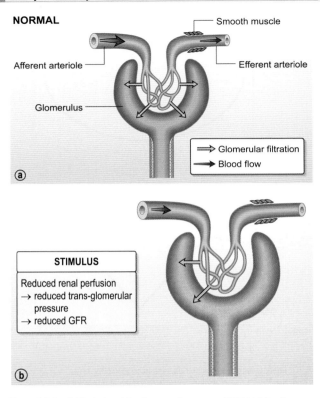

NORMAL

Smooth muscle

Afferent arteriole

Efferent arteriole

Glomerulus

⟹ Glomerular filtration
⟶ Blood flow

(a)

STIMULUS

Reduced renal perfusion
→ reduced trans-glomerular
pressure
→ reduced GFR

(b)

Figure 9.6 (a–d) Effect of angiotensin-converting enzyme (ACE) inhibitors/blockers. A I/A II, angiotensin I/II.

specificity are 70% (creatinine <150 μmol/L); however, in inpatients with severe renal impairment its sensitivity falls below 30%.

- MR angiography is increasingly used to visualise the renal arteries.
- Intra-arterial angiography: the gold standard — should be carried out by experienced radiologists with minimal contrast load.

Outcome in this patient

She responded to treatment of her AHF, her pulmonary oedema resolved and her renal function returned to normal.

She was then investigated for RAS, with MR angiography showing a narrowing of the right renal artery, thought to be due to atherosclerosis.

She was continued on diuretics and amlodipine, with good control of her BP. She is under regular review.

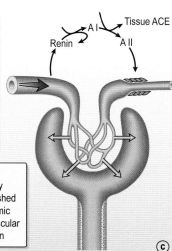

RESPONSE

Intra-renal activation of renin/angiotensin system leads to preferential efferent arteriolar vasoconstriction
→ restores trans-glomerular pressure
→ restores GFR

Note:
This process may be entirely intra-renal, but once established can spill over into the systemic vasculature. This is how vascular disease causes hypertension

©

ACE inhibitor (or A II blocker)

ACEIs block this response and can therefore abolish the trans-glomerular pressure gradient, and with it reduction of glomerular filtration

Note:
Although, in this context, blocking angiotensin II leads to decreased renal vascular resistance, any resultant increase in renal blood flow is of no benefit if no glomerular filtrate is generated

ⓓ

Figure 9.6, Cont'd

Natural history of atheromatous renovascular disease

- ACEIs/A II blockers will cause AKI only if both kidneys are affected by RAS, or if only one functioning kidney is present. However, the atheroma is diffuse and progressive. Complete renal artery occlusion with total loss of renal function on one side is usually clinically silent.
- Anatomical renovascular disease is very common and much of it is not physiologically significant (but you can't tell which is which until it is too late).
- Small vessel (intra-renal) disease behaves identically to main renal artery disease (but you can't treat it).

HYPERKALAEMIA

Don't let your patient die tonight!

Case history

A 70-year-old woman has been admitted by the vascular surgeons with an acutely ischaemic lower limb. The right leg, below the knee, was cold, the skin was mottled and there was no pulse below the knee. The patient was in agony with the pain in the limb and she was given IV morphine 10 mg. She is on an ACEI and diuretic for hypertension and also on an NSAID.

It is 2 a.m. The surgical trainee calls you because her K^+ has come back at 7.2 mmol/L and wants your help.

Remember

- This is a life-threatening condition.
- The usual symptoms of life-threatening hyperkalaemia are absent.

What do you do next?

K^+ >6.5 mmol/L

- Immediate cardioprotection:
  - 10 mL of 10% Ca gluconate over 10 min.
  - *Note:* action is relatively short-lived but dose can be replaced every 15 min.
- Get K^+ inside cells: 50 mL of 50% glucose with (or followed by) 10 U insulin. IV 50 mL sodium bicarbonate 8.4% is given over 1 h for severe acidosis, pH <6.9.
  - *Note:* if the patient has a nasogastric tube then put it on free suction because it will remove acid and potassium, causing systemic alkalosis and encouraging influx of potassium intracellularly (Fig. 9.7).

Now you have time to stop and think. The K^+ is telling you that something has gone badly wrong. Find it and treat it!

Common reversible causes of K^+

- Tissue hypoxia/damage.
- Acidosis.
- K^+-sparing diuretics.
- ACEIs.

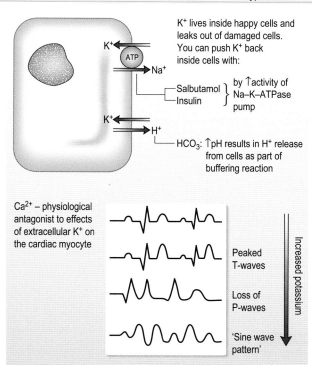

K⁺ lives inside happy cells and leaks out of damaged cells. You can push K⁺ back inside cells with:

$\left.\begin{array}{l}\text{Salbutamol}\\\text{Insulin}\end{array}\right\}$ by ↑activity of Na–K–ATPase pump

HCO₃: ↑pH results in H⁺ release from cells as part of buffering reaction

Ca²⁺ – physiological antagonist to effects of extracellular K⁺ on the cardiac myocyte

Peaked T-waves

Loss of P-waves

'Sine wave pattern'

Increased potassium

Figure 9.7 Potassium: some facts.

- Blood transfusion.
- Acute kidney injury.

Quick and simple ways to stop or reverse underlying causes of raised K⁺

- Establish a diuresis.
- Stop ACEIs/NSAIDs.
- Stop blood transfusion.
- Successfully treat sepsis.

Remember

If K⁺ is not responding, your patient might need dialysis — refer to a Nephrologist. If the patient's early U&Es suggest acute or chronic kidney disease, make arrangements to move him/her to a dialysis unit after initial resuscitative measures.

Don't sit too long on such patients — dialysis could be the only option.

While you are thinking

- Assess volume status.
- Assess ischaemic/damaged tissue. What do the surgeons think about the viability of the leg?
- Repeat ECG.
- Check arterial blood gases.
- Check drug chart.

As you can't promptly reverse the cause

- Give a loop diuretic, e.g. furosemide.
- Treat tomorrow's K^+ with Ca^{2+} resonium (15 g orally with 10 mL lactulose or 30 g PR).

Remember

1 mL of 8.4% $NaHCO_3$ = 1 mmol Na^+. Don't kill your patient with sodium overload (see Fig. 9.1).

Now go back to re-examine the patient and assess

- Fluid status.
- Peripheral perfusion.
- Acid−base status.
- Recheck U&Es.
- ECG changes.

Remember

MYTHS THAT ARE *NOT* TRUE

- A normal ECG implies your patient is not in danger.
- Ca^{2+} resonium will alter tonight's K^+.

Further management

An urgent angiogram was performed, which showed a thrombosis in the right femoral artery near the junction of the popliteal artery.

Thrombolysis was initially used, as the surgeons felt removal of the thrombus would not be feasible. The patient did not respond and gangrene occurred, so that a below-knee amputation then became necessary.

Less common causes of hyperkalaemia are listed in Box 9.3.

THE ACIDOTIC PATIENT

Case history

A 50-year-old woman with chronic kidney disease developed laryngeal oedema as an idiosyncratic reaction to a phenothiazine. She became hypotensive and oliguric. On admission, her blood gases showed:

- pH: 6.9 (Fig. 9.8)
- PO_2: 6.0

Box 9.3 Less common causes of hyperkalaemia

Endocrine

- Addison's disease
- Isolated hypoaldosteronism
- C-21 hydroxylase deficiency
- Congenital adrenal syndromes, e.g. 3-β hydroxydehydrogenase deficiency

Additional drugs

- Ciclosporin
- Succinylcholine
- NSAIDs

Others

- Tumour lysis syndrome
- Periodic hyperkalaemia paralysis
- Malignant hyperthermia
- Familial hyperkalaemia acidosis

- Remember pH is a log scale. A pH of <7.15 means that the [H⁺] (hydrogen ion concentration) has doubled.
- Before pH falls significantly, extensive buffering capacity must be consumed. Once this has happened, patients are highly unstable.

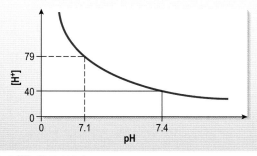

Figure 9.8 pH: some facts.

- PCO₂: 8.2
- HCO₃: 15

Following intubation, ventilation and fluid resuscitation, her BP rose to 145/70. Her blood gases returned to normal over the next 12 h.

Remember

Only <5% of patients admitted with pH 7.0 or less survive to discharge from hospital. This is because severe acidosis is usually a reflection of serious underlying problems.

How to manage severe acidosis

- Airway.
- Breathing.
- Circulation.

Problems with any of these will contribute to acidosis and must be corrected.

Identify and treat the underlying problem

Tissue damage/hypoxia is by far the most common cause of metabolic acidosis due to lactic acidosis. Examples include:

- Sepsis:
  - Hypotensive patient with warm peripheries
  - Often apyrexial and/or normal WCC on presentation, especially if very sick or elderly
  - Sometimes develop low PO_4.
- Rhabdomyolysis:
  - Areas of muscle necrosis not always clinically evident
  - $PO_4 \uparrow, K^+ \uparrow$
  - Might have a biphasic Ca^{2+} pattern (initially $\downarrow$ due to binding to damaged muscle, then $\uparrow$).
- Bowel ischaemia:
  - Severe acidosis
  - $PO_4 \uparrow, K^+ \uparrow$
  - Often have evidence of peripheral vascular disease.
- Heart failure:
  - Pump failure leading to tissue hypoperfusion
  - Often accompanied by renal hypoperfusion and impaired renal function.
- Over-production of acid or inability to excrete acid: Examples include:
  - Diabetic ketoacidosis
  - Kidney injury
  - Alcoholic ketoacidosis
  - Salicylate intoxication
  - Methanol poisoning
  - Ethylene glycol ingestion.
  Note: all the above result in metabolic acidosis with high anionic gap.
  Examples of normal anionic gap acidosis (hyperchloraemic acidosis):
- Diarrhoea
- Renal tubular acidosis
- Dehydration
- Interstitial renal disease
- Ureterosigmoidostomy
- Carbonic anhydrase inhibitors (acetazolamide)
- Arginine hydrochloride ingestion
- Ammonium chloride ingestion.

Find and treat the underlying cause.

Role of IV HCO₃ in acidosis

- The role of IV HCO_3 is not clear (Fig. 9.9)!
- Remember, 8.4% HCO_3 = 1 mmol/mL Na^+. It is very easy to precipitate volume overload.
- HCO_3 might be indicated if pH is <7.25 in an attempt to reduce the depression of myocardial function produced by severe acidosis.

Bicarbonate will not save your patient if you don't correct the underlying cause of acidosis (but it might help keep them alive until you do).

ACUTE KIDNEY INJURY

AKI is an abrupt deterioration of renal function over the course of a few days or weeks. It is usually (but not always) reversible.

Case history

A 75-year-old man has a 5-day history of anorexia, nausea, vomiting and lethargy. His doctor has noted the following findings:

- Hb: 100 g/L
- Urea: 48 mmol/L
- Creatinine: 820 μmol/L; eGFR 6 mL/min per 1.73 m².
- K⁺ 5.6 mmol/L.
  The previous history includes mild hypertension and osteoarthritis.

What are your priorities?

Safety

- Treat this man's life-threatening hyperkalaemia (see p. 224).
- Fluid assessment (see Fig. 9.1):
  - Dry: treat with fluids
  - Wet: treat with fluid restriction
  - OK.
  In this case, the patient has a K⁺ of 5.6 mmol/L and his fluid status is OK. At this stage, review/stop any drug therapy. Now, you have to consider:
- Why does this man have AKI?
- Is it reversible?
- Do you need to refer to a renal unit?

Testing the urine (and sending an MSU)

Blood + protein = 'active' urine, and suggests active glomerular disease in the absence of infection. Some hospitals provide a facility for urinary RBC morphology on fresh urine by polarising microscopy. Predominant dysmorphic RBCs are highly suggestive of glomerular pathology.

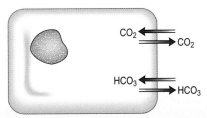

CO_2 equilibrated more rapidly between ECF and ICF than HCO_3

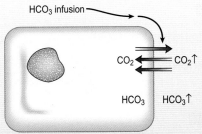

HCO_3 infusion titrates extracellular H^+ causing a rise in CO_2 which equilibrates across ECF/ICF before the HCO_3 can get into cells

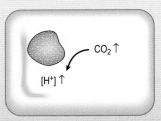

Intracellular CO_2 rises, leading to worsening intracellular acidosis

Figure 9.9 Theoretical reasons for adverse effect of HCO_3 in small rodent models of lactic acidosis. Conclusions: if you are called to A&E to see a rat with lactic acidosis, do not under any circumstances give it IV $NaHCO_3$. ECF, extra-cellular fluid; ICF, intra-cellular fluid.

Investigations

- Ultrasound (see later)
- Immunological markers: anti-nuclear antibodies (ANA), extractable nuclear antigen (ENA), anti-neutrophil cytoplasmic antibody (ANCA), anti-glomerular basement membrane (GBM) antibodies, cryoglobulins, complements, anti-streptolysin O titre (ASOT)

- Serum protein electrophoresis
- 24-h urinary protein loss

Renal tract imaging

In this case the renal ultrasound is normal. This tells you:
- There is a low probability of obstruction.
- There is potentially a reversible component.

Referral to a renal unit

- Don't delay! The most common concern expressed by renal units is that referring teams wait too long to transfer cases and patients are in a critical condition when they arrive on the unit.
- Be prepared: see Questions you will be asked (later).

Guide to indications for dialysis

There is no magic level of urea or creatinine. Dialysis is indicated:
- In uncontrolled hyperkalaemia
- In unresponsive pulmonary oedema
- When patient symptoms demand.

Outcome

In this case, the patient turned out to be taking an NSAID. He required haemodialysis for uncontrolled vomiting and subsequently had a renal biopsy. This showed tubulo-interstitial nephritis secondary to NSAID therapy. He responded well to a short course of steroids.

Questions you will be asked when referring to a renal unit

- Is the patient passing urine?
- What is the patient's fluid status?
- Have you done a renal ultrasound (Box 9.4)?
- Is the urine 'active'?
- Any nephrotoxic drugs?
- Hepatitis status?
- Any information on the patient's prior renal function?

CHRONIC KIDNEY DISEASE

Chronic kidney disease (CKD) is used to describe long-standing, usually progressive, impairment in renal function.

Case history

A 35-year-old woman registers with a new doctor and is found to be hypertensive (180/105), with blood and protein in her urine. She has no specific symptoms.

On examination, there is pallor, BP 180/105, grade II hypertension, retinopathy. On renal ultrasound, a small, non-obstructive kidney is seen.

Investigations:
- Hb: 85 g/L
- Urea: 18.0 mmol/L
- Creatinine: 310 μmol/L; eGFR: 20 mL/min per 1.73 m^2 (Box 9.5).

> **Box 9.4** Renal tract imaging
>
> **Ultrasound**
> - Non-invasive
> - Independent of renal function
> - Can measure size (renal length and cortical thickening)
> - Limited or no view of ureters
> - Low detection rate of renal calculi
> - Operator-dependent
>
> **CT**
> - Has largely replaced IVU
> - First-line investigation for cases of ureteric colic
>
> **Intravenous urogram (IVU)**
> - Good visualisation of pelvico-calyceal system and ureters
> - Gives some functional information

> **Box 9.5** Equations used to estimate glomerular filtration rate (GFR) in clinical practice
>
> **MDRD (Modification of Diet in Renal Disease) equation**
>
> - Calculates GFR from 4–6 variables (age, sex, race, serum creatinine concentration ± urea, albumin)
> - It is not valid for use in patients with malnutrition or those who have had a limb amputation. Interpret it with caution at extremes of body weight
> - The four-variable MDRD equation is the most widely used eGFR measurement in clinical practice
>
> $$\text{eGFR (mL/min per 1.73 m}^2) = 186 \times (\text{Creat}(\mu\text{mol/mL})/88.4)^{-1.154} \times (\text{Age})^{-0.203} \times (0.742 \text{ if female}) \times (1.210 \text{ if black})$$
>
> (MDRD calculator --- see www.nephron.com). Creatinine in µmol/L to mg/dL, multiply by 0.0113.
>
> **Cockcroft–Gault equation**
>
> - Well validated but the formula requires an accurate weight
>
> $$\text{eGFR (mL/min per 173 m}^2) = \frac{1.23^* \times (140 - \text{age}) \times (\text{Wt in kg})}{\text{Serum creatinine (µmol/L)}}$$
>
> *For females, multiply by 1.04 rather than 1.23.

Creatinine clearance by 24-h urine collection

Creatinine clearance = $\dfrac{\text{(Urine volume} \times \text{Urine creatinine concentration)}}{\text{Serum creatinine concentration}}$

- Corrects for normal creatinine turnover by the body and estimates GFR
- It is inconvenient for the patient, requires a simultaneous blood sample and is often inaccurate due to incomplete urinary collection

Clinical features seen in CKD are shown in Fig. 9.10 and classification in Table 9.7.

This woman has irreversible CKD and subsequent follow-up showed a progressive rise in creatinine.

Note: Not all patients with CKD have small, shrunken kidneys. Normal or larger than normal kidneys can be seen in diabetic nephropathy, amyloidosis, polycystic kidneys and hydronephrosis (here cortical thinning is the sign of irreversibility).

How do you manage this case?

Remember

Control of hypertension is the single most useful factor in CKD.

The approach should be multidisciplinary (Fig. 9.11).

Remember

- CKD is an insidious condition with no specific symptoms. In some cases, patients do not present until they have reached the stage when dialysis is required.
- Preparing the patient for dialysis is a specialist task: refer!
- CKD is a major cardiovascular risk factor: the average dialysis patient is at an approximately 20 times higher risk.

Preparing the patient

- Educate: a specialist counsellor should be consulted.
- Renoprotection (Box 9.6).

Specific conditions

Hyperparathyroidism

- Measure parathyroid hormone (PTH): X-rays become diagnostic only in advanced cases.
- Control phosphate:

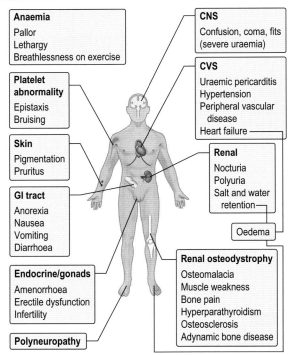

Figure 9.10 Symptoms and signs of chronic kidney disease. (From Kumar P, Clark M, eds. *Kumar and Clark's Clinical Medicine*, 9th edn. Edinburgh: Elsevier, 2017.)

- Dietitian
- Phosphate-binding drugs, e.g. calcium carbonate, calcium acetate, Sevelamer and aluminium hydroxide in selected cases.
- Vitamin D analogues (e.g. alfacalcidol).
- Monitor Ca^{2+}, phosphate, PTH and alkaline phosphatase levels.

Anaemia

- Correct iron deficiency (if present).
- Erythropoietin: can only be given IV or by SC injection × 1–3 weekly. Epoetin alfa can only be given by IV route because of increased risk of pure red cell aplasia (PRCA).
- Target Hb 115–130 g/L.
- Monitor BP.

   In summary, this woman with CKD had well controlled BP but her renal function gradually deteriorated. She eventually agreed to have haemodialysis and possible transplantation in the future.

Stage	GFR (mL/min per 1.73 m²)	Description
1	≥ 90	Normal or increased GFR with other evidence of kidney damage
2	60–89	Slight decrease in GFR with other evidence of kidney damage
3A	45–59	Moderate decrease in GFR with or without other evidence of kidney damage
3B	30–44	
4	15–29	Severe decrease in GFR with or without other evidence of kidney damage
5	<15	Established renal failure

Table 9.7 Classification of CKD

Note: The suffix 'P' can be applied to the stage of CKD if the patient has significant proteinuria, defined as a urinary albumin : creatinine ratio >65 mg/mmol or protein : creatinine ratio >100 mg/mmol.
Reprinted with permission from Kidney Disease: Improving Global Outcomes (KDIGO) CKD Work Group. (2013) KDIGO 2012 clinical practice guideline for the evaluation and management of chronic kidney disease. *Kidney International* 2013; **Suppl. 3:** 1–150.

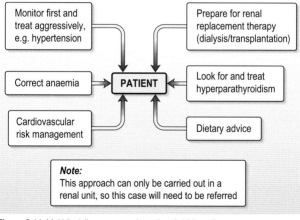

Figure 9.11 Multidisciplinary approach to chronic kidney disease.

MULTISYSTEM VASCULITIS/ACUTE GLOMERULONEPHRITIS

Case history

A 54-year-old man with a 1-month history of cough and shortness of breath (SOB), which has not responded to two courses of antibiotics from his doctor (amoxicillin, then

Kumar & Clark's Cases in Clinical Medicine

> **Box 9.6** Renoprotection
>
> **Goals of treatment**
>
> - BP <120/80
> - Proteinuria <0.3 g/24 h
>
> **Treatment**
>
> Patients with CKD and proteinuria >1 g/24 h:
> - ACE inhibitor increasing to maximum dose
> - Add angiotensin receptor antagonist if goals are not achieved*
> - Add diuretic to prevent hyperkalaemia and to help control BP
> - Add calcium-channel blocker (verapamil or diltiazem) if goals are not achieved
>
> **Additional measures**
>
> - Statins to lower cholesterol to <4.5 mmol/L
> - Smoking cessation (threefold higher rate of deterioration in CKD, if smoker)
> - Treat diabetes (HbA$_{1c}$ <7%/53 mmol/mol)
> - Normal protein diet (0.8–1 g/kg body weight)
> - Decide on mode of therapy: haemodialysis versus peritoneal dialysis versus pre-emptive renal transplantation if a live related or spousal kidney donor is willing to donate
> - Plan access surgery: an arteriovenous fistula requires at least 6 weeks before it can be used
> - In type 2 diabetes start with angiotensin receptor antagonist

clarithromycin and co-amoxiclav, re-presented to his doctor complaining of fatigue, muscle aches and pains. He requested a 'tonic'.

A week later he came to A&E, complaining of acute SOB. His CXR showed fluffy bilateral patchy alveolar shadowing, and his serum creatinine was 350 μmol/L. On further investigation, he was c-ANCA-positive. Renal biopsy showed focal necrotising glomerulonephritis. He responded well to immunosuppression with corticosteroids and cyclophosphamide.

Information

Most doctors see many patients with vague muscular aches and pains in a working day; they will see few, if any, patients with multisystem vasculitis in their working lifetimes.

To identify patients with multisystem vasculitis, dipstick the urine and don't ignore microscopic haematuria.

Inflammatory autoimmune vasculitis: microscopic polyangiitis/ granulomatosis with polyangiitis

Presentation is very non-specific: typically, vague arthralgia and myalgia with fatigue, anorexia and malaise. At a later stage, patients might develop:
- Vasculitic rash
- Mononeuritis multiplex
- Arthritis
- Ear/nose/throat symptoms, such as epistaxis or deafness.

At this point the diagnosis is more obvious but these diseases respond well to treatment if diagnosed early.

Remember

If diagnosed late, these diseases have difficult and life-threatening complications.

Pulmonary haemorrhage

- Most common disease-related cause of death in ANCA-positive vasculitis and anti-GBM disease (Goodpasture's syndrome).
- CXR appearances very variable but usually patchy alveolar shadowing (can mimic, or be accompanied by, pulmonary oedema or chest infection).
- Often precipitated by pulmonary oedema/infection/smoking.
- Can be diagnosed non-invasively by finding increased KCO; transfer factor (carbon monoxide, CO) binds to blood and gives falsely elevated KCO.

What to do

The patient requires an urgent Nephrology and ITU referral. These individuals can become very sick very quickly, and may need ventilation and plasma exchange.

How to diagnose multisystem vasculitis

If you find microscopic haematuria in a patient with non-specific malaise/myalgia:
- Enquire specifically for suggestive symptoms:
  - Nasal congestion/nose bleeds with polyangiitis (granulomatosis with polyangiitis)
  - Rash
  - Neurological symptoms.
- Examine carefully for:
  - Splinter haemorrhages
  - Nail-fold infarcts
  - Mouth ulcers
  - Rash
  - Neuropathy.
- Don't assume that microscopic haematuria is due to a urinary tract infection: send an MSU.
- If there are suggestive symptoms or signs: discuss with a Nephrologist.
- If there are no suggestive symptoms or signs but MSU is negative for a urinary tract infection: check renal function. If it is abnormal, discuss with a Nephrologist.

ANCA points (Fig. 9.12)

- False-positives occur in situations of polyclonal B-cell activation (usually on immunohistology but not against specific target antigens).
- ANCA-negative small-vessel vasculitis can be clinically and pathologically identical to ANCA-positive vasculitis.

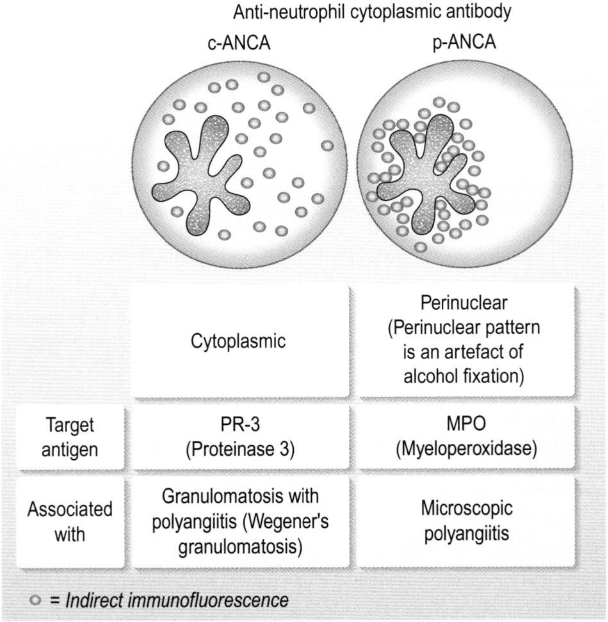

Figure 9.12 Anti-neutrophil cytoplasmic antibody.

- Changes in antibody titre might be unrelated to, lag behind or precede changes in disease activity in different patients.
- ANCA subtypes are being recognised.

Remember

These diseases will irretrievably damage your patient's kidneys in a matter of weeks. Prompt diagnosis and treatment can make a long-term difference between life on dialysis and life on a small dose of steroids.

Other markers of disease activity

↑ ESR, ↑ CRP, thrombocytosis.

Other rapidly progressive glomerulonephritides

- Goodpasture's disease is rare: it is classically described as a 'one-hit' disease and is less likely to be preceded by a non-specific prodrome than ANCA-positive vasculitis.

- IgA nephropathy, mesangiocapillary glomerulonephritis due to cryoglobulins, and diffuse proliferative glomerulonephritis in SLE can all present with a rapidly progressive, crescentic nephritis.

INTERCURRENT ILLNESS IN DIALYSIS AND TRANSPLANT PATIENTS

Case history (1)

A 72-year-old type 2 diabetic, haemodialysis patient was brought in by urgent ambulance to the A&E department, complaining of chest pain and SOB. He was due to be dialysed later that day at the nearest renal unit (5 miles away).

On admission, he had signs of mild biventricular heart failure with a tachycardia, raised venous pressure, gallop rhythm, basal crackles and peripheral oedema. His ECG showed lateral ischaemia and his Hb was 82 g/L.

He was given IV nitrates and 2 units of blood under cover of 40 mg furosemide. As the second unit of blood ran through, he complained of acute SOB and then suffered a cardiorespiratory arrest, from which he could not be resuscitated.

Remember

- Don't give blood transfusion in a dialysis patient unless a Nephrologist tells you to; you could precipitate lethal hyperkalaemia and volume overload (and the normal methods of treating these complaints will be ineffective).
- Also, even if your patient survives, you might sensitise him/her to HLA antigens in the blood, thereby removing the chance of a renal transplant.
- As a general rule, dialysis patients should not be transfused while on dialysis.

Other things *not* to do in dialysis patients

Access preservation

Dialysis access is essential for life-preserving treatment; potential sites for it are limited and easily damaged irretrievably (Fig. 9.13).

Use veins in hands or feet or the antecubital fossa. For central access use the internal jugular vein.

Fluids

Dialysis patients do *not* need 2 L/day of IV fluid or furosemide postoperatively.

Things to watch out for in dialysis patients

- Vascular disease: ischaemic heart disease is very common in dialysis patients – even young ones. It is often unmasked by anaemia.
- Infection: dialysis patients are significantly immunosuppressed functionally. They cope poorly with sepsis and rapidly become systemically unwell. Infections in access sites (lines, fistulae, peritoneal dialysis catheters) are common and might not be clinically evident, e.g. subacute infective endocarditis and osteomyelitis – always think of these complications.
- Electrolytes: haemodialysis patients are often chronically hyperkalaemic pre-dialysis (and invariably hypokalaemic immediately

Kumar & Clark's Cases in Clinical Medicine

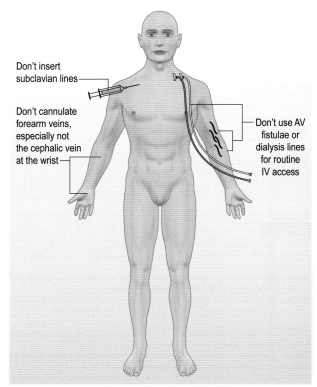

Don't insert
subclavian lines

Don't cannulate
forearm veins,
especially not
the cephalic vein
at the wrist

Don't use AV
fistulae or
dialysis lines
for routine
IV access

Figure 9.13 Things not to do in dialysis patients. AV, arteriovenous.

post-dialysis). They will often present with hypercalcaemia (too much vitamin D or Ca^{2+}-based PO_4-binders) or hypocalcaemia (too little).

- Poorly compliant patients are routinely hyperphosphataemic; if they then start taking their 'prescribed' doses of vitamin D (1-α calcidol) and Ca^{2+}-based phosphate binders, their $Ca^{2+} \times PO_4$ product might exceed 7 mmol/L, precipitating ectopic calcification.

Case history (2)

A 23-year-old renal transplant recipient (primary renal disease was reflux nephropathy), on standard triple-therapy immunosuppression (prednisolone, azathioprine, ciclosporin), presented with a hot, swollen, 'exquisitely' painful right ankle.

The joint was aspirated. The fluid contained 5000 WCC/mm^3 with negative birefringent needle-shaped crystals seen on microscopy.

Diagnosis: gout

The symptoms responded to colchicine 500 μg × 2 daily; allopurinol was started (300 mg × 1 daily) after 4 weeks, with continuation of the colchicine.

Three weeks later, the patient presented shocked with pancytopenia, developed multi-organ failure and died.

Beware drug interactions that matter in transplantation

Allopurinol and azathioprine

Azathioprine is metabolised to 6-mercaptopurine, which is metabolised by xanthine oxidase. Allopurinol inhibits xanthine oxidase and effectively trebles or quadruples the functional dose of azathioprine, leading to significant bone-marrow depression.

This was the cause of the man's pancytopenia and multi-organ failure.

Ciclosporin (CyA)

These drugs increase CyA levels:
- Macrolides, e.g. erythromycin
- Calcium-channel blockers
- Triazoles.
    These reduce ciclosporin levels:
- Rifampicin
- Anti-epileptics.

Things to watch out for in renal transplant patients

Infections

The level of immunosuppression is high initially, then reduced. A wide range of opportunistic infections can occur (Box 9.7).

Vascular disease

This remains very common after transplantation. Death (with a functioning graft) from ischaemic heart disease is the cause of death in 50% of patients.

NEPHROTIC SYNDROME

Nephrotic syndrome is not a diagnosis but a set of signs and symptoms:
- Peripheral oedema
- Proteinuria: usually >3 g per day
- Hypoalbuminaemia
- Hypercholesterolaemia: a secondary phenomenon due to increased liver synthesis associated with increased protein synthesis:
    - It can be very resistant to lipid-lowering drugs.
    - Treat the primary condition.
- Hypertension, which accompanies the fluid overload
- Thrombophilia: nephrotic syndrome is associated with an increased clotting tendency and risk of thromboembolic disease. It is also a secondary condition. However, while the patient is nephrotic, anti-coagulation is indicated, especially in membranous nephropathy.

Remember

In nephrotic syndrome there is a reduction in *relative* circulating volume in the presence of oedema.

> **Box 9.7** Opportunistic infections that can occur in renal transplant patients
>
> **Viral**
> - Cytomegalovirus
> - Epstein–Barr virus
> - Herpes simplex virus
> - Varicella zoster virus
>
> **Bacterial**
> - TB
> - *Listeria*
> - *Nocardia*
> - *Salmonella*
>
> **Protozoal**
> - *Toxoplasma*
>
> **Fungal**
> - *Pneumocystis*
> - *Candida*
> - *Aspergillus*

Case history

An 18-year-old woman presents with a 2-week history of swollen ankles and mild breathlessness on exertion.

On examination, she had dependent oedema of the lower limbs to the knee with some facial oedema. Her pulse was normal, BP 150/90. She had bilateral pleural effusions.

Investigations:
- Serum albumin 19 g/L
- 24-h urine protein 5.6 g per day confirming the nephrotic syndrome
- Fasting cholesterol 8.7 mmol/L
- Urine analysis: proteinuria, no blood or red cell casts ('bland' urine sediments).

Management

The aim in all such cases is to find the cause.

How?

Although various non-invasive tests might hint at the diagnosis, in most adult cases a renal biopsy is required.

Renal biopsy findings

Don't panic — you don't need to know about renal histopathology!

Table 9.8 lists some of the common diagnoses and therapeutic strategies.

This patient turns out to have 'minimal change' disease. She slowly responds to oral steroids (60 mg/m^2 daily) with a significant reduction in urinary protein, but only after 12 weeks of high-dose therapy.

Table 9.8 Some common diagnoses and therapeutic strategies

Diagnosis	Treatment
Minimal change disease	Steroids (first line) Cyclophosphamide
Membranous nephropathy	None *or* ACEIs to reduce proteinuria *or* Steroids Alkaloids (cyclophosphamide or chlorambucil) Rituximab
Lupus nephritis	Prednisolone + cyclophosphamide/ mycophenolate
Diabetic nephropathy	ACEIs or A II receptor antagonist Control hypertension: aim for BP <120/80 Improve glycaemic control
Vasculitis	Prednisolone ± azathioprine
Amyloid	Treat underlying condition
HIVAN (collapsing FSGS)	Anti-retroviral therapy

ACEI, ACE inhibitor; A II, angiotensin II; FSGS, focal segmental glomerulosclerosis; HIVAN, HIV-associated nephropathy.

Remember HIV-associated nephropathy (HIVAN) in high-risk patients as a cause of unexplained renal impairment. HIV patients can also develop drug nephrotoxicity and haemolytic uraemic syndrome. Modern anti-retroviral therapies have resulted in good renal outcomes in patients with nephrotic syndrome due to HIVAN.

Remember

The use of IV albumin is controversial but declining. However, where severe reduction in circulating volume threatens renal function, it might help prevent acute kidney disease.

Future progress

This woman's steroids were reduced but she subsequently relapsed and was therefore given prednisolone 15 mg daily with cyclophosphamide 2 mg/kg daily for 12 weeks. She is presently in remission.

HAEMATURIA WITHOUT ALBUMINURIA

Information

- Macroscopic haematuria (red colour urine): can be confused with bile pigments, porphyrins, Hb and myoglobin. Confirm haematuria by microscopy
- Microscopic haematuria: >3–5 RBCs per high-power field on microscopy

> ### Remember
> Haematuria cannot cause anaemia. Look for another cause of anaemia, e.g. TB, neoplasms and blood dyscrasias.

Aetiology

- Systemic: fever, anti-coagulant therapy, sickle-cell trait or disease, strenuous exercise or coagulopathies.
- Renal: glomerulonephritis (IgA nephropathy, Alport's syndrome, thin basement nephropathy), interstitial tubulonephritis, renal infarcts, TB, polycystic disease, papillary necrosis, neoplasm, trauma, vascular malformations.
- Urinary tract: calculi, foreign bodies, neoplasms, endometriosis, trauma, infections.

History

- Menstrual history to exclude vaginal cause of blood in urine.
- Frequency, urgency, dysuria or urethral discharge suggests bladder or urethral involvement.
- Pain or colic might be seen with stones, obstruction, infarction, polycystic kidney disease (PCKD).
- Bleeding at the beginning of micturition suggests urethral cause, whereas terminal bleeding is associated with prostate or bladder pathology.
- Rectal or perineal pain suggests prostatitis.
- Weight loss might suggest a neoplasm.
- History of blood dyscrasia or anti-coagulant therapy: anticoagulant therapy usage and haematuria should be investigated further for underlying lesions of the urinary tract.
- Family history of PCKD, sickle-cell disease or glomerulonephritis (Alport's or thin basement nephropathy).
- Upper respiratory tract infection or gastroenteritis suggests exacerbations of IgA nephropathy.
- History of easy bruising or vasculitic rash, arthralgia and abdominal pain suggests Henoch–Schönlein purpura. Occasionally, anti-GBM disease, SLE or vasculitis can present as isolated haematuria.

Physical examination

- Look for elevated BP or oedema (usually implies renal lesion).
- Bilaterally palpable kidneys (PCKD).
- Unilateral mass (neoplasm, cystic or hydronephrotic kidney).
- Fever and tenderness over renal angle (pyelonephritis).
- Tender prostate (prostatitis).
- Presence of atrial fibrillation or valvular heart disease suggests embolism or renal infarction.
- Presence of petechiae, ecchymosis, lymphadenopathy or splenomegaly may signal blood dyscrasia or clotting disorder.

Investigations

- Complete urinalysis: polarised microscopy may reveal dysmorphic RBCs (glomerular origin) or isomorphic RBCs (urothelial origin). Pyuria and haematuria with bacterial growth suggest UTI. No bacteriological growth triggers search for TB

- Full nephritic screen
- Imaging
- Ultrasound scan of kidneys and bladder with residual bladder volume assessment
- IVU/CT: stones and urinary tract lesions can be missed on ultrasound scan alone
- Cystoscopy is the best procedure for evaluating the urinary tract after CT-KUB (CT of kidney, ureter and bladder).

URINARY TRACT INFECTION (UTI)

Case history

You are called to see a 19-year-old woman in the MAU who is complaining of a 2-day history of frequency, dysuria and urgency. She has a temperature of 39.8°C with some right loin pain. Yesterday she had a rigor. She has a **urinary tract infection** and presumed acute pyelonephritis in view of her high fever and right loin tenderness.

Information

- **Frequency** is defined as voiding every 2 h or more than seven times per day. A variety of factors can affect voiding intervals, including fluid intake, drugs (diuretics), alcohol and caffeine. Patients with polyuria from any cause complain of frequency with an increased urine flow. By contrast, bladder inflammation can cause frequency without an increase in urine flow.
- **Urgency** is described as a powerful sensation to void, regardless of bladder volume. Typically, voided volumes of these patients are small — much less than the patient's normal maximum bladder capacity. Urgency is often caused by bladder inflammation but prostatic enlargement and external compression of the bladder by masses (as in pregnancy) can also generate the feeling of urgency.
- **Dysuria** (painful micturition) suggests irritation or inflammation in the bladder neck or urethra, usually because of bacterial inflammation.

She tells you that this is her first episode of a UTI. She has recently started to have frequent sexual intercourse with a new partner. She has no vaginal discharge and has never had a history of sexually transmitted infections.

Physical examination

A complete physical examination shows no abnormality, apart from right loin tenderness. There is no urinary bladder distension or suprapubic tenderness.

Investigations

- Urinary Dipstix are positive for both nitrite and leucocyte esterase.
- Urine microscopy: pyuria, bacteriuria and leucocyte casts are consistent with UTI.
- Mid-stream urine specimens sent for culture and sensitivity show *E. coli* 10^5 organisms/mL.
- FBC, serum U&Es and blood cultures show no abnormality.
- An abdominal ultrasound shows no abnormality of the right kidney. Ultrasound should be performed when pyelonephritis is suspected to rule out calculi obstruction and incomplete emptying.

How would you manage this patient?

The most common bacterial cause of a UTI is *E. coli*. Administer one of the appropriate broad-spectrum antibiotics IV while waiting for the culture report; pay specific attention to the patient's state of hydration:

- Cefuroxime (750 mg 8-hourly) for 3 days, then switch to oral therapy as per sensitivities
- Ciprofloxacin (500 mg oral × 2 daily if no sensitivities are available)
- Total antibiotic therapy is for 10 days.
  She made a good recovery.
  Prophylactic measures to prevent further UTIs were advised:
- A 2 L daily fluid intake
- Voiding at 2- to 3-h intervals with double micturition if reflux is present
- Voiding before bedtime and after intercourse
- Avoidance of spermicidal jellies, and bubble baths and other chemicals in bath water
- Avoidance of constipation, which may impair bladder emptying.

RENAL AND URETERIC COLIC

Case history

A 36-year-old man presented to his local A&E with excruciating right flank pain. How will you approach this case?

Likely diagnosis

Renal colic, which is often unilateral, is characterised by excruciating inter-mittent pain, usually originating in the flank or kidney area, which radiates across the abdomen towards the suprapubic region. The pain of ureteric colic has similar characteristics but typically radiates along the course of the ureter, frequently into the region of the genitalia and inner thigh.

Aetiology

- Renal colic is usually caused by stretching of the renal capsule due to acute inflammation or bleeding within the kidney. Acute pyelonephritis, an expanding cyst or an acute expansion of the renal pelvis due to pelvi-ureteric obstruction by calculus or blood clot are the usual causes.
- Ureteric colic is often caused by the passage of a calculus, sloughed papilla or blood clot.
- Renal stones are usually calcium oxalate or calcium phosphate and caused by hypercalciuric or hyperoxaluric states. Other types of stones are struvite (magnesium ammonium phosphate) stones, which are caused by urea-splitting organisms, cystine stones (the result of an inherited disorder of cystinuria) and urate stones (idiopathic or hyperuricosuric state).

What to ask about in the history

- Pain: this is usually associated with GI symptoms (nausea, vomiting, abdominal distension).

- Chills, fevers and increased frequency: common.
- Age at which symptoms of stones were first noted.
- Family history of nephrolithiasis.
- History of fractures or prolonged immobilisation.
- Previous urinary infections or manipulations.
- Intake of milk, alkali, salt and vitamins A, D and C.

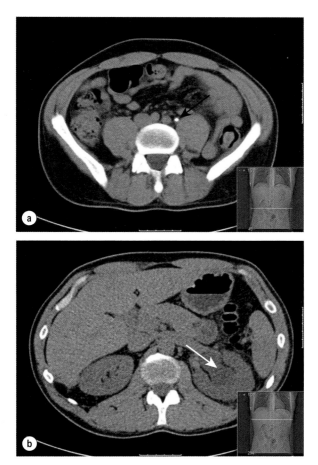

Figure 9.14 (a) Left ureteric calculus. (b) A dilated renal pelvis (arrow) proximal to the ureteric stone in (a).

Physical examination

The physical examination is usually unremarkable, except for the presence of flank tenderness.

How would you investigate this patient?

- Urinalysis: the urine might be normal despite multiple calculi. Macroscopic or microscopic haematuria is common. Pyuria with or without bacteria may be seen.
- CT-KUB is carried out during the episode of pain; a normal CT excludes the diagnosis of pain due to calculous disease. The CT-KUB appearances in a patient with acute left ureteric obstruction are shown in Fig. 9.14.

How would you manage this patient?

Give adequate analgesia, e.g. IV infusion diclofenac 75 mg, repeating as necessary. Opioids can usually be avoided.

This patient passed a small stone later in the day; it was found to be a calcium oxalate stone. He was referred to the renal physician to investigate the cause of his stone formation.

Cause of stone formation

- Urinary excretion of calcium, phosphate, oxalate, urate and cystine should be performed on at least two separate occasions.
- Morphological and biochemical analyses should be performed on all the stones that are passed.

This patient was advised to take a high fluid intake and dietary oxalate restriction (refer to a dietitian).

Further reading

Fluid balance and electrolytes: sodium problems

Sterns RH. Disorders of plasma sodium — causes, consequences and correction. *New England Journal of Medicine* 2015; **372**: 55–65.

The acidotic patient

Berend K. Diagnostic use of base excess in acid–base disorders. *New England Journal of Medicine* 2018; **378**: 1419–1428.

Chronic kidney disease

Appel LJ, Wright Jr JT, Greene T, et al. Intensive blood pressure control in hypertensive chronic kidney disease. *New England Journal of Medicine* 2010; **363**: 918–929.

Webster AC, Nagler EV, Morton RL, et al. Chronic kidney disease. *Lancet* 2017; **389**: 1238–1252.

Multisystem vasculitis/acute glomerulonephritis

Berden AE, Ferrario F, Hagen EC, et al. Histopathological classification of ANCA-associated glomerulonephritis. *Journal of the American Society of Nephrology* 2010; **21**: 1628–1636.

Nephrotic syndrome

Tervaert TW, Moovaart AL, Amann K, et al. Pathological classification of diabetic nephropathy. *Journal of the American Society of Nephrology* 2010; **21**: 556–563.

Urinary tract infection

Hooton TM. Uncomplicated urinary tract infection. *New England Journal of Medicine* 2012; **366**: 1028–1037.

Renal and ureteric colic

Wagenlehner FME, et al. Once daily plazomicin for complicated urinary tract infection. *New England Journal of Medicine* 2019; **380**: 729–740.
Worcester EM, Coe FL. Calcium kidney stones. *New England Journal of Medicine* 2010; **363**: 954–963.

SYNCOPE

Simple faints are a common and benign condition. However, anyone witnessing a faint will know that patients can look awful and it is not surprising that they are often brought to hospital for assessment. Patients who faint are often sat in a chair or even stood up — in both cases causing a recurrence or delaying recovery.

Case history (1)

A 25-year-old man is brought to hospital having fainted at work. He still appears pale but clinical examination is normal. He had a similar episode 2 years earlier. His resting 12-lead ECG is normal.

What are the key questions in establishing the diagnosis?

- Reliable eye-witness account: if not available, make a phone call to the patient's workplace.
- Prodromal symptoms: non-specific but almost always present for some minutes before a vasovagal attack (faint).
- Precipitating cause: anything from the sight of blood to a hangover!
- Circumstance of event, frequently in:
  - Pub (even without alcohol)
  - Restaurant: before or after food
  - Church, mosque or synagogue
  - Warm environment.

In the absence of any abnormal investigations, the most likely diagnosis is **vasovagal syncope** (see Table 15.6). You should be aware of some other specific forms of vasovagal syndrome:

- Carotid sinus syncope: on turning the head or shaving the chin. Due to carotid sinus hypersensitivity, usually in the elderly.
- Cough syncope: after a paroxysm of coughing, usually in a patient with obstructive airways disease.
- Micturition syncope: more common in men. Usually occurs in the night when going to pass urine or during micturition itself.

What is the differential diagnosis?

There are many other causes of syncope and all might need to be excluded.

- Cardiac:
  - Arrhythmia: associated with either profound bradycardia or tachycardia. Symptomatic palpitations can be a pointer but often are not present.
  - Structural: e.g. outflow obstruction (notably aortic stenosis or hypertrophic cardiomyopathy), ischaemia, tamponade, pulmonary embolism.
- Neurological: seizures, cerebrovascular disease, transient ischaemic attack (TIA), cerebrovascular accident (CVA) or vertebrobasilar ischaemia are the most common causes. A good eye-witness account is

key to the diagnosis. **Note:** Some jerky movements of the limbs, and even incontinence, can occur in a prolonged vasovagal attack, especially if the patient remains upright.

- Metabolic:
  - Hypoglycaemia: well known in diabetics. Spontaneous hypoglycaemia from an insulinoma is a rare cause
  - Hypoxaemia
  - Drugs/alcohol.
- Hyperventilation/anxiety (if suspected, symptoms can often be readily reproduced by voluntary hyperventilation): usually associated with a tachycardia. The patient often has symptomatic palpitations and might feel light-headed, or have a feeling of being distanced from the surroundings, chest pain and/or paraesthesiae with numbness in arms, hands or lips. Pallor and peripheral cyanosis can be striking in a full-blown attack. Circumstances provoking an attack can often be the same as for a faint (e.g. warm room, stressful situation).
- Orthostatic hypotension: especially in elderly patients. This is often caused by drugs, e.g. for hypertension, but don't forget autonomic neuropathy and Parkinson's disease.

A cardiac cause of syncope should be sought in all patients with known structural heart disease.

Progress. This man was sent home, having made a full recovery from his 'faint'.

Case history (2)

A 68-year-old man passed out suddenly at the wheel of his car and ran into the car in front. His wife reports that he was pale and sweaty but that loss of consciousness was brief and he recovered quickly.

On examination, in A&E, pulse 78/min, BP 140/85, no abnormality found on examination.

His ECG showed left bundle branch block (LBBB).

Practice points

- Sudden loss of consciousness without warning must be assumed to be a cardiac arrhythmia until proved otherwise.
- Altered consciousness when driving has legal implications and the patient must be warned not to drive again until the diagnosis is established.

Investigations

The history of the event is the key to further investigation and blanket investigations are unrewarding without some clinical pointers as to the cause.

Generally, a single faint requires no further investigation, but if there is some diagnostic doubt, the symptoms can be reproduced by a tilt test. This is usually carried out with a mechanised tilt table giving a head-up tilt of 60 degrees for 45 min, with continuous ECG and BP monitoring. Although false-positive results can occur, if the prodrome before the faint reproduces the symptoms, it provides strong support for the diagnosis.

This patient required further investigation, as the LBBB indicates cardiac disease.

Diagnosis. This man's echocardiogram (echo) showed no abnormality. However, his ambulatory ECG monitoring subsequently showed periods of asymptomatic **Mobitz type II second-degree heart block** (Fig. 10.1).

Progress. A pacemaker was implanted and he had no further problems.

Case history (3)

JR is a 26-year-old physiotherapist. Her first episode of unconsciousness occurred when she was at a party with her medical team. A nursing colleague thought she was pulseless at the time of the collapse; the possibility of excess alcohol was considered. On arrival in A&E at a nearby hospital she was intubated and ventilated, and kept ventilated overnight. The next day she was well and therefore discharged. She had two further similar episodes requiring overnight admission to hospital.

A 12-lead ECG and cardiac enzymes were normal on all three admissions. She was investigated with 24- and 48-h ECG tapes, echo and CT scanning of the head but no abnormalities were found.

An electrophysiological study was therefore performed, to exclude the possibility of tachyarrhythmia. During this study she spontaneously became bradycardic and hypotensive, but no arrhythmias were induced.

A tilt table test performed the following day produced profound bradycardia, hypotension and syncope on 60-degree head-up tilting.

Remember

In a tilt test, syncope is often accompanied by 10–20 s of asystole. This recovers as soon as the patient is returned to the flat; for this reason, a doctor should always be present.

Diagnosis

Neurally mediated syndromes are due to a reflex (called Bezold–Jarisch) that may result in both bradycardia (sinus bradycardia, sinus arrest and AV block) and reflex peripheral vasodilatation. These syndromes usually present as syncope or pre-syncope (dizzy spells).

Treatment and progress

A dual chamber pacemaker (DDD) pacing system (see p. 264) was implanted and programmed to produce a tachycardic response to counter any detected bradycardia of sudden onset. So far, she has had no more syncopal attacks.

A CLINICAL APPROACH TO PATIENTS WITH TACHYCARDIA

The main reason that people have difficulty assessing tachyarrhythmias is that they concentrate on the ECG changes without thinking about the patient to whom the ECG belongs.

Case history (1)

A 35-year-old man presents with a tachycardia at a rate of 180 bpm. He is not seriously compromised by his tachyarrhythmia and the BP is 128/64. The ECG shows narrow-complex tachycardia (Fig. 10.2).

There are three simple questions you need to ask yourself as you approach a patient with an acute tachyarrhythmia:

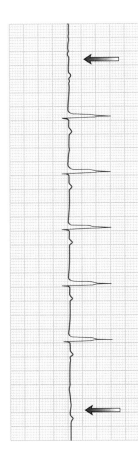

Figure 10.1 Mobitz type II atrioventricular (AV) block. The P waves that do not conduct to the ventricles (arrows) are not preceded by gradual PR interval prolongation. (From Feather A, Randall D, Waterhouse M, eds. *Kumar and Clark's Clinical Medicine*, 10th edn. Elsevier, 2021; Fig. 30.41.)

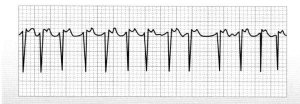

Figure 10.2 Narrow-complex tachycardia.

What is the heart rate?

That is, 180 bpm in this man.

Has the patient collapsed?

In other words, is the patient clinically compromised by the tachycardia or not? In assessing the degree of cardiovascular collapse, take the heart rate into account. Remember that the maximal heart rate you would expect a patient to achieve on the treadmill is 220 minus age.

Someone with a heart rate at this level (180 bpm) is going at the same rate you would expect if they had just hurried up several flights of stairs.

This man is not compromised by the tachycardia and so it is likely that he has a good ventricle. People with heart rates substantially above their predicted maximum, who tolerate the situation well, are more likely to be suffering from a primary electrophysiological problem than from an arrhythmia secondary to left ventricular (LV) disease.

Are the ECG complexes broad or narrow?

Divide tachycardias into broad complex (QRS complex of >120 ms or three small squares on the standard ECG) or narrow complex, rather than try to split them into supraventricular tachycardia (SVT) and ventricular tachycardia (VT) at the first glance. If you follow this approach, you will not treat VT as SVT, which is the error to avoid.

Having answered these questions, you should decide who needs admission to hospital (Table 10.1).

Take a 12-lead ECG of the arrhythmia: this is essential to distinguish VT from SVT. It is also valuable in sorting out the mechanisms in narrow-complex tachycardias; the retrograde P waves can be seen in the ST−T segments in re-entrant tachycardias, but they may be seen only in some leads. *Don't be fooled into thinking you can diagnose and manage arrhythmias with rhythm strips alone.*

Remember

Think about the underlying state of the ventricle.

To be safe:
- Always assume that a broad-complex tachycardia is VT until proved otherwise.
- If in doubt, use DC cardioversion rather than drugs.

Table 10.1 Patients with tachycardia: who to admit to the MAU

	Broad complex	Narrow complex
Collapsed	Usually need immediate cardioversion and must be admitted from A&E. Do *not* give verapamil or other negatively inotropic drugs	Usually need admission to hospital, especially if in heart failure
Did not collapse	The most difficult category to sort out	Can probably go home if tachycardia stops on treatment (Case 1)
	Probably need admission to establish diagnosis	Need outpatient assessment
	Irregular tachycardia in this group may be due to WPW with AF, so do *not* give verapamil	If this is a recurrent problem, need referral to Cardiologist to be considered for EPS, as may benefit from radiofrequency ablation of their pathway or their arrhythmia focus

AF, atrial fibrillation; EPS, electrophysiological studies; WPW, Wolff–Parkinson–White syndrome.

- Seek advice if your first drug does not work.
- Beware of verapamil (which should not be used as first-line therapy) and other negatively inotropic drugs.
- Check the electrolytes and correct them appropriately before using drugs, but do not delay treatment in a patient who is compromised because you are waiting for results. Remember, in an emergency, K^+ levels can be roughly measured using blood gas machines in A&E and used to guide replacement therapy.

The ECG and classification of tachycardias

Broadly speaking, tachycardias are classified as either supraventricular or ventricular in origin.

SVT

These are narrow-complex tachycardias (see Fig. 10.2), unless there is bundle branch block. Adenosine is very useful for their diagnosis and will terminate some SVTs:

- Atrial tachycardia: an SVT from a focus in the atrium, rather than due to re-entry.
- Atrial flutter (Afl): look for regular rhythm, often with a rate of 150. Adenosine will help in the diagnosis, often revealing underlying flutter waves.
- Atrial fibrillation (AF): look for lack of P waves, irregular rhythm and baseline; this can be very hard to see with very fast rates, in which case adenosine will help.

- Re-entrant tachycardias:
  - Wolff−Parkinson−White (WPW) is the classic example of a re-entrant tachycardia. The depolarisation wavefront 're-enters' the atrium through the bundle of abnormal conducting tissue between ventricle and atrium. In some cases a bundle is present but is not visible on the resting ECG, so that it is a 'concealed pathway'. Never treat AF in WPW with digoxin or verapamil − this can cause dangerous retrograde conduction down the accessory pathway, leading to ventricular fibrillation (VF).
  - AV nodal re-entry tachycardia (AVNRT).

Features suggesting that a tachycardia might be an SVT

- Normal LBBB or RBBB morphology but be careful: VT from right ventricular (RV) outflow tract with LBBB morphology can look like SVT. A small, stubby R wave in V_1-V_2 is characteristic of VT.
- You might be able to see evidence of both atrial and ventricular activity. A constant relationship between the P waves and the QRS complexes suggests a supraventricular origin.
- The frontal and horizontal QRS axes are in the same general direction as that in sinus rhythm.
- It slows with manoeuvres designed to increase vagal tone, e.g. carotid sinus massage.
- If the onset is witnessed, you might see a P wave that is premature.

  Diagnosis. Narrow-complex supraventricular tachycardia.

  Management. This rhythm responded to adenosine (see later), 3 mg IV going up in 3-mg aliquots to a maximum of 12 mg. IV beta-blockade (esmolol has a very short half-life of seconds and can be very useful) is also used. Synchronised DC cardioversion (start with 50 J) should be used if medication fails.

Case history (2)

A 57-year-old woman presents with a tachycardia at a rate of 132 bpm.

On examination, she is hypotensive (90/50), looks pale and distressed, and has bibasal crackles.

The 12-lead ECG shows an axis of −120 degrees and the complexes are predominantly positive across the chest leads (regular broad-complex tachycardia).

Diagnosis. This is broad-complex tachycardia with gross axis deviation, probably VT (Box 10.1). The patient needs urgent treatment (see later).

VT

This causes a broad complex regular tachycardia (Fig. 10.3), often called monomorphic VT. However, a broad complex pattern can be caused by any tachycardia if there is a pre-existing abnormality of the conduction system (usually bundle branch block). So, for example, AF with bundle branch block can cause a broad-complex tachycardia that is irregular. Although adenosine (see later) can be useful for diagnostic purposes, do not waste time using it if the patient is compromised.

Features suggesting that a tachycardia might be a VT

- A **QRS duration** of >140 ms strongly suggests a ventricular origin.

> **Box 10.1** Distinction between supraventricular tachycardia (SVT) with bundle branch block and ventricular tachycardia (VT)
>
> VT is more likely than SVT with bundle branch block where there is:
> - a very broad QRS (> 0.14 s)
> - extreme left axis deviation
> - AV dissociation
> - a bifid, upright QRS with a taller first peak in V_1
> - a deep S wave in V_6
> - a concordant (same polarity) QRS direction in all chest leads (V_1-V_6)
> - presence of capture or fusion beats
> - no response to adenosine

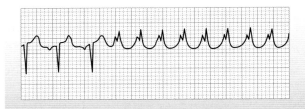

Figure 10.3 Broad-complex tachycardia after three normal beats.

- The frontal and horizontal **axes** are grossly discordant with that seen in sinus rhythm. Most people are used to looking at the frontal QRS axis in the limb leads. The horizontal axis is estimated by seeing where the predominantly negative QRS complexes become equiphasic as you look across from V_1 towards V_6. This equiphasic point is called the zone of transition and is usually at V_3 or V_4. In VT there might be no transition zone or it might be far to the right, or left, of V_4.
- **QRS morphology:** the pattern is not typical of LBBB or RBBB. These are specific appearances that strongly suggest VT, e.g. concordance; seek help if unsure.
- **Fusion beats:** these are beats where there is simultaneous activation of the ventricles from a focus of arrhythmia and from the atria via the AV node at the same time. These beats will look like a cross between the standard VT complex and the patient's normal complexes in sinus rhythm.
- **Capture beats:** occasionally the atria 'capture' a normal complex in the midst of a tachycardia.
- You might be able to see evidence of both atrial and ventricular activity. If there is no constant relationship between the P waves and the QRS complexes, it suggests a ventricular origin and this is called atrioventricular dissociation.

A word about torsade de pointes

Torsade de pointes is an uncommon form of VT with a characteristic ECG pattern (often called polymorphic VT; Fig. 10.4). The complexes appear to twist around the baseline by virtue of their changes in amplitude. It is particularly associated with syndromes involving a long QT interval. Correct diagnosis of torsade de pointes is necessary because the treatment is very different from VT and treating the underlying cause can often have a marked effect.

Acute treatment of arrhythmias

Remember

Always think about the underlying state of the ventricle when treating an acute arrhythmia.

There are problems with the use of any anti-arrhythmic drugs:

- Many arrhythmias arise as a result of pre-existing LV disease. You need to be aware of any drugs that you give which could further suppress LV function and make matters worse.
- A drug that is ineffective for the rhythm in question might also depress ventricular function without alleviating the rate-related stress on the ventricle.
- The final catch when you are treating arrhythmias with drugs (Fig. 10.5) is that ischaemia might alter the drugs' electrophysiological activity. This means that drugs that are anti-arrhythmic under normal circumstances become pro-arrhythmic in ischaemic myocardium.

This limits the use of drugs in many patients because it is often difficult to exclude the possibility of coexisting ischaemia. Because of these problems it is often safer to use DC cardioversion than drugs.

Remember

Both digoxin and verapamil can be dangerous in WPW; if you are uncertain, it is safer to cardiovert.

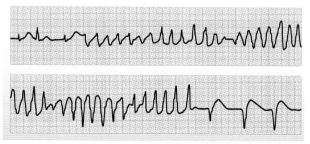

Figure 10.4 Torsade de pointes showing the complexes twisting around the baseline.

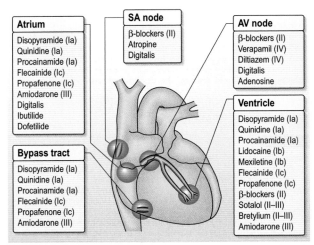

Figure 10.5 Drugs used to treat arrhythmias. The numbers in brackets refer to the Vaughan Williams classification.

A word on adenosine

IV adenosine has revolutionised the diagnosis and management of acute tachycardias. It should be used in most SVTs and is safe because of its very short half-life. The major limitation is that it should not be used in asthmatics. It will not usually cardiovert AF or flutter but will slow the rate transiently (often only one or two complexes – have the ECG running) and enable you to see the baseline, helping you make the diagnosis. It will cardiovert most other SVTs. Although it is safe to give adenosine to patients in VT, it will not usually cardiovert the problem, although it might slow the rate. Remember to give it as a rapid bolus; warn the patient he/she will feel *terrible* transiently and remember that he/she might become transiently asystolic.

Management of this patient (Case 2)

This patient has a VT with severe hypotension and pulmonary oedema. She requires emergency DC cardioversion. Measure and correct any electrolyte abnormality while preparing for DC cardioversion. If in doubt, give empirical IV magnesium sulphate, 8 mmol over 10–15 min (it is not appropriate to give K$^+$ because hypo- or hyperkalaemia can be arrhythmogenic, so you must know the serum K$^+$ before treating it). The arrhythmia did not settle with the DC shock, and IV amiodarone was started with a view to repeat DC cardioversion.

This patient has clinical evidence of poor LV function but in someone who has a good LV, a beta-blocker such as sotalol might be used. Finally, in patients refractory to treatment, remember the possibility of torsade de pointes, with low magnesium and potassium levels.

Progress. This lady settled after the repeat DC cardioversion, but as she is at risk of sudden death she was referred to the Cardiologist for further management. She was given an implantable cardioverter–defibrillator.

ATRIAL FIBRILLATION

Prevalence and risks

Atrial fibrillation (AF) remains one of the most common and challenging of arrhythmias. It is estimated that 10% of the population will suffer from AF at some stage of their lives. Patients who remain in AF after their hospital admission face a long-term risk of embolism and stroke. This is reduced by the use of anti-coagulation but long-term anti-coagulation also carries a risk. In an ideal world, all patients would be cardioverted to sinus rhythm but this might not be possible when there is underlying heart disease.

> **Case history (1)**
>
> A 76-year-old woman with a history of hypertension presents with a 6-week history of worsening palpitations accompanied by breathlessness.
>
> **On examination**, she is breathless getting undressed and has a raised JVP with bibasal crackles; BP is 116/70 and heart rate is 160 bpm. The ECG is compatible with **atrial fibrillation** (Fig. 10.6).

Management

This woman has AF in association with heart failure. The CXR shows evidence of pulmonary oedema. You need to treat the heart failure (e.g. diuretics, angiotensin-converting enzyme inhibitors [ACEIs]) and control her ventricular rate with digoxin. Remember that a tachycardia might be an indication of poorly controlled heart failure or the AF might have tipped her into heart failure. Occasionally, poor LV function is secondary to poor rate control but, more commonly, poor rate control is secondary to poor control of congestive cardiac failure (CCF). In such cases, where digoxin fails to control the rate (as in this patient), use amiodarone, which will improve rate control and the chance of cardioversion.

Progress. She was anti-coagulated and proceeded to cardioversion as an outpatient. She converted to sinus rhythm but had to continue anti-coagulation for a further 3 months.

> **Remember**
>
> AF alone, without evidence of heart failure, can cause breathlessness.

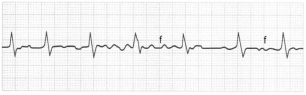

Figure 10.6 Atrial fibrillation. Note the absolute rhythm irregularity and baseline undulations (f waves). (From Kumar P, Clark M, eds. *Kumar and Clark's Clinical Medicine*, 9th edn. Edinburgh: Elsevier; Fig 23.46A.)

Case history (2)

A 70-year-old woman with a history of hypertension presented to the hospital with a history of 6 h of palpitations. She had been taking 75 mg of aspirin, prescribed by her GP, for 2 years. The ECG showed atrial fibrillation at a rate of 132 bpm. The patient looked well and had a BP of 142/78; there was no cardiomegaly on X-ray. She was clear that the symptoms started acutely 6 h previously and so anti-coagulation was not required.

Management

This patient reverted to sinus rhythm in response to a single DC shock (200 J). She remained in sinus rhythm at follow-up 6 months later.

Clinicians have several choices when faced with a patient in AF.

Should I cardiovert?

Yes, generally, DC cardioversion is always worth trying at least once, provided there are no contraindications. However, cardioablation is gaining popularity. Cardioversion can also be achieved with drugs but don't forget that there is nearly as much of a risk of a thromboembolic event as with DC cardioversion, so these patients should be appropriately anti-coagulated. Amiodarone (200 mg × 3 daily for 1 week then 200 mg maintenance per day) and class 1c drugs (e.g. flecainide) both promote cardioversion. Fig. 10.5 shows the sites of action of drugs on the heart but do not use flecainide in the presence of ventricular disease.

DC conversion (using a biphasic defibrillator) reverts AF to sinus rhythm in 80% of patients. This is the best treatment for AF of less than 24 h duration (see Case history 2).

What precautions should I take to prevent embolism at the time of cardioversion?

The risk of cerebral embolism can be markedly reduced by anti-coagulation; patients who have been in AF for more than 24 h should be adequately anti-coagulated (INR >2) for a minimum of 3 weeks before and 4 weeks after elective cardioversion.

With a trans-oesophageal echo (TOE)-guided approach, patients do not need formal anti-coagulation prior to cardioversion but should be covered with a full therapeutic dose of SC heparin before and during the procedure. If this is successful, they need another 4 weeks of formal anti-coagulation with warfarin (or dabigatran) post procedure.

Remember, a patient suffering a stroke because of lack of anti-coagulation in AF is a case of negligence. A common misconception is that aspirin is as effective as warfarin, but this is not true. You need to make a careful risk–benefit analysis of the use of warfarin in elderly patients but in most of them the benefits will outweigh the risks (Tables 10.2 and 10.3).

What should be done to promote good rate control in the long term if cardioversion fails?

Digoxin alone is often not effective in rate control and a second drug often needs to be added — beta-blockers and verapamil are usually effective. There is no good evidence that digoxin promotes conversion to sinus rhythm and it should not be used in paroxysmal AF. The only good way to assess rate control is with a 24-h tape.

Table 10.2 CHA$_2$DS$_2$-VASc scoring system for non-valvular atrial fibrillation

	Risk factors	Score/points
C	Congestive heart failure	1
H	Hypertension	1
A$_2$	Age ≥ 75	2
D	Diabetes mellitus	1
S$_2$	Stroke/TIA/thromboembolism	2
V	Vascular disease (aorta, coronary or peripheral arteries)	1
A	Age 65–74	1
Sc	Sex category: female	1
Annual risk of stroke		
0 points = 0% risk: No prophylaxis		
1 point = 1.3% risk: Anti-coagulant (oral) or aspirin		
2 + points = 2.2% risk: Oral anti-coagulant		

TIA, transient ischaemic attack. (From Feather A, Randall D, Waterhouse M, eds. *Kumar and Clark's Clinical Medicine*, 10th edn. Elsevier, 2021; Box 30.15.)

If this strategy fails, amiodarone is an excellent second-line treatment: it helps with rate control, makes cardioversion more likely and can be used with poor LV function, but remember that it does have long-term side-effects. However, it can sometimes be effectively used at a lower dose (100 mg daily), with a lower risk of side-effects, especially in the elderly.

Should I give prophylactic medication to prevent AF if sinus rhythm is achieved?

This depends on numerous clinical factors; the best drug is sotalol. You should discuss this with the Cardiologist.

Which patients should I refer to an electrophysiologist?

Patients without evidence of underlying heart disease and who have either failed drug therapy or do not want to take any medication (usually young patients) should be referred for electrophysiology (EP) studies with a view to a definitive EP procedure to prevent further AF. However, any patient might potentially benefit from this approach; if in doubt, discuss any case with your Cardiologist.

Remember

AF becomes more stable over time; it might be less easy to cardiovert, the longer you wait.

BRADYCARDIA AND PACING

Bradycardia due to increased vagal tone is a common finding in health and is also seen in an extreme form in vasovagal attacks when periods of asystole can occur.

Table 10.3 HAS-BLED score for bleeding risk on oral anticoagulation in atrial fibrillation

Clinical characteristic	Score/points
Hypertension (systolic $\geq$ 160 mmHg)	1
Abnormal renal function	1
Abnormal liver function	1
Stroke in past	1
Bleeding	1
Labile INRs	1
Elderly: age $\geq$ 65 years	1
Drugs as well	1
Alcohol intake at same time	1

(From Feather A, Randall D, Waterhouse M, eds. *Kumar and Clark's Clinical Medicine*, 10th edn. Elsevier, 2021; Box 30.16. Adapted from European Society of Cardiology Clinical Practice Guidelines. *European Heart Journal* 2012; **33**: 2719−2747.)

Bradycardia is an increasing problem in the elderly and very elderly, and can reflect degenerative disease of the conducting system at all levels:

- Sinus node: sick sinus syndrome
- AV node: complete heart block, slow AF
- His−Purkinje system: bifascicular block (left axis deviation and RBBB).

Case history (1)

A 78-year-old man without any prior cardiac disease was brought to hospital after collapsing at home with brief loss of consciousness. On arrival, he had fully recovered and the ECG showed bifascicular block. During monitoring overnight, he was shown to have periods of **complete heart block.** He subsequently had a dual-chamber pacemaker (DDD) implanted without any recurrence.

Diagnosis

- Difficulties often arise in establishing arrhythmia as a cause of dizzy spells when the condition is intermittent, as it often is in the early stages.
- 24-h ECG is the best investigation but repeat tapes might be needed to demonstrate an abnormality when the history is very suggestive. Occasionally, in a patient with persistent symptoms and no findings on repeat ambulatory ECG monitoring, an implantable ECG recording device can help.

Classification of generic pacemaker code

Notation is by the following abbreviations:

- Chamber paced (0 = none, A = atrial, V = ventricular, D = both or dual)
- Chamber sensed (0 = none, A = atrial, V = ventricular, D = both or dual)
- Response to sensing (0 = none, I = inhibited, T = triggered, D = both T + I)

- Rate response (0 = none, R = rate modulation)
- Anti-tachycardia function (0 = none, P = anti-tachycardia pacing, S = shock, D = pace and shock).

For example: VVI = ventricular pacing, ventricular sensing, inhibition of pacing when beat is sensed; DDD(R) = dual pacing, dual sensing, inhibition and triggered as appropriate when beat is sensed, rate response mode available.

Pacemakers in common use

- VVI: usually for AF with slow ventricular rate and/or pauses.
- DDD: for complete heart block.

Rate response (R) is used when a patient has lost the chronotropic response, i.e. cannot increase the heart rate with exercise/stress. The Cardiologist inserting the pacemaker will decide this but will need to know the patient's usual level of activity/independence to make this decision. AAI pacemakers are not often used in practice because a small proportion of these patients go on to develop coexisting AV nodal disease; in anticipation of this, dual-chamber pacemakers are usually implanted.

Pacemaker problems

All problems with pacemakers need to be referred to the pacing clinic; they will check the pacemaker and adjust its function as necessary. They will also refer to a Cardiologist when necessary.

Surgical problems

- Infection is potentially very serious. Even slight redness around the scar should be treated promptly with antibiotics, e.g. flucloxacillin 500 mg × 3 daily; if relevant, send swabs first. This usually occurs early after implantation.
- Haematoma can predispose to infection or technical problems.

Technical problems

- Fibrosis occurring around the pacemaker tip can cause pacemaker thresholds to rise, which can affect pacemaker function.
- Lead displacement will cause pacemaker malfunction, usually manifesting as failure to capture. It is most common in the first 6 weeks after implantation.
- Lead or pacemaker erosion through the skin usually occurs long term.
- Pacemaker syndrome refers to vague feelings of weakness or dizziness in patients with VVI pacemakers and complete heart block. This is caused by loss of synchrony between atrial and ventricular contraction, leading to episodic falls in BP and retrograde conduction of pacing impulse from ventricle to atria, which cause simultaneous atrial and ventricular contraction. It is not seen with dual-chamber pacing and is treated by upgrading to a dual-chamber system.

> **Remember**
>
> If you suspect a pacemaker problem, always send the patient to a pacing clinic — that day — to have the function checked. The clinic will consult with a Cardiologist if necessary. Out of hours, call the Cardiologist on call.

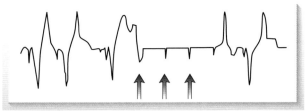

Figure 10.7 ECG showing pacing spikes (arrows) with failure to capture.

Case history (2)

A 78-year-old man is admitted for a routine hip replacement. You are quickly bleeped to the Orthopaedic ward; when you arrive, the Orthopaedic trainee tells you the patient is in 'VT'. You rush to see the patient, who is sitting up reading his newspaper. His rhythm strip from his preoperative ECG is shown in Fig. 10.7. What do you tell the trainee doctor and what do you do?

- This is a paced rhythm but there is evidence of failure to capture.
- You ask the pacing clinic to check his pacemaker; they find that the sensing threshold has risen but all other parameters are fine. They increase his pacemaker output and his pacemaker function returns to normal.

Remember

- Bradycardia and even transient conduction disturbance (first-degree and Mobitz type I or Wenckebach) can occur in healthy people during sleep. Great caution is needed when interpreting rhythm disturbances at night.
- Always take dizzy spells in a patient with a pacemaker seriously. Formal evaluation and an urgent pacing clinic check are required.

CARDIAC ARREST AND BASIC LIFE SUPPORT

Case history

You are walking alone along an isolated corridor of your hospital. Just ahead, you observe a man collapse to the ground. As you approach, you notice he is one of the hospital porters. He is lying motionless.

What should you do?

An assessment and initial resuscitation of the critically ill patient should be undertaken (ABCDE):

- **A**irway – remove any obstructing material and make sure the airway is clear.
- **B**reathing – look, listen and feel for signs of breathing.
- **C**irculation – check carotid and peripheral pulses and start external chest compression if cardiac arrest.
- **D**isability – conscious level – Glasgow Coma Scale (see Table 15.2).

- Examination/exposure – to allow a full examination to be carried out.
  The evidence emphasises that maintaining the circulation is the key factor overall. The order of resuscitation should therefore be CAB, i.e. **C**irculation, **A**irway, **B**reathing (Fig. 10.8).
- Check for danger, and then shake and shout to check responsiveness.
- If there is no response, shout for help.
- If no one responds to your call, open the airway.

What two methods could you use to open the airway?

1. Head tilt, chin lift.
2. Jaw thrust in suspected cervical spine injury.

There are no signs of breathing and you remain alone. What must you do now?

You must leave the patient and go to the nearest place where you can initiate the cardiac arrest call.

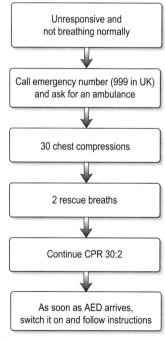

Figure 10.8 Adult basic life support (out of hospital). AED, automated external defibrillator; CPR, cardiopulmonary resuscitation. Reproduced with permission from the Resuscitation Council UK; http://www.resus.org.uk.

You have initiated the emergency call from a telephone further along the corridor.

What should be your next action?

There are no signs of circulation after your assessment. The patient is cyanosed and motionless.

Commence basic life support (see Fig. 10.8).

Chest compressions — carefully noting the following:

- Hand position: place the heel of the hand on the sternum, two fingers' breadth above where the rib margins meet.
- Arm position: lock the elbows and lean directly over the porter.
- Rate: aim to maintain a rate of 100/min.
- Depth: compress the chest by one-third of its resting diameter.
- Give CPR at a ratio of 30 : 2 (30 compressions to 2 breaths), irrespective of number of rescuers.
- Continue this until the defibrillator arrives (Fig. 10.9).

Progress. The patient showed VF on the defibrillator and was successfully brought back into sinus rhythm with DC cardioversion. He was admitted and referred to the Cardiologists.

He will need investigations to rule out structural heart disease (echo and angiogram). He will then require EP studies and an automatic implantable cardioverter—defibrillator (AICD; Box 10.2) to prevent recurrence because he has, in effect, had an 'out of hospital' VF arrest.

Information

- The chance of survival from VF is generally agreed to deteriorate by 5—10%/min. It is therefore imperative that a defibrillator is brought as soon as possible.
- Alerting the team is a priority.
- Give a praecordial thump if appropriate.

CHEST PAIN AND ACUTE CORONARY SYNDROMES

Case history (1)

You are called to assess a 73-year-old woman who gives a 40-min history of sudden-onset, tearing, severe central chest pain (see p. 270) radiating down her left arm and through to her back. She has a history of treated hypertension and has not smoked for 15 years. How are you going to manage her?

Initial assessment

Immediately, when she arrives:

- Brief history
- Risk factor profile (smoking, hypertension, lipids, diabetes, family history, age, gender, ethnic origin)
- Brief examination (BP, pulse, murmurs, chest signs)
- 12-lead ECG
- Give aspirin 300 mg orally
- Relieve pain, e.g. if ischaemic ECG, give diamorphine 5—10 mg IV and an anti-emetic
- Take blood for markers of cardiac damage (troponins).

Adult Advanced Life Support

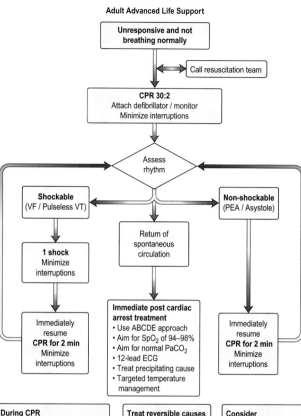

Figure 10.9 Adult advanced life-support algorithm. ABCDE, Airway, Breathing, Circulation, Disability, Exposure; CPR, cardiopulmonary resuscitation; PEA, pulseless electrical activity; VF, ventricular fibrillation; VT, ventricular tachycardia. (Reproduced with permission from the Resuscitation Council; http://www.resus.org.uk.)

> ### Box 10.2 AICDs – indications for implantation
>
> #### Primary prevention
>
> - Coronary disease, LV dysfunction (EF ≤ 35%) and inducible VT
> - High-risk, inherited or acquired conditions, e.g. long QT syndrome, hypertrophic cardiomyopathy, Brugada's syndrome
> - Chronic coronary disease, a history of myocardial infarction and LVEF ≤ 30%: from MADIT II trial
>
> #### Secondary prevention
>
> - Cardiac arrest due to VT/VF
> - Sustained VT with structural heart disease
> - Unexplained syncope with inducible sustained VT or VF with advanced structural heart disease and no other identifiable cause
>
> #### AICD plus biventricular pacing
>
> - Any of above with QRS ≥ 130 ms, LV dilatation, LVEF ≤ 30% and advanced heart failure
>
> AICD, automatic implantable cardioverter−defibrillator; EF, ejection fraction; LV, left ventricular; VF, ventricular fibrillation; VT, ventricular tachycardia.

Remember

Every year patients are inappropriately discharged from A&E departments with acute coronary syndromes because their initial ECG is normal. If in doubt, admit the patient and repeat ECG.

Causes of chest pain to consider

- Aortic dissection (see later).
- Acute coronary syndrome (ACS).
- Pericarditis: sharp central pain, related to posture and respiration.
- Pleurisy: sharp pain, usually lateral, related to respiration.
- Muscular: related to posture, localised tenderness.
- Herpes zoster: nerve root distribution, rash might appear later.
- Gastro-oesophageal reflux disease: retrosternal burning pain but can be very similar to angina.

Note: Many episodes of chest pain do not fit easily into any category and patients are often admitted and treated for acute ACS. Their symptoms should be assessed in conjunction with their risk factor profile. If in doubt, it is safer to admit.

What features would make you suspect a dissecting aneurysm?

- Pain tends to radiate to the back, starts abruptly, and is often intense and described as tearing.
- On examination: absent arm or leg pulses, murmur of aortic regurgitation, different BP in the arms, neurological signs.
- ECG might be normal or show inferior ischaemia or MI.
- As the dissection in the aortic wall extends proximally, it disrupts the origin of the subclavian arteries (affecting arm BP) first, then the carotid

arteries (causing neurological sequelae), the origin of the right coronary artery (causing inferior ischaemia), and finally the aortic valve (causing aortic regurgitation).

If you clinically suspect a dissecting aneurysm, what must you do?

- Obtain a CXR to look for mediastinal widening.
- Seek a senior opinion.
- *Never* give thrombolytic therapy, heparin or anti-platelet therapy.
- Carefully reduce BP with IV labetalol or sodium nitroprusside.
- Discuss with a cardiothoracic centre.
- Do a CT with contrast or an MRI with contrast: although TOE is an excellent investigation, it must be done by a very senior operator and should really be carried out in a Cardiothoracic centre, with surgeons on standby.

Progress. The patient's ECG now changes at approximately 20 min with 4 mm of convex up-sloping ST elevation in leads II, III and AVF. The diagnosis is, of course, an **inferior ST elevation MI (STEMI).**

Immediate medical management in A&E

All hospitals are expected to have rapid triage for chest pain to ensure that all suspected ACS patients are seen without delay. There should be an MDT approach with defined guidelines. With all ACS patients:

- IV access should be gained and bloods sent for cardiac markers, biochemistry, lipid profile, FBC and clotting profile.
- **Oxygen** is no longer recommended in the 2017 British Thoracic Society guidelines, unless the patient is hypoxaemic (check on pulse oximeter).
- **Aspirin** 300 mg chewed, then 75–150 mg daily, should be given.
- **Sublingual glyceryl trinitrate (GTN)** 0.3–1 mg should be given for pain relief, repeated as necessary (provided BP is not compromised). This can be followed by an IV infusion of 1–10 mg/h, which is titrated to pain while aiming to keep systolic BP >100.
- **IV diamorphine** 2.5–5 mg or **morphine** 10 mg is used as analgesia, with metoclopramide 10 mg as an anti-emetic.
- IV beta-blockade with **metoprolol** is given in 5 mg boluses (up to a total of 15 mg), provided the patient is not in cardiogenic shock and/or hypotensive, and there are no contraindications (e.g. asthma).
- Patients with a STEMI ideally should start beta-blockers on the first day, provided they are definitely haemodynamically stable. If there is any doubt, wait until they are stable, to avoid the possibility of cardiac shock developing.
- All ACS patients should be transferred to a coronary care unit (CCU) for continuous monitoring and further specialist care.
- Patients with ACS should have **clopidogrel** 600 mg loading dose, unless percutaneous coronary intervention (PCI) is not being done, in which case the loading dose should be 300 mg; thereafter 75 mg daily is given in addition to aspirin. It has been shown to reduce mortality and the occurrence of major vascular events without an increase in the risk of bleeding in STEMI ACS. Prasugrel 60 mg is an alternative.
- *N.B.* Proton pump inhibitors, particularly omeprazole, reduce the anti-platelet effect of clopidogrel because they are inhibitors of cytochrome p450 (CYP2C19), but have only a small therapeutic effect.
- In addition, urgent reperfusion (see later) is needed.

Kumar & Clark's Cases in Clinical Medicine

> **Box 10.3** Contraindications to thrombolytic therapy
>
> Absolute contraindications
>
> - Aortic dissection
> - Surgery or procedure within last month
> - Stroke within the last 6 months or coma
> - Recent GI haemorrhage or symptoms suggesting active peptic ulcer
> - Severe liver disease, oesophageal varices or acute pancreatitis
> - Trauma with risk of haemorrhage
> - Haemorrhagic diathesis
> - Systolic BP >200 mmHg
>
> Relative contraindications
>
> - Pregnancy or active menstruation
> - Proliferative diabetic retinopathy
> - Known aortic aneurysm or intra-cardiac thrombus
> - Known anti-coagulant therapy

Thrombolysis

This is still used in some hospitals. You must know the indications for it:
- A history of typical ischaemic chest pain, which started within the last 12 h.
- A 12-lead ECG that shows at least one of:
  - 1 mm or more of ST elevation in two or more limb leads *or*
  - 2 mm or more of ST elevation in two or more adjacent precordial leads *or*
  - New-onset LBBB.

Progress. This patient fulfils the criteria for PCI but this is not available. She should have thrombolysis, unless there is a contraindication (Box 10.3).

Thrombolytic therapy

Alteplase ('accelerated' recombinant tissue-type plasminogen activator; rtPA) 1 mg/kg over 60 min (remember you must give concomitant IV heparin or low-molecular-weight heparin [LMWH] for the first 24 h with rtPA).

Remember the other thrombolysis drugs that are available. For example, some hospitals use tenecteplase, which is an easy-to-administer, single-bolus thrombolysis agent of proven benefit in large trials. If a patient has any type of contraindication to thrombolysis, you must discuss the case with a Cardiologist immediately.

Don't forget pericarditis!

ST changes in pericarditis are often widespread, involving inferior as well as anterior leads (Fig. 10.10), but the ST changes are concave with peaked T waves and there is often associated widespread PR depression (a feature specific to pericarditis).

Also beware

- LBBB: if this is known to be old, the diagnosis will rest on the history and cardiac enzymes; it can be difficult to distinguish acute changes on

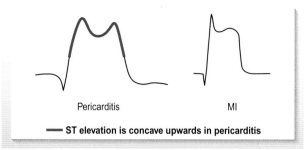

Figure 10.10 ECG changes in pericarditis and myocardial infarction (MI). AST, aspartate aminotransferase; CK, creatine kinase; LDH, lactate dehydrogenase.

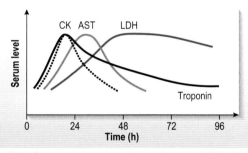

Figure 10.11 Enzyme and troponin profile in acute myocardial infarction.

a background of LBBB. If it is known to be new, it can be used to support the diagnosis.
- Other (non-ischaemic) causes of ST elevation:
  - High ST take-off is seen more commonly in certain racial groups, e.g. Afro-Caribbean.
  - There are other causes you should be aware of, e.g. the ST elevation seen in leads $V_1–V_3$ in patients with Brugada's syndrome.

Cardiac markers in the early assessment of a patient with chest pain (Fig. 10.11)

Troponins start to be released within minutes of myocardial damage and are very useful. Apart from in the patient with known LBBB, though, they rarely play a role in initial management decisions at the time of admission in patients with ACS. They should, however, be measured both at admission

---

Box 10.4 Definition of myocardial infarction (MI)

Both of the following definitions satisfy the diagnosis of an acute, evolving or recent MI:
1. Typical rise and gradual fall of troponin with at least one of the following:
   - Ischaemic symptoms (chest pain)
   - ECG changes indicative of ischaemia (e.g. ST depression or elevation, T-wave changes)
   - Development of pathological Q waves on the ECG
   - Following coronary artery intervention, e.g. angioplasty
2. Pathological findings of an acute MI (usually dead patient)

---

and at 4–12 h in all patients with a suspected ACS. Most other cardiac markers take several hours to rise and might be misleading; they are therefore used much less, given the availability of troponin assays.

Progress. This 73-year-old lady with a STEMI was given thrombolysis with alteplase. She was seen by the coronary rehabilitation team.

Classification of ACS

The term 'acute coronary syndrome' covers the spectrum from unstable angina to MI. This has been a rapidly evolving area (Box 10.4). With this in mind, the decisions to make, using this definition, are:
1. Is this a STEMI or a non-ST elevation MI (NSTEMI)?
2. Or is this unstable angina?

This helps you direct your therapy; patients with a STEMI should receive PCI or thrombolysis. It is easy to appreciate from the pathogenesis (Fig. 10.12) how failure to treat unstable angina can allow progression to an MI. All the patients should initially be admitted to the CCU for management.

Symptoms suggestive of an ACS

- Angina occurs at rest, at night or on minimal effort.
- The pain might require escalating doses of GTN.
- It might be associated with sweating, nausea or breathlessness, especially in an MI.
- There might be a background of worsening exertional symptoms prior to the admission episode of pain.

Case history (2)

You are about to finish your hours on duty when the doctor in A&E asks you, 'while you are here', to look at the ECG of a patient who is about to be sent home. The patient is a 44-year-old male smoker who has had anterior central chest pain on and off at rest for the past 2 days. The first ECG shows some subtle T-wave changes in the anterior leads but his repeat ECG is normal and he is now pain-free, having had GTN. The A&E doctor has told him he can go home with a GTN spray and come back to clinic in 6 weeks. The patient is pleased and is sitting, fully dressed, waiting for his GTN spray, because he is keen to get home to watch the football. Can he go home?

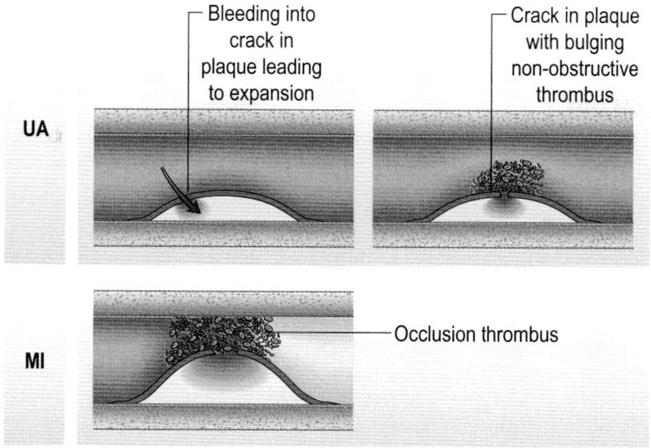

Figure 10.12 The pathology of unstable angina (UA) versus acute myocardial infarction (MI).

What do you say and do?

This patient absolutely cannot go home! He needs admission, treatment for **unstable angina** and risk stratification. This is exactly the type of patient who, if sent home, will go on to have an MI. Admit him to the CCU.

Remember

Management of MI depends on a fast-track approach: 'time is muscle'.
 Therapy consists of:
- **Aspirin** 300 mg loading dose then 75 mg daily thereafter; in addition, give the patient a 300 mg loading dose of **clopidogrel** and 75 mg daily thereafter (CURE trial).
- Start him on SC **LMWH**, usually enoxaparin (1 mg/kg × 2 daily).
- Start him on a **beta-blocker**, e.g. metoprolol 25 mg × 3 daily (unless contraindicated); patients with a sinus tachycardia or hypertension will benefit most from this and should be given early IV beta-blockade.
- Put him on an IV **GTN infusion** (0–10 mL/h, titrated according to pain and BP).
- Assess and correct **risk factors** (smoking, lipids, hypertension, diabetes).
- Ensure a **troponin** is sent at the time of admission and at 12 h.

Remember

- If the initial ECG is normal: do not discharge the patient. It is possible to have a normal ECG in an ACS.
- Repeat the ECG every 20 min for at least 1 h.
- Consider other causes of chest pain.
 Further management will depend on risk stratification using the patient's troponin (at 24 h), symptoms and ECG. Should his symptoms settle:
- If he is troponin-positive (high-risk), he should be referred for immediate inpatient PCI.

- If he is troponin-negative (low-risk requiring further investigation, e.g. coronary artery imaging), he can initially be managed medically but the case will need discussion with the Cardiology department.

Remember

There are many other causes of a raised troponin, e.g. pericarditis, pulmonary embolism, myocarditis.

If his symptoms do not settle:

- He will need urgent inpatient angiography; in the mean time, his medical therapy should be increased.
- If he is troponin-positive and has dynamic ECG changes, he should be referred for angiography that day.

Note: IIb/IIIa antagonist infusions have not been proven to be of benefit as medical therapy alone. A GP IIb/IIIa antagonist, e.g. abciximab, should be given before PCI and for 12 h post PCI. If a patient does not go straight away for a PCI, he should receive an infusion of either tirofiban or eptifibatide. The dosing is complex and you need to look it up (e.g. in a National Formulary).

A brief note on glucose and statins

Any patient with an abnormal admission glucose should be started on an IV insulin on a sliding scale (see p. 405); there is evidence that this improves outcome. High-dose statins (e.g. atorvastatin 80 mg daily) should be started on admission because there is evidence that they improve prognosis above and beyond their lipid-lowering effects, by stabilising the acute plaque.

Remember

- Do not miss an aortic dissection! Giving such a patient thrombolysis is dangerous and likely to be fatal.
- If in doubt about whether to give thrombolysis, discuss the patient with a Cardiologist immediately.

Progress. In this patient the troponins were normal. As his symptoms had settled, he was sent home with medication and an angiogram as an outpatient was arranged.

Case history (3)

A 62-year-old man with type 2 diabetes was admitted to hospital with a 6-h history of central chest pain radiating to both shoulders and to his jaw. The ECG in A&E showed 2 mm of ST segment depression in the inferior leads. His troponin T was elevated at 0.9; a negative predictive value of 99.4% has been shown with a serum troponin of <0.5 ng/L. The diagnosis was an NSTEMI. The pain settled with medical therapy and he was referred for PCI.

His angiogram showed a single tight mid-right coronary artery stenosis but no other significant disease. He went on to have a successful angioplasty and a stent, with excellent results.

Acute MI: who needs acute intervention?

This is a very rapidly evolving field because of constant advances in techniques and biomechanical engineering, i.e. stent technology. As a result, there is a lot of clear evidence from numerous large trials showing improved outcome with percutaneous intervention in certain groups of patients (FRISC II, Tactics-TIMI 18, GUSTO IV ACS, RITA III — to name just a few). Broadly speaking, these can be put into one of three groups:

1. STEMI:
   - Primary intervention: there is clear evidence that PCI is better than thrombolysis for acute STEMI. There is no doubt that, given appropriate resources, infrastructure and staff, this is the treatment of choice. In many parts of the world, thrombolysis is still used, although PCI is now more readily available.
   - Secondary intervention: patients who are re-infarcting, in whom thrombolysis has failed to resolve the ECG findings and symptoms, have post-infarct angina or have VT after the first 24 h should be discussed urgently with a Cardiologist with a view to urgent PCI.
2. **NSTEMI**: these patients should be referred for immediate PCI. If PCI is not available, give fondaparinux 2.5 mg SC daily with aspirin 75 mg, as they represent a high-risk group for further subsequent events.
3. **Unstable angina**: patients with ongoing symptoms and evidence of ischaemia, despite medical treatment, should be discussed with a Cardiologist for consideration of PCI.

In the long term, the value of revascularisation — whether by surgery or PCI — in relieving persistent symptoms is beyond doubt. Revascularisation should be considered in all outpatients, taking into account their symptoms, lifestyle and investigation results. Generally, bypass surgery is used in left main stem disease, three-vessel disease, diffuse disease with a poor ventricle and diabetics.

CARDIOGENIC SHOCK

Information

DEFINITION

Persistent hypotension (<90 mmHg systolic) associated with reduced end-organ perfusion due to low cardiac output.

This is usually the result of acute MI and is manifested by poor peripheral perfusion and low urine output, often associated with clinical/radiological evidence of left ventricular failure (LVF). Mortality approaches 80% with treatment and is much higher without. Predisposing factors include:

- Old age
- Previous MI
- Large anterior MI
- Prior hypertension/diabetes
- Inadequate or late thrombolysis.

Case history

You are called at 2 a.m. to see a 68-year-old diabetic woman who was admitted with a 12-h history of chest pain and ECG changes of an extensive anterior MI. She was treated with alteplase at 2 p.m. the previous day. She has previously had an inferior MI. She has remained hypotensive with a poor urine output since admission and is now feeling very unwell. Her current CXR is clear. What do you do?

Management (see Fig. 10.16 later)

- Get a repeat ECG to look for evidence of reperfusion or continuing ischaemia.
- Check that the patient is not volume-depleted; this must be done using at least a CVP line and preferably a Swan–Ganz catheter on the CCU (see p. 369).
- Check that there is no structural cause by performing an urgent transthoracic echo:
  - Ventricular septal rupture (murmurs at left sternal edge – may be inaudible if large); usually occurs after 2–3 days
  - Papillary muscle rupture giving severe mitral regurgitation (usually murmur but might be silent).

Remember

An urgent echo should be performed in every patient with cardiogenic shock.
- Give inotropes IV if there is no response to volume replacement:
  - Dobutamine and/or low-dose dopamine
  - If possible, try to avoid adrenaline (epinephrine) or noradrenaline (norepinephrine) because they will worsen any ischaemia.
- Discuss with Cardiologists immediately with a view to transfer for PCI:
  - This is particularly appropriate in the patient with an anterior MI and no previous history of ischaemic heart disease where cardiac stunning might be present.
  - In the SHOCK trial, patients referred for early intervention (within 24 h of onset) had an improved prognosis – time counts.
- Insert an intra-aortic balloon pump (IABP), if available: this is a highly effective way of improving cardiac perfusion, and should be used in any patient in whom there is a reasonable prospect of further definitive treatment (e.g. revascularisation/repair ventricular septal defect). It cannot be used in the presence of significant aortic regurgitation.

Progress. This patient was treated with IV dobutamine with some initial improvement in BP and peripheral perfusion, but 24 h later she remained anuric and developed acute pulmonary oedema and shock unresponsive to increasing inotropic support. By the time she was discussed with the Cardiologists she had been anuric and shocked – with a systolic BP of 65 despite inotropes – for 36 h. She was too unstable to transfer and died shortly after.

Remember

Do not go to bed when you have a patient in cardiogenic shock (who is appropriate for aggressive treatment). Stay up, get on the phone to the Cardiologists quickly and sort it out. It is hopeless referring a patient 36 h later: by this time, he/she will not be treatable.

Remember

- There is *never* a role for renal-dose dopamine in any patient with renal failure.
- In patients on prior beta-blockers, competitive blockade may persist for 24 h or more and will require much higher doses of dobutamine/dopamine.
- It is probably simpler in this situation to use milrinone/enoximone, which bypasses the beta-adrenoceptor.

MYOCARDIAL STUNNING AND HIBERNATING MYOCARDIUM
- When heart muscle is subjected to acute ischaemia, it might cease to contract but remain viable. This is a potentially reversible cause of haemodynamic problems in acute MI.
- **Myocardial stunning.** If the blood supply to the relevant area is restored as a result of natural recanalisation of occluded arteries, pharmacological thrombolysis or angioplasty, the functional capacity might return relatively quickly — over a matter of a few hours. Such myocardium is called stunned myocardium.
- **Hibernating myocardium.** A similar state of affairs might occur on a more chronic basis, usually in severe three-vessel disease. In this case the cellular ultrastructure might become seriously deranged, even though the ischaemic myocytes are still potentially viable. This is known as hibernating myocardium; such myocardium can be restored by revascularisation.

These major changes, which have occurred at the cellular level, mean that the period of recovery might be over weeks or even months. PET scanning, stress echocardiography and radionuclide myocardial perfusion scanning can all be used to identify hibernating myocardium.

RIGHT VENTRICULAR INFARCTION

Right ventricular infarction is often associated with volume-dependent hypotension that responds well to fluid replacement.

Case history

A 58-year-old man is admitted with an inferior MI (Fig. 10.13) and is given successful thrombolysis within 2 h of the onset of pain. Although ST elevation and pain largely resolve within 1 h, he remains hypotensive with a systolic BP of 70–80 associated with a low urine output.

A further ECG with right-sided chest electrodes (Fig. 10.14) suggests RV infarction with ST elevation in V_3R–V_4R. A fluid challenge of 1 L of 5% glucose, given over half an hour IV, restores the BP to 110 systolic with a good urine output.

IV fluids in an acute MI should be given using an appropriate measure of the patient's filling status, such as CVP (via a central line) or Swan–Ganz (pulmonary artery) catheter readings.

RV infarction is:
- Diagnosed readily by elevation of ST segment in V_3R–V_4R on right-sided ECG
- Associated with volume-dependent hypotension
- Often associated with elevation of JVP without other evidence of heart failure
- Associated with a higher incidence of all post-MI complications, e.g. arrhythmias, cardiac rupture

Heart failure and cardiogenic shock usually reflect extensive cardiac damage, but cardiac 'stunning' might be present and active treatment can save lives.

Progress. The patient was given medical therapy with aspirin, clopidogrel, beta-blockers and LMWH, and was stable after 5 days. He was referred for urgent PCI.

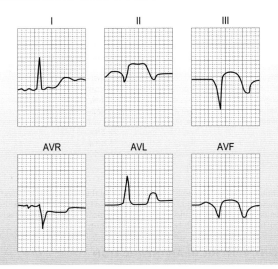

Figure 10.13 An acute inferior wall myocardial infarction. Note the raised ST segment and Q waves in the inferior leads (II, III and AVF).

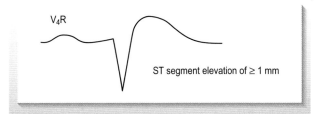

V₄R

ST segment elevation of ≥ 1 mm

Figure 10.14 Right ventricular infarct.

HEART FAILURE FOLLOWING AN MI

Case history

A 63-year-old man has been on the CCU for 5 days following his second MI. He has been managed with PCI and on this occasion has had two eluting stents in his left anterior and circumflex arteries.

You are asked to see him because he has felt breathless over the last hour.

On examination, he is tachypnoeic with a pulse of 90/min and a BP of 140/80. His venous pressure is raised and he has a gallop rhythm and basal crackles. You diagnose **acute heart failure.**

The presence of heart failure, even if transient or only evident on CXR or echo, places the patient with an MI in a far worse prognostic group.

Acute heart failure in the context of an acute MI is associated with a very high inpatient mortality.

Treatment

- IV diamorphine boluses 2.5−10 mg.
- An IV nitrate infusion (0−10 mL/h), titrated to BP and symptoms.
- Boluses of IV furosemide 40−80 mg, although an infusion is better in severe heart failure.
- Invasive monitoring to help guide therapy.
- IV inotropes if patient remains hypotensive despite these measures.

Treatment of underlying poor ventricle

- Introduce an ACEI (or angiotensin receptor antagonist) as soon as possible: ACEIs have been shown to reduce the mortality of this high-risk group by 20−30%. Initiate this therapy as soon as the patient is off inotropes and haemodynamically stable, and has stable renal function. Ramipril (1.25 mg initially) is a good choice, given its simple dosing regimen. A slight deterioration in renal function (up to 30%) might be seen; if this happens, do not increase the dose. If, despite this, renal function continues to worsen, withdraw the ACEI and reconsider at a later date.
- Introduce a beta-blocker as soon as it is safe: there is a wealth of evidence supporting the use of beta-blockers in heart failure to improve prognosis. Evidence from the CAPRICORN and COPERNICUS trials showed that even patients with severe heart failure benefit from the cautious introduction of beta-blockers (provided the patients are not on IV inotropes or vasodilators), e.g. carvedilol, starting at 3.125 mg × 2 daily or bisoprolol, starting at 2.5 mg daily.
- Give spironolactone 12.5−25 mg daily (if the heart failure is moderate to severe).
- Consider further revascularisation: remember patients will benefit from revascularisation if part of their poor ventricular function is due to viable stunned or hibernating myocardium. All patients with post-infarct cardiac failure should be seen by a Cardiologist.

Progress. The patient was treated intensely with diuretics, an ACEI and a beta-blocker. He made a very slow recovery but was able to be discharged in 2 weeks and followed up by the Cardiologists.

POST-INFARCTION ARRHYTHMIAS AND HEART BLOCK

Case history (1)

A nurse on the CCU calls you at 5 a.m. A 56-year-old man without previous heart disease was admitted with an inferior MI and had had successful thrombolysis at 11 p.m. the previous evening. The nurse had been looking at the monitor and noticed that the patient kept having ectopics and has had two short five-beat bursts of non-sustained VT. The nurse wants you to 'review' the patient. When you arrive, the patient is lying flat, fast asleep with a heart rate of 50 (sinus rhythm) and haemodynamically stable. He was given a beta-blocker on admission, and when you look at his results, all his electrolytes (including Mg^{2+} and Ca^{2+}) are normal. You reassure the nurse, who, however, is 'just not happy' and wants you to prescribe something.

What do you do?

- Reassure the nurse that anti-arrhythmics are not indicated. In the CAST trial, post-MI patients with asymptomatic ventricular arrhythmias were randomised to anti-arrhythmic drugs or placebo; the patients given anti-arrhythmics had a worse outcome.
- There is no role for giving empirical IV Mg^{2+} to all patients with an acute MI, as shown by the MAGIC trial.

Arrhythmias — atrial and ventricular — are common in the first 24 h after an MI and might be life-threatening. For this reason, all these patients must be in monitored beds on the CCU. Late arrhythmias (after the first 24 h) are of more prognostic significance and will require specialist evaluation.

Early ventricular arrhythmias

- Ectopics and non-sustained VT are very common, particularly in the 1–2 h after thrombolysis ('reperfusion arrhythmias') and usually require no treatment. Check K^+, Mg^{2+} and Ca^{2+}, and correct if needed.
- With sustained VT or after VF, standard practice is IV bolus 100 mg over 5 min, then infusion of 2–4 mg/min) for 24 h after cardioversion. Amiodarone is also used.
- Early use of IV beta-blockers, e.g. metoprolol, often reduces the incidence of ventricular arrhythmias.

Progress. This patient's arrhythmias settled without the need for anti-arrhythmics. He was discharged with an outpatient appointment with the Cardiologist.

Case history (2)

A 72-year-old woman with diabetes was admitted with an anterior MI and received thrombolysis 8 h after the onset of pain. The CXR demonstrated pulmonary venous congestion. The ECG after thrombolysis is shown in Fig. 10.15.

During the night, the nurses observed isolated non-conducted P waves but no action was taken. The next morning the patient collapsed with a heart rate of 28 bpm and complete heart block; she had not passed urine since admission. A wire was passed via the internal jugular route and she was successfully paced. Despite this, she developed increasing heart failure and died 2 days later.

Heart block

Management is usually very different for inferior and anterior MI. In inferior infarcts a conduction disturbance is common. Provided the patient is not haemodynamically compromised, temporary pacing is usually not required and the problem resolves within 2 weeks; permanent pacing is rarely required. However, heart block in anterior infarcts invariably represents extensive myocardial damage and nearly always needs pacing (temporary and permanent).

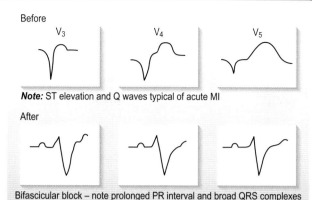

Before

V₃   V₄   V₅

Note: ST elevation and Q waves typical of acute MI

After

Bifascicular block – note prolonged PR interval and broad QRS complexes

Figure 10.15 ECG following thrombolysis in this patient.

Information

INDICATIONS FOR TEMPORARY PACING POST MI

- Mobitz II heart block with anterior MI.
- Third-degree (complete) heart block (CHB) with inferior MI if hypotensive or cardiac failure, *always* with anterior MI.
- Bifascicular block (RBBB with left or right axis deviation): usually anterior MI and at risk of CHB.
- Trifascicular block (long PR interval and either LBBB or RBBB with axis deviation): usually anterior MI and at risk of CHB.
- Alternating LBBB and RBBB: usually extensive myocardial injury and high risk of CHB.
  Note: Do not use the subclavian route after thrombolysis; instead, choose either the jugular or the femoral route because there is less risk of haemorrhagic complications.

Management of late arrhythmias

- AF/SVT: commonly associated with pericarditis or heart failure. Usually self-limiting or responds to digoxin. Consider cardioversion if this fails or the patient is compromised. Treat pericarditis or cardiac failure actively.
- VT: as a late event carries a bad prognosis.
- Beta-blockers: all patients should be on these unless contraindicated.
- IV amiodarone: if there is recurrent VT that has not settled with beta-blockers.
- All patients must be referred for early inpatient angiography, appropriate EP investigations and management as necessary (usually implantation of an internal defibrillator).
- Avoid other anti-arrhythmics, especially those that are negatively inotropic, e.g. flecainide.

> **Remember**
>
> Ventricular 'escape' rhythms are common in bradycardia due to increased vagal tone, and usually respond to atropine.

> **Information**
>
> Anterior MI and CHB carry a very high in-hospital and 1-year mortality.

MYOCARDIAL INFARCTION – SECONDARY PREVENTION

The greatest concern of patients who have recovered from a heart attack is whether they will have another. As well as lifestyle changes, a wide range of drugs is available for secondary prevention, with strong evidence to support their use. The following should be undertaken:

- Smoking cessation
- Strict control of BP
- Diet modification with a view to appropriate weight loss: low fat, low salt, fish oils, high vegetable content
- Exercise
- Drug therapy.

Drug therapy

Antiplatelet therapy
Aspirin
- Dose: 75 mg daily.
- Contraindications: clear history of type 1 allergic reaction (angio-oedema, anaphylaxis), in which case give clopidogrel 75 mg daily. If there is a history suggestive of peptic ulceration disease, give a proton pump inhibitor. *Note:* check later for the presence of *Helicobacter pylori* and eradicate.

Clopidogrel
- Dose: 75 mg daily for 12 months after acute episode.
- Alternatively, prasugrel 10 mg daily can be used.

Beta-blockers
- Should be used in all patients.
- Evidence: 20–25% mortality reduction; greatest benefit in the high-risk group (prior MI, diabetes, transient heart failure). Probably a class effect but documentary evidence for propranolol, timolol, metoprolol, acebutolol (not atenolol, although this is the most widely used drug in British practice).
- Contraindications: reversible airways disease.

Calcium-channel blockers
- Non-dihydropyridines: should not be routinely used and in STEMI have not been shown to improve mortality (INTERCEPT trial).

However, they can be given when beta-blockers are contraindicated and rate control is needed.
- Dihydropyridines, e.g. nifedipine: have no place in secondary prevention and might be harmful.

Angiotensin-converting enzyme inhibitors (ACEIs)

Should be given to all patients with post-ACS (HOPE trial); those with reduced ventricular function obtain most benefit. There are many large trials to show this. Although it is probably a class effect, ramipril, lisinopril and trandolapril are most commonly given; captopril is less used because it causes more severe first-dose hypotension.

Monitor BP and renal function (see earlier). If ACEIs are contraindicated or not tolerated due to cough, an angiotensin receptor antagonist such as losartan is given. In the VALIANT trial it was shown that valsartan is equivalent in efficacy to, but no better than, an ACEI.

Lipid-lowering drugs

'Statins' should be given to all patients because there is a huge amount of evidence backing their use in primary (WOSCOPS) and secondary prevention (4S trial) in ischaemic heart disease. This is highly likely to be a class effect. Pravastatin has the best side-effect profile but atorvastatin is more powerful in reducing cholesterol. According to UK National Service Framework (NSF) guidelines, you should aim for a total cholesterol of less than 5, or a 25% reduction – whichever produces the best effect. These should be started on the day of admission (ensure a lipid profile has been sent; see earlier). Occasionally, myalgia/myositis can occur in the first few weeks in some patients. Do not forget to look at and treat low high-density lipoproteins (HDLs).

Anti-coagulation

There is no evidence that this is routinely of any benefit. However, it might be valuable in:
- Patients with proven LV thrombus, those at risk of LV thrombus (large ventricle and LV dysfunction)
- Those with AF (see p. 261).

Summary of drugs required for secondary prevention

- ACEI for all, unless contraindicated or not tolerated.
- Calcium antagonists for selected patients, e.g. intolerance to beta-blockers.
- Anti-coagulation for selected patients.

Identifying 'high-risk' survivors of MI

- Prior ischaemic heart disease, hypertension, diabetes mellitus.
- Heart failure (even transient).
- Late arrhythmias (> 24 h after MI).
- Age >60 years.
- Impaired ventricular function.
- Inability to perform exercise tolerance tests because of cardiac symptoms.

Remember

- All patients should be offered cardiac rehabilitation.
- Strict blood sugar control improves prognosis in diabetics; a 3-month regimen of SC insulin is often needed.
- After MI, the lipid levels might fall for up to 2 months. Ideally, check the lipid profile at this stage, although statin therapy is given (after a random cholesterol has been sent) at presentation.
- High-risk patients benefit most!

HEART FAILURE RECOGNITION AND ACUTE MANAGEMENT

Differentiating heart failure from lung disease as a cause of breathlessness can be difficult because there is often coexisting cardiac and respiratory disease. In the case of smokers, this usually consists of ischaemic heart disease and COPD. There is thus a tendency to give a concoction of therapy to cover both cardiac failure and an exacerbation of COPD, often with antibiotics added in to cover infection, especially in the elderly. This section will attempt to provide a diagnostic route to clarify the problem and seek therapeutic solutions.

Case history

At 3 a.m., a doctor in A&E refers to you an 80-year-old man with a 4-day history of increasing breathlessness, wheeze and non-productive cough. He lives alone in a first-floor flat and smokes 10 cigarettes a day. The doctor is not sure what the diagnosis is but thinks it might be a 'chest infection'.

Is it heart failure?

Remember that wheeze and cough occur in heart failure, as well as respiratory disease. Although the onset of breathlessness is often rapid in heart failure, it can also be rapid in respiratory disease. Clinical examination might help you further differentiate the two but you often need the results of investigations to help distinguish the causes.

- In heart failure the ECG will almost always be abnormal.
- The echo will invariably show depressed systolic function (but beware of a small percentage of patients with diastolic heart failure and normal systolic function).
- The CXR will help, as will respiratory function tests (but remember respiratory function tests may be of no help in the acute phase).
- Serum natriuretic peptides are useful in the diagnosis of heart failure; serum brain natriuretic peptide (BNP) >200.
- Assess response to therapy.

Progress. The patient gives you a history of sudden onset of breathlessness, preceded by dull chest pain, which started 4 days ago. *On examination,* he is apyrexial, tachypnoeic and sitting up; he has crackles at both his lung bases, a small left-sided pleural effusion, a raised JVP and a BP of 160/95. His ECG showed an old anterior MI.

He clearly has **left ventricular failure**, the aetiology of which is likely to be ischaemic heart disease with hypertension.

Common causes of acute cardiac failure include:
- Ischaemic heart disease
- Hypertension
- Valvular heart disease
- Profound tachy- or bradycardia
- Myocarditis
- Myocardial depression by drugs
- Cardiac tamponade.

Practice point

If you can't identify an aetiology for the cardiac failure and the ECG is normal, reconsider your diagnosis; don't forget the possibility of constrictive pericarditis or diastolic ventricular dysfunction. This latter diagnosis is difficult to make but is more common in elderly hypertensives and can be diagnosed with echo.

When cardiac failure appears, consider what has precipitated it and treat this, as well as the failure itself. Such precipitating factors include:
- Arrhythmia: tachycardia or bradycardia (e.g. AF, CHB)
- MI
- Excess fluid intake (e.g. postoperative IV fluids)
- Excess fluid retention (e.g. NSAIDs, acute kidney injury)
- Anaemia, thyrotoxicosis or any precipitating illness, such as infection in the elderly
- Either precipitating drugs or poor medication compliance in a patient on anti-failure drugs.

Rule out the above with the appropriate investigations and correct them if possible.

Progress. The patient remained breathless despite an initial bolus of furosemide 80 mg. His CXR confirmed that he had pulmonary oedema.

Management (Fig. 10.16)

He needs rapid therapy to improve his clinical condition, with acute treatment to correct his breathlessness, followed by further therapy to maintain and improve LV function.

The acute phase of therapy consists of:
- **IV nitrates** (e.g. GTN 10–200 µg/min titrated to reduce systolic BP by 10–15% and not <90 mmHg): these provide excellent and rapid symptomatic relief by offloading the ventricle, and should be first-line therapy. Continue IV diuretics, initially as boluses (e.g. furosemide 40 mg), but this patient might need a furosemide infusion.
- **IV diamorphine** (5 mg slowly): this not only relieves symptoms, by offloading the ventricle, but is an excellent anxiolytic.
- **ACEI or angiotensin receptor antagonist:**
  - Start after acute symptoms have settled and patient is haemodynamically stable.
  - Remember to watch renal function.
  - Use an appropriate dose of ACEIs, or they will be ineffective.
  - Sacubitril, a nephrolysin inhibitor *plus* valsartan, an angiotensin receptor, are a useful combination in the treatment of symptomatic heart failure.
- **Beta-blockers:**
  - There is excellent evidence to back their use (e.g. CIBIS II, MERIT) and they should be started as soon as the patient is haemodynamically stable and

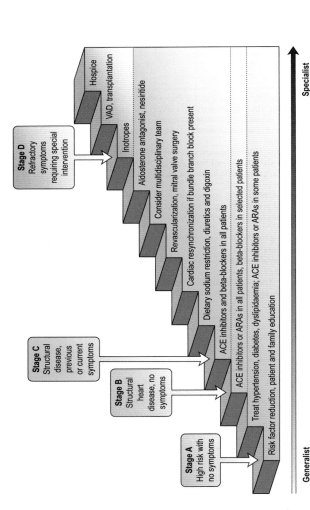

Figure 10.16 Stages of heart failure and treatment options for systolic heart failure. ACE, angiotensin-converting enzyme; ARA, angiotensin II receptor antagonist; VAD, ventricular assisted device. (From Feather A, Randall D, Waterhouse M, eds. *Kumar and Clark's Clinical Medicine*, 10th edn. Edinburgh: Elsevier; Fig. 30.57.)

Within the figure:

Stage A High risk with no symptoms

Stage B Structural heart disease, no symptoms

Stage C Structural disease, previous or current symptoms

Stage D Refractory symptoms requiring special intervention

Generalist — Specialist

Risk factor reduction, patient and family education

Treat hypertension, diabetes, dyslipidaemia; ACE inhibitors or ARAs in some patients

ACE inhibitors or ARAs in all patients, beta-blockers in selected patients

ACE inhibitors and beta-blockers in all patients

Dietary sodium restriction, diuretics and digoxin

Cardiac resynchronization if bundle branch block present

Revascularization, mitral valve surgery

Consider multidisciplinary team

Aldosterone antagonist, nesiritide

Inotropes

VAD, transplantation

Hospice

off IV inotropes and IV vasodilators. There is now evidence to support their use even in patients with severe heart failure. Either carvedilol or bisoprolol is the first-line drug (see starting dose, mentioned earlier).

- Up-titration of the drugs must be very gentle (every 2 weeks). Warn patients that they might initially feel worse. If their symptoms worsen, do not increase the dose; if they continue to worsen, reduce or stop the beta-blockers.

- **Spironolactone:** 12.5–25 mg daily should be given to all patients with moderate to severe heart failure (RALES trial); check the potassium because of the risk of hyperkalaemia.

- **Digoxin:**
  - Valuable in AF.
  - Shown to reduce rate of hospitalisation, not mortality (VA study).

- **Non-invasive ventilation (NIV):** patients often respond very well to just continuous positive pressure ventilation (CPAP) alone, but might need bilevel positive airway pressure (BIPAP). You should be aware that positive pressure ventilation might cause hypotension: monitor the patient appropriately.

Other lifestyle changes

- Reduce alcohol intake.
- Reduce weight.
- Reduce salt intake.
- Take moderate regular exercise.

This patient's breathlessness and pulmonary oedema resolved after 2 days and plans were made to discharge him when his condition was stable.

Practice point

Patients are often left on excessively high doses of diuretics and can easily become dehydrated on discharge, unless their therapy is reduced. However, patients developing heart failure while on diuretics usually require to be discharged on a higher dose than on admission.

The trend would be to increase the dose of the ACEI while reducing the diuretic dose, assessing the response by monitoring symptoms, signs and weight. Ideally, this should be done by a heart failure clinic; these are often nurse-led and are excellent for such patients.

Remember

- Heart failure may be difficult to diagnose, especially with diastolic dysfunction.
- A proportion of elderly patients are on diuretics but have no objective evidence of heart failure (systolic or diastolic).
- Echo should be performed in all patients to identify an aetiology.
- ACEIs should be given to all patients unless contraindicated (i.e. renal impairment, aortic stenosis, renal artery stenosis).

Information

- Systolic heart failure is associated with a decreased LVEF. The heart is enlarged and there is frequently accompanying diastolic heart failure. The cause is often ischaemic heart disease.
- In diastolic heart failure there is normal LV systolic function with a small heart and impaired LV filling. It often occurs in the elderly in association with hypertension. At present there are no data from large trials on treatment of diastolic failure but the expert consensus opinion is that it should be treated in the same way as systolic failure.

Progress. This 80-year-old man was treated according to the algorithm in Fig. 10.16. He made a gradual recovery but was unable to go home. He was placed in a nursing home but was re-admitted with a recurrence of pulmonary oedema and died.

VALVULAR HEART DISEASE

Aortic stenosis

In the UK the most common cause of aortic stenosis in the elderly is degenerative calcific disease; in younger patients it is more often on the basis of a congenital bicuspid valve. Although it is now less common, don't forget rheumatic heart disease as a cause.

Case history (1)

A 75-year-old man is brought to hospital after he had blacked out when running for a bus. He had fully recovered when he reached hospital.

Cardiac examination revealed normal pulse, with normal rhythm and BP 180/90. The heart sounds were soft with an ejection systolic murmur heard all over the praecordium.

The CXR was normal and the ECG showed LBBB.

A clinical diagnosis of **aortic stenosis** was made. The trainee doctor has seen him and has asked you to review him.

How should you manage this patient?

- You *must* admit him to the MAU; you need to quantify the severity of his aortic stenosis with an echo.
- Patients with severe aortic stenosis have a very high 1-year mortality.
- If he has severe aortic stenosis, he should be referred for consideration of aortic valve replacement as an inpatient.

Progress. His echo showed a gradient across the aortic valve of 70 mmHg with good LV function. He had an aortic valve replacement on that admission without complications, and was well at follow-up 18 months later.

Remember

If in doubt, refer for echo *and* cardiac assessment.

Practice points

In aortic stenosis the physical signs can be misleading and do not necessarily correlate with severity:

- Post-exercise syncope in someone with a systolic murmur is suggestive of significant aortic stenosis.
- A diagnosis of aortic sclerosis should not be made without full echo assessment.
- Soft heart sounds in the context of an aortic murmur often suggest significant stenosis.
- Although the pulse might be useful in diagnosing aortic valve lesions (Fig. 10.17), you should note that in elderly patients the pulse might not be reduced because of loss of arterial tree elasticity.
- Severe aortic stenosis with symptoms needs referral for inpatient surgery.

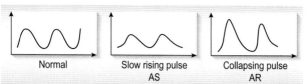

Figure 10.17 Pulse patterns in aortic valve disease. AR, aortic regurgitation; AS, aortic stenosis.

- Elective aortic valve replacement for aortic stenosis either at surgery or via a trans-catheter implantation with a balloon-expandable stent valve (TAVR, transcatheter aortic valve replacement) is associated with a very low mortality and is excellent curative surgery for symptomatic aortic stenosis with good ventricular function.

Aortic regurgitation (AR)

There are many causes of aortic regurgitation, including both valve and aortic root disease. Degenerative disease, rheumatic disease, congenital valvular diseases and infective endocarditis are some of the more common aetiologies.

> **Remember**
>
> In acute AR (e.g. endocarditis) the murmur might become inaudible and be replaced by a third heart sound. If this happens, the patient needs *urgent* surgical referral.

Practice points

In aortic regurgitation the physical signs do tend to correlate with its severity, i.e. the worse the lesion, the more marked the collapsing pulse, the wider the pulse pressure and the longer the murmur:

- Carry out echo to quantify the severity and LV size, and monitor these parameters on a regular basis thereafter.
- When the ventricle begins to dilate, referral for consideration of surgery is necessary.
- Medical therapy with an ACEI may delay the time until surgery is needed.

Mitral valve disease

> **Case history (2)**
>
> A 64-year-old man was admitted in heart failure with signs of mitral regurgitation. He had been in hospital 6 months earlier with heart failure but had been well since then on maintenance medical therapy, including an ACEI. He had cardiomegaly on CXR but the ECG showed no ischaemic changes. Echo assessment confirmed papillary muscle dysfunction causing posterior valve leaflet prolapse with resultant severe mitral regurgitation; the LV was dilated and had some impairment of function. Cardiac catheterisation showed normal coronary arteries and confirmed the echo findings. He had an intraoperative TOE and then mitral valve repair, and made a good recovery.

In MR the underlying cause must be adequately treated; this alone can cause a marked improvement in the severity of the MR. Surgery should be considered in all patients with functional disability (despite adequate medical therapy) and/or worsening LV function documented by echo. The threshold for surgery is constantly dropping with improving technique. Outcome often depends on LV function, so refer early. All patients with MR should be discussed with a Cardiologist to arrange appropriate follow-up, investigation and surgical referral.

When should you consider surgery in valvular disease?

- **Aortic stenosis:** this is usually well compensated but deterioration is rapid once symptoms have developed. Refer for operation if there is dyspnoea, chest pain or syncope. *Note:* do this as an inpatient if stenosis is severe.
- **Aortic regurgitation:** refer for operation when the LV starts to dilate (end-systolic dimension >5.5 cm).
- **Mitral stenosis:** refer for an opinion when symptoms are uncontrolled on medical treatment. Remember that percutaneous valvuloplasty may be a first-line option. Generally, when the valve area is <1 cm^2 intervention is needed.
- **Mitral regurgitation:** refer if there are progressive symptoms despite medical therapy and/or LV dilatation.

> **Remember**
>
> Age is not a barrier to valvular surgery if LV function is good and no major coronary disease is present.

Prosthetic valve problems

All of these should be referred urgently to a Cardiologist:

- Heart failure: must be assumed to be due to valve malfunction until proved otherwise.
- Murmurs: paraprosthetic leaks are common but should be formally assessed by urgent echo followed by TOE.
- Infection: blood cultures must be taken for any febrile illness before giving antibiotics. Endocarditis of the prosthetic valve should be referred to a Cardiothoracic centre.
- Anti-coagulants: control is essential (INR 3.5). *Always* take specialist advice before any surgical intervention. *Don't stop a patient's warfarin or reduce the dose until he/she is fully anti-coagulated with IV heparin.*

INFECTIVE ENDOCARDITIS

Infective endocarditis is an endovascular infection of cardiovascular structures, including cardiac valves, atrial and ventricular endocardium, large intra-thoracic vessels, and intra-cardiac foreign bodies, e.g. prosthetic valves, pacemaker leads and surgical conduits. The annual incidence in the UK is 6–7 per 100 000, but it is more common in developing countries. Without treatment the mortality approaches 100%, and even with treatment there is a significant morbidity and mortality.

Delay in the diagnosis of infective endocarditis might:
- Make medical treatment more prolonged

- Increase the risk of death
- Promote the need for surgery, which might have been avoided had treatment been started earlier.

It follows that endocarditis is a diagnosis that needs to be kept in mind when dealing with any pyrexial or constitutional illness in patients with valvular or congenital heart disease.

Remember

The main problem with endocarditis is delay in the diagnosis. *Never* delay empirical antibiotic therapy; take the appropriate cultures and start treatment.

Diagnosis is made using the modified Duke criteria (Box 10.5).

Case history

One of your colleagues hands over a patient who has just been admitted. He is a 28-year-old man who presented with a pyrexia and history of feeling unwell for 6 weeks. His doctor had prescribed amoxicillin for a flu-like illness 3 weeks previously. He has a pyrexia of 38.5°C and looks unwell. There is a mid-systolic murmur radiating to the neck and the apex. Careful inspection of the nail beds showed some splinter haemorrhages. Blood cultures were taken in A&E on arrival. Your colleague wants you to look these up tomorrow and, depending on the results, start antibiotics.

What do you do and what else do you want to ask the patient?

- If you have good clinical grounds for a diagnosis of endocarditis you must start empirical treatment as soon as you have taken at least three sets of cultures (from different sites). You take blood for an FBC and a further blood culture *now* so that he can have his first dose of antibiotics without delay.
- You will ask him if he has had any recent dental work, is an IV drug user or has ever been told he has a murmur (pre-existing lesion).
- You will send off baseline U&Es, CRP, ESR, urinalysis and microscopy, and arrange an ECG.

While taking the cultures you ask him a few questions and he tells you someone mentioned he had a murmur when he was a child but nothing further was done. He also says he had root canal work 8 weeks ago. You start him on a slow injection of benzylpenicillin (1.2 g, to be given 4-hourly thereafter) and gentamicin (80 mg 12-hourly) for the first 2 weeks. You must subsequently discuss anti-microbial therapy with a microbiologist.

All sets of his cultures subsequently show he has *Streptococcus viridans*, and his echo demonstrates a vegetation on a bicuspid aortic valve but no significant gradient (stenosis) or regurgitation.

Progress. He makes an uneventful recovery on 2 weeks slow IV therapy penicillin 1.2 g 4-hourly plus gentamicin 80 mg 12-hourly, followed by oral penicillin for a further 4 weeks.

What advice do you give him?

You tell him that prophylactic antibiotic therapy is unnecessary for dental procedures unless there is an infective process already present.

Kumar & Clark's Cases in Clinical Medicine

Box 10.5 Modified Duke criteria for endocarditis*

Major criteria

- A positive blood culture for infective endocarditis, as defined by the recovery of a typical microorganism from two separate blood cultures in the absence of a primary focus (*viridans* streptococci, *Abiotrophia* species and *Granulicatella* species; *Streptococcus bovis*, HACEK[†] group, or community-acquired *Staphylococcus aureus* or enterococcus species); or
- Persistently positive blood cultures, defined as the recovery of a microorganism consistent with endocarditis from either blood samples obtained more than 12 h apart or all three or a majority of four or more separate blood samples, with the first and last obtained at least 1 h apart; or
- A positive serological test for Q fever, with an immunofluorescence assay showing phase 1 IgG antibodies at a titre >1 : 800; or
- Echocardiographic evidence of endocardial involvement:
  - An oscillating intra-cardiac mass on the valve or supporting structures, in the path of regurgitant jets, or on implanted material in the absence of an alternative anatomical explanation; or
  - An abscess; or
  - New partial dehiscence of prosthetic valve; or
- New valvular regurgitation

Minor criteria

- Predisposition: predisposing heart condition or IV drug use
- Fever: temperature ≥38°C (100.4°F)
- Vascular phenomena: major arterial emboli, septic pulmonary infarcts, mycotic aneurysm, intracranial haemorrhage, conjunctival haemorrhages, Janeway's lesion
- Immunological phenomena: glomerulonephritis, Osler's nodes, Roth's spots, rheumatoid factor
- Microbiological evidence: a positive blood culture but not meeting a major criterion as noted earlier, or serological evidence of an active infection with an organism that can cause infective endocarditis[‡]
- Echocardiogram: findings consistent with infective endocarditis but not meeting a major criterion as noted earlier

*The diagnosis of infective endocarditis is definite when: (a) a microorganism is demonstrated by culture of a specimen from a vegetation, an embolism or an intra-cardiac abscess; (b) active endocarditis is confirmed by histological examination of the vegetation or intra-cardiac abscess; (c) two major clinical criteria, one major and three minor criteria, or five minor criteria are met.

[†]HACEK denotes *Haemophilus* species, *Actinobacillus actinomycetemcomitans*, *Cardiobacterium hominis*, *Eikenella corrodens* and *Kingella kingae*.

[‡]Excluded from this criterion is a single positive blood culture for coagulase-negative staphylococci or other organisms that do not cause endocarditis. Serological tests for organisms that cause endocarditis include tests for *Brucella*, *Coxiella burnetii*, *Chlamydia*, *Legionella* and *Bartonella* species.

After Raoult D, Abbara S, Jassal DS, Kradin RL. Case records of the Massachusetts General Hospital. Case 5-2007. A 53-year-old man with a prosthetic aortic valve and recent onset of fatigue, dyspnea, weight loss, and sweats. *New England Journal of Medicine* 2007; **356**: 715–725.

A few practical points

- Prosthetic valve endocarditis is very difficult to manage and must be referred to a Cardiothoracic surgical centre.
- Haemodynamic deterioration might precipitate the need for surgery in endocarditis. The difficulty is that operative results are clearly better if the surgeons can wait to allow adequate antibiotic therapy to enable them to operate in a field that is no longer infected. However, in some cases this might not be possible because fatal haemodynamic deterioration can be prevented only by early surgery.
- Endocarditis often needs surgical intervention. *Always* involve the Cardiologists as soon as possible.
- Transthoracic echocardiography does not always exclude a diagnosis of endocarditis and TOE will often help; the Cardiologist will give appropriate advice.
- Development of first-degree AV block strongly suggests an aortic root abscess: hence the need for regular ECGs in all cases.
- A fever as a result of antibiotic sensitivity can develop after a prolonged course of IV antibiotics (especially penicillins). This can lead to a false suspicion that the endocarditis is not successfully treated: always liaise closely with the microbiologist.
- Always discuss cases that are either not responding or worsening with the surgeons, via the Cardiologist.
- Right-sided endocarditis is a disease that is characteristic of IV drug users. The condition presents with cardiac signs such as a murmur or evidence of tricuspid regurgitation on the JVP. However, there might be few signs at the outset and the major abnormality could be on the CXR, with areas of apparent consolidation suggestive of a bronchopneumonia. The condition can present with a 'white-out' of the two lung fields.

Remember

Always involve the Cardiologist early in patients with endocarditis.

PULMONARY HYPERTENSION

Case history (1)

A 54-year-old woman presents with increased breathlessness over 2 weeks. She is a heavy smoker with a chronic productive cough. She recently developed a cold, followed by a cough with purulent sputum and increased breathlessness.

  On examination, she is cyanosed and tachypnoeic at rest. Her pulse is 120/min, irregularly irregular (atrial fibrillation).

  Her JVP is raised by 5 cm. She has a systolic murmur at the left sternal edge with an enlarged pulsatile liver and bilateral leg and ankle oedema.

  On examination of her chest, she had generalised wheezing with bilateral basal crackles.

Investigations

ECG confirms atrial fibrillation with RV hypertrophy.

CXR shows evidence of **pulmonary hypertension** with prominent pulmonary arteries.

Echo shows an enlarged right ventricle. Doppler shows pulmonary artery pressure to be 25 mmHg.

Diagnosis. Cor pulmonale – pulmonary hypertension, secondary to COPD.

Pulmonary hypertension/cor pulmonale

Pulmonary hypertension/cor pulmonale is defined as fluid overload secondary to lung disease in hypoxic patients with COPD. Pulmonary hypertension can be present for years without causing symptoms.

Cor pulmonale is enlargement of the right ventricle secondary to increased afterload due to primary lung disease in patients who have no other cause of ventricular dysfunction. Symptoms include worsening exertional dyspnoea, fatigue and chest pain. On examination, JVP is raised and there is a RV parasternal heave, a loud pulmonary component of the second heart sound, fluid retention and peripheral oedema.

Pathophysiology of cor pulmonale

Pulmonary hypertension leads to the elevation of RV pressure and dilatation of both the right ventricle and the right atrium. This produces the physical findings of peripheral oedema, raised JVP, hepatic enlargement (which might be pulsatile because of the tricuspid regurgitation) and ascites. The cause of the fluid retention in cor pulmonale is still debated because there is little evidence that it is truly due to haemodynamic dysfunction of the right ventricle. The most likely explanation is that hypercapnia – an almost invariable feature of cor pulmonale – interferes with the humoral mechanisms controlling sodium and water balance, leading to fluid retention.

In practice, it is relatively common to encounter patients in whom there is evidence of fluid retention, RV hypertrophy and LV problems. Presumably, this occurs because of coexistent primary problems such as ischaemic heart disease and hypertension.

How would you manage a case of cor pulmonale?

You must treat the underlying disease process, hopefully with the aim of avoiding this final common pathway. Some of these patients are at risk of pulmonary emboli and need anti-coagulation: discuss with the Cardiologist. Otherwise, treatment of cor pulmonale is symptomatic, with diuretics for fluid retention. There is not yet any direct evidence of benefit from ACEIs for RV dysfunction alone. However, patients will often have coexisting LV disease that benefits from ACEIs.

In COPD, a PaO_2 of <7.3 kPa is an indication for home oxygen treatment. This has been shown to reduce mortality, pulmonary resistance and hypoxia, and might produce symptomatic relief.

What is the prognosis?

In COPD the development of cor pulmonale is always a sinister sign because it invariably represents the final common pathway. The prognosis of cor pulmonale in COPD without treatment is poor (5-year survival is about 30%) compared with treatment (5-year survival of about 60%). Although cor pulmonale is not an invariable feature of COPD, it usually heralds the terminal phase of the illness in those who develop it.

Remember

Patients with long-standing lung disease may develop pulmonary hypertension.

Investigations

COR PULMONALE

- Arterial blood gases
- CXR: showing large pulmonary arteries $\pm$ evidence of underlying lung disease
- ECG: showing RV strain pattern with right axis deviation and often P-pulmonale
- Echo: showing large right ventricle and atrium, tricuspid regurgitation and high pulmonary artery pressures
- CT chest with contrast: to delineate underlying lung disease and pulmonary vasculature further

Progress. This patient's underlying COPD was treated with bronchodilators, and she was given antibiotics and told to stop smoking. After recovery from the acute episodes, her blood gases showed a PO_2 of 7.1 kPa and arrangements were made for domiciliary oxygen. She was continued on anti-coagulation with warfarin and her AF was controlled with digoxin 0.125 mg. She is being followed by the pulmonary rehabilitation nurse and Outpatients.

Case history (2)

A 21-year-old man presents with an 8-week history of increasing breathlessness; he is now able to walk less than 20 m, having previously been able to keep up with his peers at weekly soccer games. He has no past medical or drug history and has never smoked.

On examination, he is cyanosed, and has a JVP raised to his ears with 'cv' waves, an RV heave, pansystolic murmur at the right sternal edge and peripheral oedema.

His CXR shows strikingly enlarged pulmonary arteries but clear lung fields. His echo demonstrates an enormous right heart with torrential tricuspid regurgitation but no significant left-sided problems.

What is the likely diagnosis and prognosis?

Primary pulmonary artery hypertension is the most likely diagnosis. This is an aggressive disease process with a very poor outlook. Heart–lung transplantation is usually the only chance for survival. Prostacyclin, high-dose calcium-channel antagonists, bosentan (an oral antagonist of endothelin-1 receptors) and sildenafil have all been shown to be of limited benefit as medical therapy.

Progress. This man was assessed in the Transplantation Centre and is awaiting heart–lung transplantation.

CARDIOMYOPATHIES

A cardiomyopathy is a primary disease of the heart muscle. Generally, these fall into three functional categories: dilated, hypertrophic and restrictive cardiomyopathies.

Remember

- Cardiomyopathies are rare in acute medical practice but don't forget them.
- Echo is essential in defining the problem.

Case history (1)

A 42-year-old man is admitted to the MAU with increasing breathlessness and signs of pulmonary oedema. There is no history of chest pain or palpitations. He had a severe episode of flu 3 months ago and since then has not been able to return to his marathon running. He has never smoked and drinks less than 10 units per week.

On examination, he is tachypnoeic. His pulse is 120/min and regular, with BP 100/60. His venous pressure is raised and he has a gallop rhythm on auscultation. He also has bilateral basal crackles but no peripheral oedema. His CXR confirms cardiomegaly and pulmonary oedema.

Diagnosis. Acute heart failure with pulmonary oedema. He is given immediate treatment for this (see p. 287). He has a dilated cardiomyopathy.

Dilated cardiomyopathy (DCM)

There are a number of causes of DCMs. This case history is suggestive of either a post-viral or idiopathic cardiomyopathy. A thorough history, examination and investigations will enable you to rule out many causes of cardiomyopathy, e.g. alcohol-induced cardiomyopathy.

Further investigations show no ischaemia on the ECG and global ventricular systolic dysfunction on his echo. Cardiac MR shows dilatation. Viral titres to enteroviruses are positive.

Treatment is as for acute heart failure (see p. 287). He recovers well and is able to return to normal activities after 4 months.

Some tips on the management of DCMs

- In principle, the treatment is the same as the treatment of heart failure, but you should ask for Cardiology input early for advice on specialist investigations and further treatment.
- Define an aetiology if possible, as this might identify a reversible/treatable cause, e.g. alcohol excess:
  - An echo is essential.
  - An endocardial biopsy might be helpful.
- It is possible to make a complete recovery from a DCM, especially those of viral aetiology (remember to check viral titres).
- Some acute DCMs run an aggressive course with rapidly worsening ventricular function, and cardiac transplantation might be required. Surgically implanted left ventricular assist devices (LVADs) are becoming increasingly common as a bridge to either recovery or transplantation.

Remember

Ischaemic heart disease can present as a DCM; it can respond well to treatment with secondary prevention and, where appropriate, revascularisation.

Case history (2)

You are a doctor in clinic and see a new and urgent GP referral. She is a 35-year-old woman who presented to the A&E department with syncope and palpitations. She was noted to have a soft systolic murmur. She was sent home by A&E, as her palpitations had settled and her ECG was thought to be normal. The GP is concerned and has asked you to see her because the patient's sister, age 28, 'dropped dead' while ironing. The patient's ECG shows LV hypertrophy with an S in V_1 of 21 mm plus an R wave in V_6 of >35 mm (see Fig. 10.19 later).

What are you concerned about?

Hypertrophic cardiomyopathy.

Hypertrophic cardiomyopathy (HCM)

This is an autosomal dominant condition with variable penetrance. There is disorganisation of myocytes and myofibrils, which often results in ventricular hypertrophy that most often affects the septum. The septal hypertrophy can cause LV outflow obstruction, resulting in symptoms such as exercise-induced syncope. The main risk that should concern you is sudden death.

Some practice points for HCM

- On echo (which all patients must have) cardinal features include asymmetrical septal hypertrophy, systolic anterior motion of the mitral valve and an outflow gradient.
- The degree of outflow obstruction and hypertrophy does not correlate reliably with risk of sudden death.
- Screening of family members and referral to a geneticist are essential because certain HCM mutations are associated with a higher risk of sudden death. Don't forget, HCM can be sporadic as well as hereditary.
- Beta-blockers are the mainstay of medical therapy but amiodarone can be useful. However, certain patients will benefit from an AICD.
- Patients with outflow obstruction might benefit from septal reduction by either percutaneous alcohol ablation or surgical myomectomy.
- Sometimes, differentiation of HCM from aortic stenosis can be difficult (Fig. 10.18; Table 10.4) — seek specialist advice!

   Progress. This patient was treated with beta-blockers but had further episodes of syncope. She has been fitted with an AICD.

HYPERTENSION (HT)

Case history (1)

An anxious 33-year-old woman comes to A&E with a bad migraine. Her BP has been recorded as 180/120 on a number of occasions while she is waiting to be seen by the medical team.

How will you assess her?

First you need to decide on the significance of the BP reading:

- Relevance of anxiety: a raised BP is a common response to stress, more so in some individuals than in others. Twenty-four-hour ambulatory BP monitors can be of help in these situations.

Kumar & Clark's Cases in Clinical Medicine

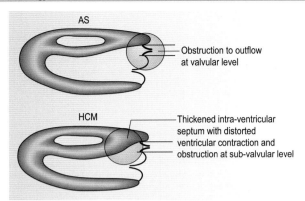

Figure 10.18 The difference between aortic stenosis (AS) and hypertrophic cardiomyopathy (HCM).

Table 10.4 Differentiation of aortic stenosis (AS) and hypertrophic cardiomyopathy (HCM)

	AS	HCM
Murmur	Ejection systolic	Ejection systolic There may be additional MR murmur
Pulse/ Additional heart sounds	May be slow-rising	Described as jerky fourth sound possible (associated with double apical pulsation)
ECG	LVH in later stages. May be normal even when AS severe	LVH (including early stages) There may be bizarre changes, including large septal Q waves
CXR	Heart size may be normal even when AS severe	Heart size may be normal
Echo	Aortic valve thickened Gradient on Doppler across valve LVH if severe	Characteristic: Asymmetric septal hypertrophy Systolic anterior motion of mitral valve Mid-systolic closure of aortic valve

LVH, left ventricular hypertrophy; MR, mitral regurgitation.

- Prior history of high BP: adds significance to the present reading.
- Presence of family history HT: probably the single most useful determinant in essential HT.
- Relationship to migraine: no direct link between this and HT has been established.
- Relationship to age: BP does rise with age but still carries an adverse cardiovascular risk. The WHO/International Society of Hypertension classify hypertension as a systolic pressure of >130 mmHg and a diastolic of >85 mmHg.
- Relationship to lifestyle: high alcohol intake, obesity and lack of exercise are common contributory factors in patients with high BP.

What should you be looking for?

- Clinical signs of end-organ damage:
  - Fundoscopy: hypertensive retinopathy grades I–IV
  - LVH: forceful/displaced apex beat, loud A2
  - Proteinuria.
- Causes of secondary HT:
  - Coarctation of the aorta: have you felt the femorals, especially in the young patient?
  - Renal disease: renal bruits, proteinuria, U&Es
  - Cushing's syndrome: obesity, striae; might have low K^+
  - Conn's syndrome: no signs; usually low K^+ and high normal Na^+
  - Phaeochromocytoma: presentation often atypical (e.g. acute pulmonary oedema, sweating attacks) rather than textbook flushing/palpitations.
- Baseline investigations:
  - U&Es, eGFR and glucose: look for electrolyte imbalances (e.g. Conn's, renal disease and diabetes)
  - ECG: a very insensitive detector of LVH but when voltage criteria are present this carries considerable prognostic risk and should not be ignored. Fig. 10.19 shows LVH with S in lead V_2 and R in V_5 >35 mm
  - CXR: cardiomegaly might be present but rarely adds much to good clinical examination (rib notching exciting but coarctation should not have been missed clinically!).
- Echo: a more sensitive indicator of LVH.

When should you look for secondary causes?

- Young patient (under 45) and no family history of hypertension.
- Those with HT resistant to treatment.
- Those with accelerated HT.

Investigations in this group

These include:
- Renal ultrasound: non-invasive, readily available, excludes major renal pathology.
- Isotope renogram (+ captopril stress): reasonable screening test for renal artery stenosis but not very sensitive (might miss some).
- MR angiography with contrast: will give a definitive diagnosis in renal artery stenosis. Although renal angiography is the gold standard, this tends to be used only when intervention (renal angioplasty) is considered.
- 24-h urine collection: catecholamines and cortisol: these require separate bottles! Plasma catecholamines are most accurate for phaeochromocytoma, if available.

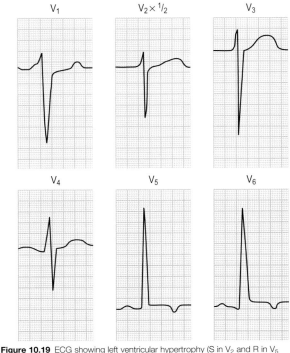

Figure 10.19 ECG showing left ventricular hypertrophy (S in V_2 and R in V_5 >35 mm).

- CT/MRI abdomen: when adrenal disease is suspected/confirmed. Perform CT and MRI angiography for reno-vascular disease.

Remember

- High BP is a significant risk factor for future cardiac events and should be followed up, especially in diabetics.
- Secondary causes, apart from renal disease, are rare — but you will see a few cases.

Progress. This patient's hypertension was treated with candesartan 8 mg daily. Her BP fell to 160/100 and therefore bendroflumethiazide 2.5 mg daily and amlodipine 5 mg daily have been added to her treatment. She was also prescribed a statin. Her BP is now controlled at 140/85.

Case history (2)

A 50-year-old man is visiting from Ghana and is brought to A&E by his relatives after behaving oddly. His BP is recorded by the nurses as 220/140 in both arms. This is **accelerated hypertension.**

What is your immediate management?

Clinical assessment:

- CNS: orientation, focal neurological signs (differentiation of hypertensive encephalopathy and a small stroke might be difficult).
- Fundi: haemorrhages/exudates and/or papilloedema indicate accelerated hypertension.
- LVH: clinical and ECG. Most patients with severe HT have ECG evidence of LVH.
- Urinalysis: to look for renal disease and diabetes.
- Remember to look for secondary causes and treat as appropriate.

Investigations

- Renal function: renal impairment likely in severe HT and may be accompanied by electrolyte disturbance
- CT head scan: if focal signs present to exclude stroke

What drugs are available for treatment in this case?

- Oral:
  - ACEIs (Fig. 10.20)
  - Diuretics, e.g. thiazides
  - Calcium-channel blockers, e.g. nifedipine, diltiazem.
- IV treatment (labetalol, nitroprusside) should be reserved for a real emergency, e.g. aortic dissection, when minute-to-minute control is needed. But lower BP *cautiously.*
- In this man, a reasonable approach would be 10 mg capsule of nifedipine intra-buccally, which will gradually reduce his BP over the next half an hour or so.

Information

- Lowering BP is crucial in the management of accelerated HT. Be cautious because of the risks of causing a stroke if you lower BP too quickly.
- Very high BP readings can occur in an ischaemic stroke and should be treated *very cautiously* because of the risk of extending the stroke.

Long-term treatment of hypertension

Don't forget non-pharmacological measures, including weight loss, diet, smoking cessation and regular exercise; these are often glossed over and can have a significant impact. Current practice includes all major classes of anti-hypertensive drug as first-line therapy. The ANBP2 trial showed that diuretics were as effective as any other treatment for first-line therapy. However, in many patients, an ACEI would be a sensible choice. Remember, strict control is of paramount importance in diabetic patients.

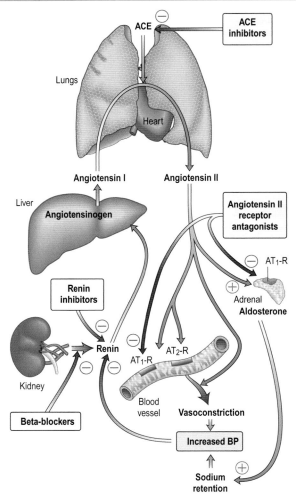

Figure 10.20 The renin–angiotensin–aldosterone system. ACE, angiotensin-converting enzyme.

Side-effects of anti-hypertensive medication that might present acutely to hospital

- Beta-blockers:
  - Asthma
  - Symptomatic bradycardia (especially in the elderly)
  - Cardiac failure
  - Masking of hypoglycaemic symptoms
  - Worsening of peripheral vascular disease symptoms.
- Diuretics:
  - Gout
  - Hypokalaemia (if severe, i.e. <2.5 mmol/L: consider Conn's syndrome)
  - Diabetes (often overlooked).
- ACEIs:
  - Cough (often overlooked)
  - Hypotension/falls (especially in the elderly)
  - Renal failure (especially in diabetics and claudicants, where renal artery stenosis is more common).
- Calcium-channel blockers:
  - Non-dependent ankle oedema (especially nifedipine, amlodipine)
  - Constipation (especially verapamil).

  Progress. This patient was started on lisinopril 5 mg daily, increasing to 15 mg over 3 weeks, along with bendroflumethiazide 2.5 mg daily. Six months later the BP was still not adequately controlled at 150/88 and he has just been started on aliskiren (a renin inhibitor).

THE SWOLLEN/PAINFUL LEG

Common causes of a swollen leg include:
- DVT
- Acute rupture knee joint/Baker's cyst
- Trauma, e.g. rupture of tendon/muscle
- Infection: cellulitis, osteomyelitis.

Case history (1)

A 36-year-old woman on the oral contraceptive pill developed pain in her left calf 3 days ago; it had become increasingly swollen since. Examination revealed oedema of the lower leg without any change in colour or prominence of the veins; there was tenderness along the line of the deep veins. Doppler studies showed early thrombus in the popliteal veins. She was anti-coagulated with heparin and warfarin for 6 months and given alternative contraceptive advice.

Many hospitals now have an excellent DVT service run by specialist nurses.

Investigation of DVT

- D-dimer assay:
  - Has a high negative predictive value, i.e. if low (<500 ng/mL), a DVT is unlikely

- Is often used in conjunction with a clinical risk score to decide if a patient needs treatment and ultrasonographic studies.
- B mode venous compression ultrasound: is generally the first-line investigation of choice. It detects clot reliably only in the popliteal/ femoral vein, not in calf veins. However, 30% of patients with calf vein clots will have an extension and anti-coagulation is now recommended.
- Venography: although probably the gold standard, can be misleading if there is a past history of venous thrombosis and is no longer used as a first-line investigation.

Treatment

The patient should be started on subcutaneous LMWH, continued until formal anti-coagulation with warfarin is at target level. Current recommendations for warfarin are:

- 6 months: proximal DVT $\pm$ pulmonary embolus
- 3 months: localised calf DVT (6 weeks is probably enough for a first DVT with no persisting risk factors).

Target INR is 2.5. With recurrent DVT, rivaroxaban or apixaban (Xa inhibitor drugs), plus screening for thrombophilia, are necessary.

Dabigatran, a direct thrombin inhibitor, is now being used as it does not require therapeutic monitoring.

Case history (2)

A 78-year-old man developed sudden pain and weakness of the left hand. The hand was cold and pulseless, indicating **acute limb ischaemia.** He was in sinus rhythm but a systolic murmur was noted at the apex. Successful embolectomy was performed. Echo showed a mass in the left atrium, which proved at surgery to be an atrial myxoma and was removed.

Some practical points

- AF (even when paroxysmal) is the most common cause of embolisation but don't forget rare causes such as endocarditis, ventricular thrombosis and atrial myxoma.
- If you suspect a peripheral embolus, involve a vascular surgeon early because minimising time to embolectomy is as vital as 'door to needle' time in an MI.
- In a patient with acute abdominal pain and AF, whom the surgeons say is not 'surgical', don't forget mesenteric ischaemia.

Progress. This patient's hand recovered following embolectomy. He was left with a mild sensory loss but has had no further problems.

Further reading

Atrial fibrillation

Kirchhof P, Benussi S, Kotecha D, et al. Guidelines for the management of atrial fibrillation. European Society of Cardiology Guidelines. *European Heart Journal* 2018; **39**: 2893–2962.

Link MS. Paradigm shift for treatment of atrial fibrillation in heart failure. *New England Journal of Medicine* 2018; **378**: 468–469.

Marrouche MF, Brachmann J, Andresen D, et al. Catheter ablation for atrial fibrillation with heart failure. *New England Journal of Medicine* 2018; **378**: 417–427.

Redfield MM. Heart failure with preserved ejection fraction. *New England Journal of Medicine* 2016; **375**: 1868–1877.

Cardiac arrest and basic life support

Brady WJ, Mattu A, Slovis CM. Lay responder care for an adult with out-of-hospital cardiac arrest. *New England Journal of Medicine* 2019; **381**: 2242–2251.

Valvular heart disease

Otto CM. Informed shared decisions for patients with aortic stenosis. *New England Journal of Medicine* 2019; **380**: 1769–1770.

Infective endocarditis

Rajani R, Klein JL. Infective endocarditis: a contemporary update. *Clinical Medicine* 2020; **20**: 31–35.

Heart failure

Velazquez EJ, Morrow DA, DeVore AD, et al. Angiotensin–neprilysin inhibition in acute decompensated heart failure. *New England Journal of Medicine* 2019; **380**: 539–548.

Respiratory Disorders 11

ACUTE BREATHLESSNESS

Case history (1)

You are called by the nurses to see a 63-year-old man who has become breathless. As you walk over to the ward, you consider what the causes might be on this rather scanty history.

Remember

Respiratory diseases can cause breathlessness within minutes or hours, or slowly over days, weeks or months.

The systems involved would most probably be cardiac or respiratory. You go through the list in Box 11.1 as you walk to the ward.

Box 11.1 Causes of breathlessness

Sudden-onset breathlessness

- Inhaled foreign body
- Pneumothorax
- Pulmonary embolus

Breathlessness developing over a few hours

- Asthma/chronic obstructive pulmonary disease (COPD)
- Pneumonia
- Pulmonary oedema
- Respiratory muscle disease, e.g. Guillain−Barré

Intermittent breathlessness

- Asthma
- Pulmonary oedema
- Pulmonary emboli

Breathlessness developing over a few days

- Pleural effusion
- Carcinoma of the bronchus
- Pneumonia, including pulmonary tuberculosis

Breathlessness developing over months or years

- Fibrosis alveolitis
- COPD
- Sarcoidosis
- Chest wall or neuromuscular disease
- Occupational lung disease
- Non-respiratory causes: anaemia, hyperthyroidism

Despite the long list, the chances are that this 63-year-old man has chronic pulmonary disease (COPD), chest infection or heart failure; if the onset was sudden, it could also be a pulmonary embolus (PE).

Initial assessment

- What does the patient look like? Is he in shock?
- What is the severity of the problem?
  - Tachypnoea?
  - Is the patient using his accessory muscles?
  - Is there any respiratory distress?
  - Colour: is the patient cyanosed?
- Pulse: rate, type, volume?
- BP?

Then make a full cardiac and respiratory examination. Is there any evidence of deep vein thrombosis (DVT)?

This vague history shows the vast number of diagnostic possibilities (see Box 11.1), but a shorter differential diagnosis can be made in the context of the age of the patient, the past medical history and the current clinical situation. This man turned out to have **heart failure**.

Progress. He was treated with furosemide 40 mg daily, and 3 days later was discharged for follow-up with his own doctor.

Upper airways obstruction

Case history (2)

A 29-year-old male had been at a party, where he had consumed a lot of alcohol. He managed to get home with the help of his friend but he then vomited and fell to the floor. He was holding his throat and had great difficulty in breathing. The friend realised that he was in great distress and called an ambulance.

Diagnosis

Upper airways obstruction. *This is an emergency!*

- Stridor
- Respiratory distress
- Cyanosis ± shock.

Fortunately, the emergency team recognised the problem and tried to clear the airway. There was no improvement so the Heimlich manoeuvre (also called abdominal thrusts) was performed and a large bone was expelled with immediate relief of the man's respiratory distress. He was taken to A&E for assessment but discharged after 2 h.

Remember

HEIMLICH MANOEUVRE

This is used to expel an inhaled foreign body:
- Stand behind the patient.
- Encircle the upper part of the abdomen, just below the patient's rib cage, with your arms.
- Give a sharp, forceful squeeze, forcing the diaphragm sharply into the thorax.

This should expel sufficient air from the lungs to force the foreign body out of the trachea. If this fails, urgent assessment by an experienced ENT or Cardiothoracic clinician is

Table 11.1 Causes of upper airways obstruction (with management strategies)

Cause	Action
Anaphylaxis: laryngeal oedema	Adrenaline (epinephrine) 0.5 mg IM Antihistamine, e.g. chlorphenamine 10–20 mg by slow IV injection Hydrocortisone IV 100 mg slowly O_2
Carcinoma of upper airway	Call ENT for laryngoscopy
Tracheal compression, e.g. bleeding post thyroidectomy	Tracheal decompression, e.g. release skin sutures
Inhaled foreign body	Heimlich manoeuvre

required. Fibre-optic or rigid bronchoscopy will be required if the obstruction is beyond the vocal cords.

Causes of upper airway obstruction are shown in Table 11.1. All of these require emergency management, which is also shown.

COUGH

Cough is common and, when persistent, can cause considerable fear and distress. Apart from the immediate discomfort of coughing, paroxysmal cough can interrupt sleep, provoke retching or vomiting and, if severe, result in rib fractures or syncope. Always enquire about sputum and its colour.

Case history

A 67-year-old man was admitted to hospital with a myocardial infarct. Following successful coronary intervention, he was discharged on anti-platelet therapy, atorvastatin and enalapril. When seen again 2 weeks later, he was very well but complained of a persistent hacking cough. This had been keeping him awake at night.

In this case, as the patient has only a cough and is not breathless, the cause is very likely to be the angiotensin-converting enzyme **(ACE) inhibitor (enalapril)**. This should be stopped and an ACE receptor antagonist, e.g. valsartan, started. Unlike ACE inhibitors, angiotensin receptor antagonists do not affect bradykinin metabolism and do not produce a cough.

Cough is provoked by stimulation of mucosal and stretch receptors that are present in the larynx, carina and proximal airways of the lung. Accordingly, it has a number of causes.

Acute cough

- Inhalation of direct irritants, e.g. smoke, chlorine gas, ozone and other air pollutants.
- In the asthmatic, inhalation of specific allergen, e.g. pollen or non-specific low-concentration irritants, e.g. perfume, tobacco fumes.
- Upper and lower respiratory tract infections (yellow/green sputum).

Chronic cough

- Large airway obstruction, e.g. carcinoma of the bronchus or inhaled foreign body (*Note:* peanuts and other inhaled food will not be radio-dense).
- Persistent bronchial inflammation, e.g. asthma, bronchiectasis, COPD, smoking.
- Persistent infection, e.g. tuberculosis, lung abscess.
- Interstitial lung disease, e.g. pulmonary fibrosis, asbestosis.
- Raised left atrial pressure, e.g. mitral stenosis, left ventricular failure.
- Gastro-oesophageal reflux disease (GORD) and bulbar dysfunction. (Laryngopharyngeal reflux disease – cough, hoarse voice, postnasal drip.)
- Iatrogenic, e.g. ACE inhibitors, radiation pneumonitis.

Enquire about associated features

- Haemoptysis.
- Pleuritic pain.
- History of myocardial infarction (suggesting cough is due to left ventricular failure).
- Post-nasal drip.

Investigations

All patients with persistent cough should have a CXR. Other investigations will depend on the likely cause, e.g. serial peak flow in asthma, or contrast studies if GORD or aspiration is suspected and sputum culture, including a request for *Mycobacterium tuberculosis* isolation if the cough is productive.

BREATHLESSNESS AND WHEEZE

Asthma causes breathlessness, cough and wheeze. However, all that wheezes is not asthma.

Information

- Asthma provocation tests might be required to exclude mild–moderate and variable bronchial irritability.
- Bronchoscopy will be required in all chronic cases remaining undiagnosed.

The differential diagnosis of asthma includes:
- COPD:
  - Patient usually >40 years of age
  - Heavy smoker: >20 pack years. (*Note:* patients with asthma might also smoke)
  - History of variable wheeze: in patients with asthma, chest wheeze is usually worse at night and may only be episodic.
- Upper airway obstruction with stridor:
  - Occurs when there is a mechanical obstruction in the larynx or trachea
  - Is heard during inspiration and expiration, but inspiratory sound when mouth open is most typical
  - Might be associated with vigorous accessory muscle activity and obvious distress.

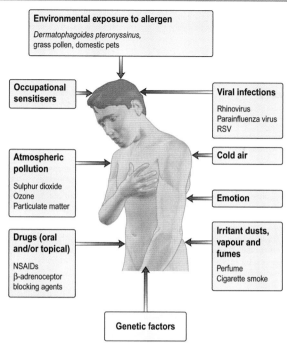

Figure 11.1 Causes and triggers of asthma. NSAIDs, non-steroidal anti-inflammatory drugs; RSV, respiratory syncytial virus.

- Left ventricular failure (LVF):
  - Acute LVF can be difficult to differentiate from asthma
  - Nocturnal symptoms are common to both.
  Fig. 11.1 shows causes and triggers of asthma.

Information

CAUSES OF STRIDOR
- Tumour
- Foreign body
- Bilateral vocal cord palsy
- Laryngeal oedema
- Thyroid goitre

Case history

A 24-year-old female was admitted to the MAU with breathlessness for 6 h. She has had a 'cold' for 2 days. Past history revealed her being 'chesty' as a child. It was noticed that she could not complete sentences easily. Heart rate was 126 bpm and respiratory rate was 30/min. There was expiratory wheeze over the lung fields. This patient has **severe acute asthma**.

Remember

SEVERE ACUTE ASTHMA
- Increased breathlessness/cannot complete sentences
- Respiratory rate >25/min
- Heart rate >100 bpm
- Peak expiratory flow rate (PEFR) 30–50% of best
- Arterial oxygen saturation (SaO_2) <92%

How would you manage this patient in A&E?

Immediate management should be:
- Reassurance that treatment will be effective
- Oxygen 40–60% (keep SaO_2 >90%)
- Nebulised short-acting β_2 agonist (SABA), e.g. salbutamol 5 mg or terbutaline 10 mg, with oxygen (*N.B.* Only 10% of drug reaches the lungs)
- Systemic corticosteroids:
  - Prednisolone 30–40 mg daily or
  - IV hydrocortisone 200 mg 8-hourly
- Monitoring of SaO2 by oximetry
- Arterial blood gases (ABGs):
  - Initially if SaO2 <90%
  - Recheck (2-hourly) if PaO2 <8 kPa or PaCO2 >5 kPa until PaCO2 is stable and saturation is >90%
- PEFR 4-hourly. Note: performing PEFR might be distressing for patient: do not demand unnecessary repeat testing
- ECG
- CXR.
  Normal ranges are shown in Table 11.2 later.
  Thirty minutes later there has been no significant improvement in her breathlessness and PEFR.

What would you do next?

- Call for senior help.
- Continue with nebulised β_2 agonist, now with added ipratropium (500 µg). Repeat every 30 min if necessary.
- IV aminophylline infusion can be used if patient does not respond to repeated nebulisation with β_2 agonist and ipratropium. However, *do not use this* if oral aminophylline has been taken.

Information

IV AMINOPHYLLINE
- Ensure patient is not on oral theophylline (don't give IV aminophylline if patient is on oral aminophylline)
- Monitor BP and heart rate
- Loading dose 250–500 mg over 1 h

INFUSION

- 1 mg/kg over 4 h
- 0.5 mg/kg per hour thereafter
- Check aminophylline level at 6–8 h after start of infusion and adjust dose

Other therapy

- IV β_2 agonist, e.g. salbutamol 3–20 µg/min, is an alternative in most cases.
- Magnesium sulphate 1.2–2 g IV infusion over 20 min with cardiac monitoring.

Remember

LIFE-THREATENING ACUTE ASTHMA

- Silent chest, feeble respiration, cyanosis
- Bradycardia/hypotension, arrhythmia
- Exhaustion/confusion
- PEFR <33% of best
- Arterial oxygen saturation <92%

Indications for HDU or intensive care

- Presence of life-threatening features *and*
- PaO_2 <8 kPa on 60% oxygen
- $PaCO_2$ >6 kPa
- Previous history of requiring ventilation.

Remember

Beware of the *silent chest!*

If asthma is very severe, air entry will be minimal and breath sounds quiet or absent.

There is now an improvement in PEFR and breathlessness with the nebulised β_2 agonist and ipratropium.

What treatment should be offered to the patient now?

Continuing management should be:

- Keeping SaO_2 >90% with oxygen supplementation
- Corticosteroids: prednisolone 20–40 mg daily, on a reducing dose
- 2–4-hourly nebulised SABA therapy and tiotropium.

When could she be discharged?

The patient can be discharged when:

- Symptoms, particularly nocturnal symptoms, have improved
- Ideally, PEFR is 75% of best and diurnal variation (i.e. 'morning dips') <25%. If the patient is improving and compliance is expected to be good, an earlier discharge is reasonable.

24–48 h before discharge

- Add inhaled corticosteroids, e.g. beclometasone, to oral steroids.
- Replace nebulised bronchodilators with inhalers.

- Introduce inhaled long-acting β_2 agonists (LABAs), e.g. salmeterol.
- Check inhaler technique (? might need spacer).
- Determine the cause of this attack (non-compliance, infection, allergen exposure).

Talk to asthma nurse

At discharge, the patient should have:

- Oral and inhaled corticosteroids and LABA. LABAs should be administered as fixed-dose combinations with corticosteroids (e.g. salmeterol/fluticasone or formoterol/budesonide) in the same inhaler. SABAs can be used on an 'as required' basis.
- Peak flow meter and diary.
- Management plan if condition deteriorates.
  Progress. This patient was discharged after 7 days on treatment as above. She requires close follow-up because of the severe acute attack.
  The discharge letter to her GP should include:
- Admission and discharge PEFR
- Recommended GP follow-up in 1 week
- Asthma clinic follow-up, preferably within 4 weeks.

HYPERVENTILATION

Case history

A 15-year-old schoolgirl is brought by her teacher to the A&E department feeling dizzy and faint. You notice that she is anxious and sighing, and has erratic ventilation. There are no other physical signs on examination. Her teacher volunteered that the girl was anxious about impending examinations.

What should you do?

- Full examination
- CXR
- PEFR or spirometry
- ABGs (even if oximetry is normal).

You have decided that her symptoms are due to hyperventilation. This should be confirmed by demonstration of a respiratory alkalosis with a low $PaCO_2$ and $[H^+]$ in the arterial blood. Reassure the patient and ask her to breathe into a closed paper bag: when settled, she can be discharged with further reassurance. *Note:* mild asthma is a common provocative cause and might require further investigation.

Hyperventilation syndrome refers to a condition of recurrent attacks of anxiety, sometimes phobic in nature, and provoking profound hyperventilation such as to cause a reduction in arterial pCO_2 and ensuing tetany. Other features include perioral and digital paraesthesia, carpopedal spasm, muscle weakness, dizziness and a sense of impending loss of consciousness or fear.

An attack of hyperventilation can be induced by a strong emotional experience in otherwise normal individuals, e.g. witnessing an accident.

In many patients, the label of hyperventilation syndrome is inappropriately given when mild asthma or other conditions, such as heart failure, lie behind the respiratory sensation. Indeed, hypocapnia resulting from hyperventilation might further provoke bronchoconstriction.

Clinically obvious hyperventilation can also result from a metabolic acidosis and will be recognised by ABG analysis: a reduced pH and bicarbonate, contrary to the alkalosis of respiratory hyperventilation.

Tetany (see p. 427): overbreathing can cause tetany.

Progress. This patient settled quickly. She was reassured that there was nothing seriously wrong with her. She was taken home to her parents with a pamphlet explaining the hyperventilation syndrome.

HAEMOPTYSIS

Case history

A 63-year-old male smoker presents with a 4-month history of cough. Recently, he has been coughing up blood in his sputum. He has also been breathless on exertion.

Coughing up blood is a dramatic symptom and can be frightening for patients and their families.

Colour of blood

This can differ with different causes.
- Pink frothy sputum: pulmonary oedema.
- Rusty sputum: pneumonia.
- Make sure it is not haematemesis, which would be suggested by:
  - History of retching
  - Altered blood (resembling coffee grounds)
  - Low pH of contents.

Enquire about epistaxis, which may cause confusion. Blood-stained saliva suggests bleeding from gums.

Common conditions presenting with haemoptysis

- Carcinoma of the bronchus:
  - Smoker
  - Age >40 years
  - Usually abnormal CXR.
- Pulmonary embolism:
  - Risk factors for DVT
  - CXR often negative
  - History of acute breathlessness.
- Pulmonary tuberculosis:
  - More common in Africa and Asia, people drinking alcohol in excess, patients with HIV infection
  - Age often <40 years
  - CXR usually shows patchy opacities in the upper lobes.
- Bronchiectasis:
  - History of purulent sputum and/or possibly recurrent haemoptysis over years
  - Cystic lesions on CXR at lung bases in some but not all patients
  - High-resolution CT scan of the lungs is diagnostic, with bronchial dilatation, loss of airway tapering at the periphery, bronchial wall thickening and cysts at the end of the bronchioles
  - Bronchiectasis is also a feature of cystic fibrosis.

Less common causes of haemoptysis are:
- Vasculitis (both of the following are anti-neutrophil cytoplasmic antibody [ANCA]-positive):
  - Granulomatosis with polyangiitis
  - Microscopic vasculitis.
- Pulmonary haemorrhage:
  - Goodpasture's syndrome
  - Idiopathic pulmonary haemosiderosis.
- Chronic venous congestion of lungs:
  - Mitral stenosis
  - LVF.
- Aspergilloma: seen in association with cavitatory lung disease.

Management of this case

A CXR was taken (Fig. 11.2 and Information box) and showed a pleural effusion and a hilar mass. The pleural effusion was aspirated and sent for cytology. A pleural biopsy was taken under ultrasound control and showed no evidence of malignancy on histology.

Video-assisted thoracoscopy was then performed and this allowed visualisation of the pleura. The biopsy showed a **squamous cell carcinoma**.

The patient was referred to the MDT for discussion of treatment options.

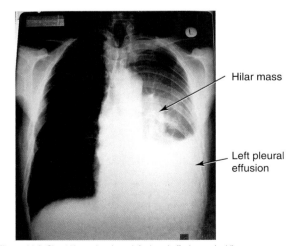

Hilar mass

Left pleural effusion

Figure 11.2 Chest X-ray showing a left pleural effusion and a hilar mass.

Information

CHEST X-RAYS

A standard chest X-ray (CXR) is taken posteroanteriorly (PA), with the patient facing the X-ray plate; the beam is directed at the patient's back at a standard distance.

An emergency department film is often taken anteroposteriorly (AP), with the patient lying down (supine) on the X-ray plate; the beam is directed at the patient's front; the distance from X-ray source can vary.

In an AP:

- Heart AP size and mediastinum are magnified.
- A pleural effusion that lies along the back of the chest cavity when the patient is supine might be missed.
- Film quality may be poor.

Don't request an AP 'portable' film unless it would be unsafe for the patient to have a PA film.

Management of massive haemoptysis

As little as 250 mL can fill the bronchial tree and be life-threatening. Happily, this is uncommon but it is nevertheless frightening for everyone involved:

- Monitor oxygen saturation with oximetry, BP and pulse rate.
- Perform CXR. Exclude coagulation defects.
- Endotracheal intubation and suction might be required.
- Urgent bronchoscopy by an experienced doctor is sometimes needed.
- A cuffed tube can be employed to protect the unaffected lung. It is inserted into the bronchus via a bronchoscope.
- Bronchial artery embolisation is highly effective if the bleeding vessel can be identified.

Information

Massive haemoptysis can occur in the following conditions:

- Tuberculosis
- Bronchiectasis
- Aspergilloma
- Carcinoma of the bronchus

Remember

Only a minority of patients have a malignant cause of massive haemoptysis.

CHEST PAIN

Diagnosing the cause of a chest pain can be straightforward but is often difficult, taking days to diagnose correctly. A careful history (eliciting site, character and radiation of the pain) is often more useful than tests:

- Exercise-induced central chest pain is usually cardiac in origin.
- Rest pain might be cardiac, pleuritic, musculoskeletal, nerve root irritation, oesophageal, mediastinal or referred pain from the abdomen.
- Lung diseases cause pain only if the pleura, mediastinum, intercostal nerves or bones are involved.

Is it cardiac pain?

See also page 268.

Central chest pain radiates to the arms and neck. There is a dull ache, with a severe, heavy, 'constricting' character. It may be associated with breathlessness.

Typical angina

Occurs on exercise and is eased by rest.

Acute coronary syndrome

Pain at rest or on minimal exertion, sometimes very severe with sweating; pain persists.

Pericarditis

Dull or sharp, central; eased by sitting forwards, may be worse with breathing.

Aortic dissection

Severe sudden onset, might be described as 'tearing' pain in the back or anterior chest; patient often shocked.

Is it pleurisy?

Sharp pain in the sides of the chest, which 'catches' with breathing. This is often accompanied by fever, cough with or without sputum or haemoptysis, indicating underlying lung disease.

Think of:

- Pneumonia and pleurisy
- Pulmonary infarction/embolism
- Pneumothorax
- Malignant invasion of pleura.

Is it musculoskeletal?

- Trauma:
  - Rib fracture: 'point' tenderness
  - Crushed vertebra: pain often referred around the chest.
- Chronic pain:
  - Osteoarthritis (OA): long history with acute episodes; look for spinal deformity
  - Rib or spine disease: might be metastatic cancer; local tenderness and swelling, lumps, history of cancer.
- Muscles: Bornholm's disease. Follows an upper respiratory tract infection; a low-grade fever can occur. Ache in muscles. Might be tender. Definite cases rare.
- Costochondral junction: Tietze's disease; local pain on pressure over costochondral junctions. Responds to NSAIDs.

Is it nerve root irritation?

- Typically in a dermatome distribution around the chest. Might be unilateral.
- Vertebral OA, osteomyelitis, prolapsed disc.
- Malignant nerve root compression.
- Herpes zoster (shingles): is there a vesicular rash (pain may precede rash)?

Is it oesophageal?

Reflux causes retrosternal burning pain, usually after food. Worse lying flat and eased by antacid. Can be severe and mimic myocardial infarction.

Oesophageal rupture

Central pain with shock. Might have associated pleural effusion. Occurs after severe vomiting or more commonly endoscopy at which dilatation has been performed for a malignant lesion.

Is it referred pain from outside the chest?

Diaphragm irritation may cause shoulder tip pain. Localisation might be difficult for the patient. Several abdominal emergencies might have chest pain with or without abdominal pain.

Think of:

- Acute cholecystitis
- Acute duodenal ulceration
- Subphrenic abscess
- Perforated bowel
- Peritonitis
- Pancreatitis.

Is it genuine?

Yes – nearly always. Exclude organic disease in *all* cases.

A tiny minority might be attention-seeking or have psychiatric disease. Even patients with Munchausen's syndrome might have genuine disease.

What tests do you need to do for chest pain?

After a good history and examination do the following (as a minimum):

- ECG – repeat if first ECG normal
- CXR
- Serum cardiac troponins
- FBC, including ESR and CRP.
  Many diagnoses will now be obvious but remember:
- A normal ECG does not exclude cardiac pain.
- A normal CXR does not exclude PE.
  If still in doubt:
- Retake the history, re-examine the patient and consider unusual causes.
- Is WCC or ESR raised?
- Is the patient pyrexial?
- Arrange further investigations, e.g. CT, MRI scan.

RESPIRATORY FAILURE

Respiratory failure (PaO_2 <8 kPa) is a common medical emergency, often presenting with non-specific symptoms such as mild confusion or agitation. Recognition requires ABG analysis (see later).

Oximeters that estimate arterial oxygen saturation from the finger or ear lobe are useful in assessment or monitoring. Oximeters might, however, be falsely reassuring in the patient breathing oxygen. Importantly, they will not detect alveolar hypoventilation, producing high pCO_2.

> **Remember**
>
> All breathless patients should have oximetry checked at triage in A&E.

Respiratory failure commonly results from either a problem with the respiratory pump or intrinsic lung disease.

> **Remember**
>
> All unconscious patients should have ABG analysis at initial assessment.

In respiratory pump failure the arterial pCO$_2$ (PaCO$_2$) is raised

You should think of:
- Severe air-flow limitation, e.g. COPD
- Neurological depression, e.g. coma, sedatives, overdose
- Chest wall problems, e.g. flail chest, pneumothorax
- Neuromuscular disease, e.g. Guillain–Barré syndrome, old poliomyelitis.

In intrinsic lung disease (apart from COPD) hypoxaemia is often combined with a reduced PaCO$_2$

The hypoxaemia arises primarily from a mismatch of ventilation and perfusion in the pulmonary alveolar bed. Hypoxic stimulation of ventilation, coupled with abnormal respiratory sensation, then leads to a reduced arterial pCO$_2$ (alveolar hyperventilation). A raised PaCO$_2$ indicates impending respiratory arrest, as it suggests either a reduction in ventilatory effort or failure of the respiratory pump.

In hypoxaemia with reduced PaCO$_2$

Consider:
- Infection, e.g. pneumonia
- Shock, e.g. sepsis, hypovolaemia, acute respiratory distress syndrome (ARDS)
- Asthma
- Cardiac disease, e.g. LVF, pulmonary hypertension
- PE.

In respiratory failure

ABG sampling is necessary to:
- Assess severity
- Identify type, i.e. alveolar hypo- or hyperventilation
- Appreciate the degree of compensation (i.e. the chronicity of the condition)
- Recognise the base excess (BE) value (see later), as a coexisting metabolic acidosis commonly causes confusion.

> **Information**
>
> ABG sampling is painful. Contrary to common belief, the use of local anaesthetic does not make the procedure more difficult. Heparin has a low pH and should be expelled from the syringe. Heparin-bonded microsamplers are available and small-diameter needles make local anaesthetic unnecessary. When taking ABG samples it is essential to note the inspiratory O$_2$ concentration (F$_i$O$_2$).

Summary of acid–base changes (Fig. 11.3)

In a respiratory acidosis
Carbon dioxide clearance is reduced – there is alveolar hypoventilation. The $PaCO_2$ and $[H^+]$ rise. The HCO_3 is also increased due to renal compensation.

Examples include exacerbation of COPD, flail chest injury and Guillain–Barré syndrome.

In a respiratory alkalosis
There is alveolar hyperventilation and both the $PaCO_2$ and $[H^+]$ are decreased. The HCO_3 is slightly decreased.

Examples include acute asthma and anxiety attack.

In a metabolic acidosis
There is disturbance of bicarbonate regulation or excessive H^+ production. The HCO_3 is reduced and the $PaCO_2$ falls because of respiratory compensation.

Examples include diabetic ketoacidosis, chronic kidney disease and shock.

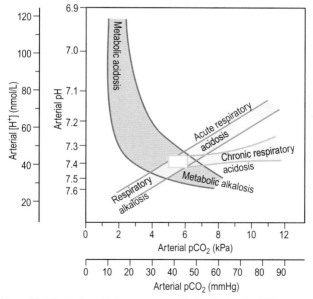

Figure 11.3 The Flenley acid–base nomogram. The bands show the 95% confidence limits representing the individual varieties of acid–base disturbance. The central white box shows the approximate limits of arterial pH and pCO_2 in normal individuals.

In a metabolic alkalosis

The HCO_3 is increased and relative hypoventilation leads to a small compensatory increase in the $PaCO_2$.

Examples include excessive vomiting and profound hypokalaemia.

Information

The base excess value provided by the ABG analyser is calculated by back-titration to normal values for $PaCO_2$ and HCO_3.

Common ABG abnormalities

Normal blood gas values are shown in Table 11.2.

Life-threatening asthma

- pH: 7.2.
- PaO_2: 15.4.
- $PaCO_2$: 6.
- HCO_3: 16.2.
- BE: -7.3.

Supplemental O_2 is being provided (note the high PaO_2). There is a metabolic acidosis (note the pH and BE) as a result of metabolic demands exceeding O_2 delivery and producing a lactic acidosis. Airflow limitation limits the normal respiratory compensation to this profound acidosis.

Acute or chronic respiratory failure in a patient with COPD

- pH: 7.3.
- PaO_2: 25.8.
- $PaCO_2$: 12.6.
- HCO_3: 42.1.
- BE: $+4.3$.

This is acute or chronic respiratory acidosis exacerbated by a high F_iO_2 using a variable-performance mask (40–60% O_2) (note high PaO_2 and $PaCO_2$). The high HCO_3 results from renal compensation. The patient was changed to 28% oxygen.

Table 11.2 Normal blood gas values (with F_iO_2 21%)

Analysis	NORMAL RANGE	
	SI units	Non-SI units
PaO_2	10.6–13.3 kPa	80–100 mmHg
$PaCO_2$	4.5–6.0 kPa	34–45 mmHg
Hydrogen ions	37–45 nmol/L	pH 7.35–7.43
Bicarbonate	24–28 mmol/L	24–28 mEq/L

To convert kPa to mmHg, multiply by 7.5.
The pH changes by approximately 0.1 per 1 kPa change in $PaCO_2$.

Severe pneumonia (F_iO_2 60%)

- pH: 7.15.
- PaO_2: 4.8.
- $PaCO_2$: 3.5.
- HCO_3: 12.5.
- BE: −9.3.

Despite high F_iO_2 this patient is hypoxaemic because of ventilation–perfusion mismatch. The profound hypoxia despite oxygen and the associated metabolic acidosis indicate the need for urgent intubation and intermittent positive pressure ventilation (IPPV), and are a reflection of circulatory failure resulting from septic shock.

Management

Respiratory failure can be difficult to assess or manage. Always review the CXR. Discuss with your consultant or other more senior staff. If you feel that the situation is unstable, do not hesitate to call an anaesthetist. Semi-elective intubation is much preferred to a respiratory arrest. It should be performed in the ward before transfer of the patient to the ICU.

How do I recognise impending respiratory arrest?

- Tachycardia >120.
- Tachypnoea, respiratory rate >30.
- Hypotension.
- Sympathetic activation: pale and sweaty, agitation, confusion.
- Progressive increase in $PaCO_2$ or fall in PaO_2.
- Rapid desaturation on disconnection from O_2, e.g. when drinking or coughing.

Evaluation is often at the 'end of the bed'. Is the patient getting tired? Be sensitive to subtle changes or a failure to improve.

Treating the cause

- Individual causes will require different actions: e.g. an intercostal drain for a tension pneumothorax or large pleural effusion (see p. 346).
- In neurological coma, intubation might be necessary for airway protection or to manage raised intracranial pressure by hyperventilation.
- Drug-induced respiratory failure can be confirmed by a therapeutic trial with a specific antidote, i.e. a bolus injection of naloxone for opiates and flumazenil for benzodiazepines. Infusions will be required if a positive response is obtained, as antidotes have a short half-life.
- Oxygen supplementation should be aimed at raising the PaO_2 to beyond the steep part of the oxygen dissociation curve (Fig. 11.4). Very high PaO_2 values are unnecessary but controlled O_2 therapy via a fixed-performance mask is necessary only in chronic respiratory failure resulting from COPD.

Case history

A 65-year-old man with advanced COPD was admitted with a 1-week history of cough, breathlessness and purulent sputum. In the previous 24 h he had become mildly confused. He was agitated with a respiratory rate of 35 and BP of 170/90, and was sweaty with an oximeter reading on air of 72%. There was widespread wheeze and coarse

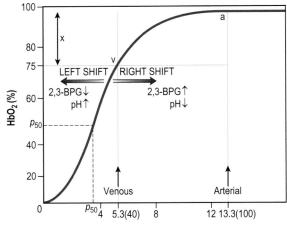

Figure 11.4 Oxygen dissociation curve. BPG, bisphosphoglycerate; a, arterial point; v, venous point; x, arterial venous difference; HbO₂, oxygen saturation of haemoglobin.

crackles suggestive of retained secretions. ABG analysis revealed pH 7.32, PaO$_2$ 5.8, PaCO$_2$ 8.1 and HCO$_3$ 28.

What do these blood gases mean?

Hypoxaemia with mild acute respiratory acidosis. There is no evidence of chronic respiratory failure with chronically elevated pCO$_2$, as HCO$_3$ is normal, i.e. there is no compensation.

The initial treatment in A&E was:

- Nebulised bronchodilators (salbutamol 5 mg nebulised + ipratropium bromide 500 μg).
- 28% O$_2$ by controlled mask.
- IV amoxicillin (erythromycin if patient penicillin-allergic).
- IV steroids (this is conventional treatment although there is limited evidence for effectiveness): hydrocortisone 100 mg × 3 daily.
- Encouragement to clear secretions, including sitting patient up and asking the physiotherapist to attend.
- CXR to exclude pneumothorax or demonstrate associated pneumonia.

Information

Controlled oxygen via Venturi mask commonly leads to intermittent therapy, as the mask is poorly tolerated by agitated, breathless patients. Oxygen via nasal prongs at 1 or 2 L/min is more effective and continuous, but is not 'controlled'.

Repeat ABGs were requested: pH 7.20, PaO_2 6.5, $PaCO_2$ 12.5, HCO_3 30.

These results show further CO_2 retention and a deteriorating situation. Oxygen should not be removed, as this will precipitate severe hypoxaemia. Alveolar ventilation must be increased. Despite using a nasal airway to stimulate cough and aid suction of respiratory secretions, there was no improvement. Furosemide was given because it was difficult to exclude coexistent LVF. Intubation was considered appropriate but a trial of non-invasive ventilation (NIV), bi-level positive airway pressure (BiPAP) with tight-fitting facial mask, was first tried with repeat gases at 1 h. On NIV the respiratory rate slowed and the acute respiratory acidosis resolved.

Non-invasive ventilatory support employs a nose or face mask to provide ventilatory assistance to breathing (this is termed 'spontaneous pressure support') or timed breaths ('pressure-controlled ventilation'). An exhalation valve reduces rebreathing. NIV is successful in approximately 70% of patients with respiratory failure resulting from COPD. It should not be employed if intubation would be more appropriate.

Information

CONTRAINDICATIONS/CAUTIONS TO NIV
- Unconscious or uncooperative patient
- Vomiting
- Large amount of respiratory secretions
- Cardiovascular instability (beware hypotension)
- Recent facial or upper airway surgery
- Recent upper GI tract surgery
- Inability to protect airway

Mechanical ventilation

In an unstable situation it is essential to maintain oxygenation. As intubation of an acutely unwell patient requires experience, refer to the ITU outreach team.

Aims of intubation and mechanical ventilation
- Immediate correction of hypoxaemia.
- Slower correction of hypercapnia.
- To allow effective suctioning of respiratory secretions.

Hypotension after intubation
This is very common and relates to:
- High airway pressures limiting venous return and causing a fall in cardiac output
- Vasodilatation directly caused by sedatives
- A fall in sympathetic tone.

Progress. This patient was seen by the ITU team, who felt, despite his confusion, that he should first be tried on non-invasive ventilatory support. He was put on BiPAP and his blood gases were monitored. These gradually improved on this regimen and antibiotics. He was discharged and advised to see his doctor as soon as he develops a chest infection.

Kumar & Clark's Cases in Clinical Medicine

COPD – ACUTE EXACERBATION

Chronic obstructive pulmonary disease (COPD) is used to describe a number of clinical syndromes associated with destruction of the lung and airflow obstruction.

Case history (1)

A 63-year-old male ex-smoker has had a chronic productive cough for 20 years. For 10 years he has had gradually increasing breathlessness on exertion. His usual exercise tolerance is 200 m on the flat. One week previously he became breathless on walking between rooms and his sputum became purulent. His normal medication is salmeterol, tiotropium and beclometasone inhalers.

On examination, his chest expanded poorly and he was wheezy, but there were no localising signs, and no evidence of cor pulmonale or heart failure.

His usual forced expiratory volume in 1 s/forced vital capacity (FEV_1/FVC) was 1.9/3.2 (predicted 3.4/4.4) but on arrival was 0.9/2.6. His CXR showed no acute lesion.

It was decided not to admit him to hospital because:
- He was able to cope at home with the aid of his wife.
- He was not cyanosed: oximetry showed SaO_2 97%.
- His general condition was good and he had a normal level of consciousness.

He was discharged home with:
- Amoxicillin 500 mg $\times$ 3 daily for 1 week
- Prednisolone 30 mg daily for 2 weeks
- Advice to use inhaled SABAs in addition to normal medication bronchodilators 4-hourly via a spacer
- A follow-up appointment at the chest clinic for 2 weeks.

Key points

- The patient did not need admission because:
  - There was no evidence of respiratory failure.
  - There was no evidence of cor pulmonale.
  - He was able to cope at home.
- The antibiotic was broad-spectrum and, in particular, covered the majority of *Haemophilus influenzae* and *Streptococcus pneumoniae* organisms (the most common causes of acute exacerbation). Erythromycin was unnecessary because *Mycoplasma* was unlikely.
- Oral steroids were used as an adjunct to antibiotics because the patient was already on inhaled steroids and possibly had a degree of steroid responsiveness. This is conventional treatment but there is limited evidence to support it.
- The patient was given a spacer (and shown how to use it) in order to increase the lung deposition of aerosol.
- The salbutamol dose was given 4-hourly because the effect lasts only 4–6 h and is partly dependent on dose.
- Follow-up at the chest clinic was arranged because the patient had moderately severe COPD and had never been assessed:
  - Advise pneumococcal and influenza vaccination.
  - Consider referral for pulmonary rehabilitation.

However, the patient's doctor, when seeing the patient 1 week later, cancelled the outpatient appointment, believing it unnecessary. He wrote to the chest physician, saying that he was able to manage the patient himself. He had a spirometer in the surgery and, when well, the patient had an FEV_1 of >50% predicated normal. Furthermore, the doctor said that the patient:

- Had a definitive diagnosis
- Had only moderately severe COPD
- Had no cor pulmonale
- Had no respiratory failure and did not need oxygen
- Did not have bullous lung disease
- Did not have a rapidly declining FEV_1.

The patient's doctor was arranging to perform bronchodilator tests himself using a spirometer and checking the response to both salbutamol and ipratropium inhalers. He would arrange vaccination.

Remember

Spirometry is required to assess the severity of COPD. Most COPD patients can be satisfactorily managed in the community.

Prognosis of COPD

Predictors of a poor prognosis are increasing age and worsening of airflow limitation, i.e. a fall in FEV_1.

A patient with a BODE index (Table 11.3) of 0–2 has a mortality rate of 10%; one with a BODE index of 7–10 has a mortality rate of 80% at 4 years.

Case history (2)

A 68-year-old female smoker, with a chronic productive cough and 5 years of gradually increasing breathlessness on exertion, had a usual exercise tolerance of 40 m on the flat and was breathless bending and washing. She was virtually housebound and lived alone. She developed a cough with purulent sputum and had been breathless at rest for 2 days. She was sent as an emergency to the A&E Department. She was admitted to the MAU immediately.

On examination, the following were noted:

- Signs of respiratory failure: drowsiness and cyanosis, CO_2 flap
- Pulse 130/min; atrial fibrillation; BP 100/60
- Cor pulmonale with tricuspid regurgitation:
  - JVP raised up to the level of the ear
  - Mid-systolic murmur at the left sternal edge

Table 11.3 BODE index[a]

Variable	POINTS ON BODE INDEX			
	0	1	2	3
FEV_1 (% of predicted)	≥ 65	50–64	36–49	≥ 35
Distance walked in 6 min (m)	≥ 350	250–349	150–249	≤ 149
MMRC dyspnoea scale[b]	0–1	2	3	4
Body mass index	> 21	≤ 21		

[a]Body mass index, degree of airflow Obstruction, Dyspnoea and Exercise capacity.
[b]Scores on the modified Medical Research Council (MMRC) dyspnoea scale range from 0 to 4, with a score of 4 indicating that the patient is breathless when dressing.

- Enlarged pulsatile liver
- Bilaterally oedematous legs to knees
- Respiratory rate 30, shallow breaths using accessory muscles of respiration, generalised wheezing and bilateral basal crackles.

Investigations showed:

- ABGs: pH 7.32, PaO_2 5.6, pCO_2 8.2 on air
- FBC: Hb 178 g/L, haematocrit (Hct) 54%, WCC 12 300
- Urea 9.0, K^+ 3.5, creatinine 102
- ECG 130 (ventricular rate); atrial fibrillation and right heart strain
- CXR: over-inflated lungs with prominent pulmonary arteries (indicating pulmonary hypertension) and normal-sized heart.

Key points

- The patient is in respiratory failure with raised $PaCO_2$: give oxygen via fixed-performance mask 24%, initially increasing to 28% or 35% if no rise in $PaCO_2$.
- Cor pulmonale (right heart failure secondary to lung disease) is difficult to improve while the patient remains hypoxic.
- Atrial fibrillation may only be secondary to hypoxaemia and might revert to sinus rhythm when PaO_2 improves.

Immediate treatment

- Oxygen 28% via Venturi mask and repeat ABGs.
- Patient to sit upright to help breathing.
- Nebulised bronchodilators:
  - Salbutamol 5.0 mg with ipratropium 0.5 mg 6-hourly via nebuliser
  - Air rather than high-flow O_2 is safer for nebulising bronchodilators.
- Chest physiotherapy to help sputum expectoration.
- Amoxicillin 500 mg × 3 daily IV until condition improves and then oral for 1 week in total.
- IV hydrocortisone 100 mg × 3 daily until patient improves and then oral prednisolone 20 to 30 mg daily for 2 weeks. If not on oral theophyllines, start aminophylline infusion.
- Monitor oximetry and mental state, respiratory rate and pulse until improvement. Daily weights.

What should you do if there is no improvement?

This patient did not improve and she was therefore given:

- Doxapram as a respiratory stimulant (1.5–4 mg/min infusion), which sometimes helps
- Non-invasive intermittent positive pressure ventilation (NIV) (see p. 327). The best technique is using a tight-fitting facial mask to deliver BiPAP ventilation support.

Progress

- Patient more alert.
- PaO_2 8.0, $PaCO_2$ 8.4, pH 7.35 now on 2 L nasal oxygen.
- In sinus rhythm.

Key points (Fig. 11.5)

- Oxygen should be prescribed on the treatment sheet and given continuously, not 'as required'.

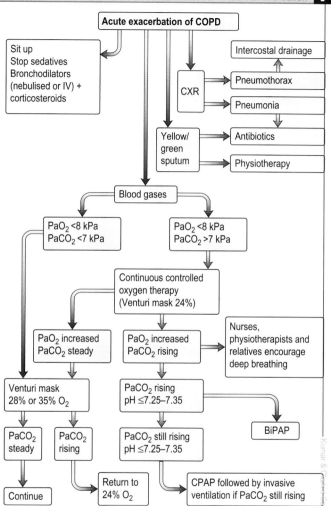

Figure 11.5 Algorithm for the treatment of respiratory failure in COPD. BiPAP, bi-level positive airway pressure; CPAP, continuous positive airway pressure; CXR, chest X-ray. (From Kumar P, Clark M, eds. *Kumar and Clark's Clinical Medicine*, 9th edn. Edinburgh: Elsevier, 2017; Fig. 24.24.)

- Management of oxygen is the most helpful and difficult component of treatment.
- Although oxygen by Venturi mask gives a known concentration, it is uncomfortable and claustrophobic. The mask has to be removed to eat, talk and cough, and for nebulised treatment.
- Oxygen by nasal spectacles is more comfortable and can be kept on continuously.
- Nasal oxygen gives variable F_iO_2, depending on pattern of breathing and flow rate between 24% and 35%. It worked on this patient, but in many with COPD 24% oxygen via a mask is preferable when $PaCO_2$ >8.0 kPa.
- It takes 30–40 min to equilibrate blood gases with any change in F_iO_2, and blood gases should not be checked earlier.
- It is unnecessary to restore the PaO_2 to normal: aim for it to reach the top of the steep slope of the oxygen saturation curve (see Fig. 11.3).
- If PaO_2 is >7.5 kPa, a small fall in PaO_2 has little effect on O_2 saturation: this is safe.
- If PaO_2 is ≤6.5 kPa, a small fall produces a dangerous fall in SaO_2. *Note:* the oxygen dissociation curve is sigmoid in shape (see p. 326).
- Increasing the inspired oxygen may cause a small rise in $PaCO_2$ (mostly because of relaxation of hypoxic vasoconstriction in relatively poorly ventilated alveoli). A pH change of <0.1 or $PaCO_2$ <1 kPa is not significant, so do not reduce or remove the oxygen.
- On increasing F_iO_2, this patient had not clinically improved and ABGs showed PaO_2 6.8 and $PaCO_2$ 12.0:
  - Action: the patient still needs oxygen but at a more controlled concentration. Increase F_iO_2 to 35%.
  - Get help from a senior, preferably from the respiratory team, and discuss transfer to HDU for non-invasive ventilation or to ITU for assisted ventilation.

Progress. Over the next few days the patient improved and felt well by 1 week. Her Hb came back as 180 g/L and Hct 55.

What would you do now?

Venesect cautiously under Haematology guidance: 3–4 units venesected over the next few weeks, starting before discharge from hospital and aiming for an Hct of 50. Continue bronchodilators as inhalers via a spacing device; oral steroids are continued for 2 weeks and diuretics, e.g. furosemide, are given.

Key points

Before discharge, blood gases were checked on air and showed a PaO_2 of 7.0 and $PaCO_2$ of 6.3. The respiratory nurse was asked to visit to:

- Discuss disease/risk factors, especially to urge smoking cessation and refer to smoking cessation clinic
- Explain mechanism of action of drugs
- Explain use of aerosol devices and spacers
- Arrange chest clinic follow-up for 2 weeks.

Follow-up in chest clinic

This was arranged to:
- Optimise bronchodilator treatment

- Monitor for polycythaemia and cor pulmonale
- Assess for long-term domiciliary oxygen (indication PaO_2 <7.3 on two occasions 3–4 weeks apart when patient stable)
- Consider obstructive sleep apnoea in view of marked polycythaemia.

PNEUMONIA

Pneumonia is an inflammation of the substance of the lungs. It can be classified by site (e.g. lobar, diffuse, bronchopneumonia) or by aetiological agent (e.g. bacterial, viral, fungal, aspiration, or radiotherapy or allergic mechanisms). Pneumonias can be community-acquired (CAP; commonest organism *Strep. pneumoniae*), hospital-acquired (often Gram-negative bacteria) or ventilator-associated (multiple organisms, e.g. *Pseudomonas*, *Klebsiella* and *Acinetobacter*).

Information

RECENT GLOBAL RESPIRATORY VIRUSES

- **SARS**. In November 2002 a new lower respiratory tract disease occurred in China. Severe acute respiratory syndrome (SARS) was a bronchopneumonia caused by a coronavirus (SARS-CoV), probably spread by bats.
- **MERS**. In 2012 a new disease caused by a coronavirus, Middle East respiratory syndrome (MERS-CoV), was identified in patients who died of respiratory failure, the virus being spread via camels.
- **SARS-CoV-2**. In 2020 a new **Coronavirus** was identified in the Wuhan district of China. This virus spread widely around the world and was declared a pandemic in March 2020. People can be asymptomatic, but infective, or develop symptoms. The symptoms include a high temperature, a new continuous cough with shortness of breath, a loss of taste and smell, and fatigue. Patients have required admission to intensive care and ventilator support. Complications include respiratory, cardiac and renal failure, and metabolic problems. A small number of children have been shown to have a multi-system inflammatory syndrome. Spread is via exhaled droplets and particles, as well as contact. High-risk patients include those with co-morbidity, the elderly, the immunosuppressed and the obese. In the UK, black, Asian and ethnic minority (BAME) people have had a higher incidence. Measures were taken by many countries to ban large gatherings and to enforce social distancing of 2 metres. All non-essential shops and workplaces were required to close during 'lockdowns', with people being encouraged to work at home and online where possible. The implications have been horrendous, with on-going job losses and economic recessions worldwide.

  Regular hand washing has been recommended to reduce contamination. Testing and contact tracing have been shown to slow the spread of the virus in many countries. Facial masks have also been recommended for confined spaces, and in some countries, on leaving home. Treatment is largely supportive, but dexamethasone and hydrocortisone have been shown to be of benefit in severe cases. Anti-virals, e.g. remdesivir, have shown some efficacy. By the end of August 2020, over 26 million cases had been reported worldwide, with deaths in excess of 870,000. Vaccines are under development but large-scale production of these will take time.

Case history (1)

A 33-year-old female non-smoker was admitted to the medical assessment unit with a 2-day history of fever, sweating and cough, productive of yellow, lightly blood-stained sputum. She had pleuritic pain in the left axilla. Herpes labialis was present.

This is the typical history of community-acquired pneumonia (CAP).

Signs

- Fever 39°C.
- Respiratory rate 28/min.
- Dullness to percussion left lung base; consolidation.
- Bronchial breathing left lung base; consolidation.

Likely infecting organisms

- *Streptococcus pneumoniae:* the most likely cause (35–80% of cases).
- *Haemophilus influenzae:* especially in smokers with COPD.
- *Mycoplasma* (4-yearly epidemics).
- *Legionella.*
- *Staphylococcus aureus.*
- Viral: influenza.
- *Chlamydophilia psittaci.*

Investigations

- CXR
- ABGs
- FBC, WCC + differential
- U&Es
- Urinalysis for sugar (is patient diabetic?)
- Blood and sputum culture
- Blood for viral serology and *Legionella/Mycoplasma*
- Serology for pneumococcal antigen (blood, sputum and urine)
- Rapid urine test available for *Legionella*

Box 11.2 CURB-65 criteria for the diagnosis of severe community-acquired pneumonia

- *C*onfusion*
- *U*rea >7 mmol/L
- *R*espiratory rate ≥30/min
- *B*lood pressure (systolic <90 or diastolic ≤60 mmHg
- *A*ge >65 years

    Score 1 point for each feature present:

    Score 0–1 — Treat as outpatient

    Score 2 — Admit to hospital

    Score 3 + — Often require ICU care

    Mortality rates increase with increasing score.

Other markers of severe pneumonia

- CXR — more than one lobe involved
- PaO_2 <8 kPa
- Low albumin (<35 g/L)
- WCC (<4 × 10^9/L or high >20 × 10^9/L)
- Blood culture — positive

* Confusion is described as new disorientation in person, place or time.

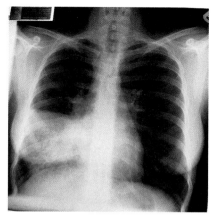

Figure 11.6 Right lobar pneumonia.

How ill is this patient?

The CURB-65 criteria (Box 11.2) indicate the severity of CAP.

Progress. This patient was young, previously fit, and not breathless or shocked. The CXR (Fig. 11.6) showed a right lower lobe pneumonia. The WCC was 11 500; normal urea; PaO_2 10.5 kPa.

This pneumonia is not severe on the CURB criteria.

The patient was treated with oral antibiotics and was discharged in 24 h (see Antibiotic choices, p. 336).

Case history (2)

A 73-year-old man was brought to A&E by his very anxious wife. He had had winter bronchitis for the last 5 years and was currently smoking 20 cigarettes/day. One week ago he had had the 'flu' and this morning became increasingly breathless, sweaty, pale and confused. A diagnosis of angina was made 2 years ago.

   Bedside assessment summary:
- *C*onfusion
- *R*espiratory rate >30/min
- *B*P 110/40
- *73 years old*
- Dehydrated
- Pre-existing COPD
- Pre-existing angina
  i.e. CURB-65 score of 4 + (no blood tests done yet for urea).

   Investigations showed:
- CXR (Fig. 11.7):
  - Diffuse opacification in both lungs
  - Ring opacities in right lung
- Urea 9 mmol/L
- WCC 28 000
- ABGs: PaO_2 9.0 kPa, $PaCO_2$ 5.3 kPa, on FiO_2 40%.

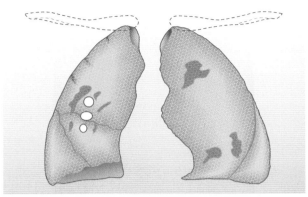

Figure 11.7 Diagram of chest X-ray showing bilateral diffuse opacities and ring opacities in the right lung.

This is a high-risk case. The patient has influenza and a superinfection with *Staphylococcus aureus*, causing **severe community-acquired pneumonia** with early abscess formation (ring opacities on the CXR). He needs:

- Rehydration: IV fluid
- IV antibiotics (see Antibiotics choices later): severe CAP
- Pulse oximetry: give O_2 to try to keep O_2 saturation >90%
- Nursing: where he can be easily observed or in an HDU (hourly BP, pulse, respiratory rate)
- Watching: for respiratory failure, as IPPV might be needed
- Physiotherapy: if he has difficulty coughing up sputum.

Information

INDICATIONS FOR INTENSIVE CARE MONITORING AND ASSISTED RESPIRATION
- PaO_2 <8 kPa on 60% O_2
- $PaCO_2$ >6.4 kPa
- Patient exhausted, drowsy or unconscious
- Shock
- Hypotension or circulatory failure

Antibiotic choices for CAP

Consult your hospital formulary or select from the following:

Remember

Clarithromycin resistance is a significant problem and it should be used with care.

Uncomplicated mild CAP

- Treat for 5 days with oral medication unless patient not swallowing or not absorbing.
- Oral amoxicillin 500 mg × 3 daily + erythromycin 500 mg × 4 daily (or clarithromycin).
- In **penicillin-allergic patient with underlying lung disease** (*Haemophilus influenzae* suspected) give clarithromycin 500 mg × 2 daily.

Severe CAP

- IV antibiotics until significant improvement. Co-amoxiclav 1.2 g IV × 3 daily and clarithromycin 500 mg IV × 2 daily.
- Antibiotics for up to 10 days.

Staphylococcal pneumonia

- Treat for 10–14 days.
- Flucloxacillin 2 g × 4 daily IV + fusidic acid oral 0.5–1 g × 3 or gentamicin 3.0–5.0 mg/kg IV daily as single dose (check gentamicin levels before second dose).

Legionnaire's disease

- Treat for 3 weeks.
- Clarithromycin 500 mg × 2 daily (for severe cases IV).

Mycoplasma pneumonia

- Treat for 2 weeks.
- Erythromycin 500 mg × 4 IV or oral daily.
- If **allergic to erythromycin**, give doxycycline 200 mg orally then 100 mg daily or ciprofloxacin 500 mg × 2 daily.

Q fever and psittacosis

- Tetracycline 500 mg × 3 daily for 10 days.

Progress. This patient made a significant improvement on his IV antibiotics. He was switched to oral antibiotics and made a slow recovery.

Case history (3)

A 24-year-old male, recently arrived in the UK from East Africa, presented with breathlessness of 2 weeks' duration, gradually increasing in severity, with a dry cough and sweats. He had a diarrhoeal illness 6 months ago and has recently noticed swollen glands in his neck.

Bedside assessment summary:

- Worried-looking patient
- Respiratory rate 34/min
- Tachycardia 120 bpm
- Temperature 41°C
- No abnormal signs in chest
- Pre-existing illness: HIV infection
- ABGs: PaO_2 9.0 kPa; on F_iO_2 60% $PaCO_2$ 3.2 kPa
- WCC 23 × 10^9/L
- Normal serum urea.

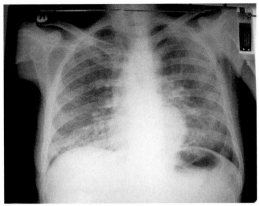

Figure 11.8 Chest X-ray showing bilateral perihilar shadowing in *Pneumocystis jiroveci* pneumonia.

You should think this patient may have HIV infection with a *Pneumocystis jiroveci* pneumonia because of country of origin, 6-month history of illness, lymphadenopathy, low WCC and appearance on CXR (Fig. 11.8).

On *investigation*, the CXR had:
- Ground glass appearance of lung fields
- Bilateral and perihilar shadowing.

Remember

OTHER PNEUMONIAS
- Inhalation pneumonia (Gram-negative organisms): heavy alcohol users
- Infected emboli to lungs (*Staphylococcus aureus*): drug users — 'dirty' needles and syringes
- Tuberculosis: a sputum smear for acid-fast bacilli (AFB) is quick and easy to do; can coexist with other pneumonias
- Cytomegalovirus
- Fungal: *Aspergillus, Candida albicans*
  These last two are seen in immunocompromised patients, e.g. those with:
- HIV infection
- Leukaemia and lymphoma
- Chemotherapy
- Transplantation
- Steroid therapy
- Chronic kidney disease.

What treatment should be started in this patient?

Treatment should start in this patient for *Pneumocystis jiroveci* infection:
- Give high-dose IV co-trimoxazole.

- Add IV cefuroxime and erythromycin if in doubt as to the cause of the pneumonia.
- Refer to an HIV specialist.
- Patient may need high-dose steroids IV if his condition deteriorates.
- Give O_2 to keep O_2 saturation >90%.
- Arrange for induced sputum collection next day.

Progress. This patient improved on antibiotics and his care was taken over by the HIV team.

Case history (4)

A 68-year-old female smoker was admitted by the surgical team 9 days previously with intestinal obstruction. A laparotomy showed severe diverticulitis with a pelvic mass, and a defunctioning colostomy was performed. She has been very slow to mobilise postoperatively and developed a troublesome cough. Two days ago she developed a fever and has now become breathless and tachycardic, with right-sided pleurisy.

Bedside assessment summary:
- Ill-looking patient
- Respiratory rate 24/min
- Pulse 112 bpm regular
- Temperature 40°C
- Coarse crackles right lung base, patchy bronchial breathing
- Pleural rub
- No evidence of DVT
- Recent vomiting
- Recent surgery
- The surgeons gave her 5 days of IV amoxicillin postoperatively. Her NEWS score (see p. 6, Fig. 1.1) has increased to 4.

Investigations revealed:
- CXR: patchy opacification right lung base
- ABGs: PaO_2 7.3, $PaCO_2$ 4.6
- WCC: 16×10^9/L
- Urea: 10 mmol/L
- ECG: sinus tachycardia

What is the diagnosis?

Severe hospital-acquired pneumonia. However, for all cases, remember that:
- DVT with pulmonary emboli might coexist
- Inhalation of vomit causes aspiration pneumonia
- Previous antibiotics could have selected out Gram-negative organisms
- The IV cannula may be infected
- There may be pre-existing lung disease – smoker.

Bacteriology in hospital-acquired pneumonia

There is a wide range of possible organisms:
- Gram-negative bacilli (50%):
  - *Acinetobacter* spp.
  - *Escherichia coli*
  - *Proteus* spp.
  - *Klebsiella* spp.

- *Pseudomonas* spp.
- *Haemophilus influenzae*
- Gram-positive cocci:
  - *Staphylococcus aureus*
  - *Streptococcus pneumoniae*
- Anaerobes:
  - *Bacteroides* spp.
  - *Clostridia* spp.

Management

- Give O_2 to raise O_2 saturation >90%.
- Rehydrate intravenously.
- Give IV antibiotics to cover a wide spectrum:
  - Ceftazidime 2 g × 2 daily and gentamicin 800 mg initially with checks on the blood level.
- If improving after 48 h and able to swallow, switch to:
  - Co-amoxiclav (500/125) 625 mg × 3 daily + oral metronidazole 400 mg × 3 daily.
- Patient is at high risk of PE: low-molecular-weight (LMW) heparin, e.g. enoxaparin 40 mg SC × 1 daily if not already prescribed.
- Watch for deterioration.
- Arrange physiotherapy to encourage cough.
  Progress. She responded slowly and was discharged a week later.

LUNG ABSCESS

This is a severe localized suppuration in the lung. The CXR shows cavity formation, often with the presence of a fluid level (not due to tuberculosis).

The causes of lung abscess include aspiration, particularly amongst alcohol users. Lung abscesses also frequently follow the inhalation of a foreign body into a bronchus. They can also occur when the bronchus is obstructed, e.g. by a bronchial carcinoma. Chronic or subacute lung abscesses can also follow inadequately treated pneumonia.

Case history

A man of 74 presented with a 1-month history of a productive cough with offensive-tasting sputum, malaise and weight loss. His dentition was very poor. He had just stopped smoking.

On examination, he had a temperature of 39.8°C, a few crackles at the right base but no other respiratory signs. A CXR (Fig. 11.9) showed a cavity.

Differential diagnosis

- Lung abscess.
- Cavitating lung cancer.
- Tuberculosis.
  Bronchoscopy showed thick secretions in the right lower lobe. There was no bronchial obstruction and cytology was negative.

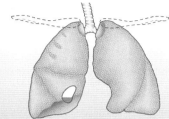

- Thin-walled cavity with fluid level in right lower lobe

Figure 11.9 Diagram of chest X-ray showing a cavity (lung abscess).

Diagnosis

Pyogenic abscess.
   Progress. The patient responded to antibiotics (cefuroxime and metronidazole) and the abscess resolved in 6 weeks. It probably resulted from aspiration, with mouth anaerobes contributing to the unpleasant smell and taste of the sputum. Aspiration usually occurs on the right side, as the right bronchus is more vertical.

TUBERCULOSIS (TB)

Case history (1)

An 18-year-old man who came to the UK 2 years ago from the Indian sub-continent presented with general malaise, photophobia, unproductive cough, weight loss and night sweats.
   On examination, his temperature was 39.5°C. He looked unwell and appeared rather vague. There was no neck stiffness or any abnormal chest signs.
   Investigations revealed Na 120, K 2.6 and urea 2.8, Hb 104 g/L and WCC 6.4; serum ALT and alkaline phosphatase were slightly raised. A portable AP chest film appeared normal.

The patient was admitted with a diagnosis of **pyrexia of unknown origin**. He had blood and urine cultures and CSF examination. CSF showed an increased cell count, mostly lymphocytes, raised protein and low glucose. No organisms were seen but cultures were sent. A departmental PA CXR was performed after 2 days and showed miliary mottling.

This patient has **miliary tuberculosis with meningitis** (TBM). It carries a high morbidity if not treated early. The hyponatraemia is dilutional secondary to inappropriate secretion of anti-diuretic hormone.

What does treatment consist of?

Treatment is with anti-tuberculous drugs – rifampicin, isoniazid and pyrazinamide. These must commence before cultures are available and are continued for at least 9 months. Ethambutol should not be used because of its eye complications. Corticosteroids, e.g. prednisolone 60 mg, are given for the first 3 weeks, as they reduce mortality. Relapses and complications (e.g. seizures, hydrocephalus) are common in TBM. The mortality remains over 60%, even with early treatment.

Progress. This patient was started on anti-tuberculous therapy as described. His mental state improved and temperature settled. He was discharged after 3 weeks with an appointment for 3 weeks later in outpatients.

Case history (2)

A 50-year-old man, who was a heavy drinker with no fixed abode, was brought to A&E 'collapsed'. He had stopped drinking alcohol 1 week previously because he had run out of money. He was confused, hallucinating and coughing, and was transferred to the MAU.

On examination, he was unkempt, emaciated, confused and jaundiced:
- Temperature: 37.9°C
- Pulse: 100 bpm
- BP: 100/60.

On further examination, right upper chest, bronchial breathing + coarse crackles; trachea deviated to the right. The liver was enlarged 3 cm below the costal margin and there was ascites.

Investigations revealed:
- Hb 180 g/L; MCV 106; WCC 8500
- Urea: 1.3
- K⁺: 3.5
- Creatinine: 60, eGFR 98 mL/min
- Na: 126
- Bilirubin: 40
- Alkaline phosphatase and ALT: raised
- CXR: Fig. 11.10.

A provisional differential diagnosis was made of:
- Delirium tremens
- Pulmonary tuberculosis
- Alcoholic liver disease.

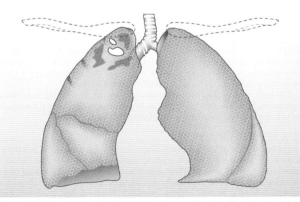

Figure 11.10 Diagram of chest X-ray — patchy opacification with cavitation in right upper lobe and trachea deviated to the right in tuberculosis.

Urgent sputum was sent for staining with auramine—phenol fluorescent test plus culture and sensitivities for AFB (if no organisms are found, send at least three more good sputum specimens). TB bacilli were found in the third sputum specimen (smear-positive).

Risk factors for developing TB reactivation

- Heavy alcohol or other drug use.
- Diabetes mellitus.
- Malnutrition.
- Immunosuppression (any cause, including steroid therapy).

Management

- Isolate patient as smear-positive.
- Treat delirium tremens (see p. 495). *Note:* always give thiamine too.
- Start anti-TB therapy (see later) as soon as possible.
- Notify infection control about the patient and ask the TB health visitor to do contact tracing.

Progress. The patient was started on anti-TB therapy and treatment for his delirium tremens. He needed directly observed treatment (DOT) because he was unlikely to comply with treatment otherwise. He was also referred to the Respiratory and Gastroenterological teams.

Case history (3)

A 64-year-old white male smoker was treated by his doctor with antibiotics for bronchitis 3 months ago. As his cough had not resolved, he was admitted to hospital (MAU) 1 week ago. Initial assessment showed a right upper lobe pneumonia and he was treated with oral amoxicillin and erythromycin. Blood and sputum cultures were negative. He had a persistent low-grade fever and the CXR still showed patchy right upper lobe consolidation. You have been called to see him because he has just had a haemoptysis.

Why is this pneumonia slow to resolve?

Consider:
- Obstructing carcinoma of right upper lobe bronchus:
  - Is there a hilar mass?
  - Should he be bronchoscoped?
- Unusual infecting organism.

Further history

It is always worth retaking the history.
- The patient's mother was treated for pulmonary TB in 1941. He was seen in a chest clinic as a child but does not think that he had drug treatment. He does not recall having BCG vaccination and does not have a BCG scar.
- Pulmonary TB is a possible diagnosis.
- Look carefully at a new PA CXR (Fig. 11.11).

Action

This is TB until proved otherwise.
- Send urgent sputum for auramine staining and TB culture.
- Send at least three sputum specimens.
- Check blood count, liver biochemistry and renal function.

Kumar & Clark's Cases in Clinical Medicine

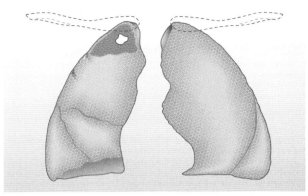

Figure 11.11 Diagram of chest X-ray — right upper lobe consolidation with small apical cavity. This was probably obscured by the clavicle on the previous chest X-ray.

Results

The microbiologist calls you urgently:

- The patient has AFB seen on sputum smear.
- Sputum is being cultured for TB.
- Culture results will be available in 6—8 weeks.
- Sensitivities perhaps may not be available for 12 weeks.

Progress and action

This patient was isolated in a side room (smear-positive).

- Treatment for TB was given (see later).
- TB is a notifiable disease in the UK and allows contact tracing to be initiated.

Case history (4)

A 34-year-old Ugandan refugee presented to A&E with high fever, diarrhoea and weight loss. She omitted to inform the staff that she had been found to be HIV-positive 6 months previously (with a CD count of 250) and had declined further investigation or treatment at that time.

On examination, she appeared unwell and cachectic, and was coughing continuously.

Investigations revealed:

- CXR: right lower lobe shadowing and possible right hilar lymphadenopathy
- Hb 75 g/L; WCC 4.2; lymphocytes 0.8; platelets 156
- Na$^+$ 128; K$^+$ 2.5; urea 11.8; albumin 18.

Blood, stool, sputum and urine cultures were taken and she was admitted to the MAU unit and commenced on amoxicillin and erythromycin. She failed to improve and after 3 days the antibiotics were changed to ciprofloxacin, although sputum culture was unhelpful. On day 5 the microbiologist was consulted: examination of sputum for AFB was positive and *Mycobacterium tuberculosis* was subsequently isolated from blood and stool.

Key points

- Many patients do not volunteer their HIV status.
- You must indicate that *Mycobacterium tuberculosis* is a possibility when requesting sputum examination.
- Atypical radiological changes are common in TB in the immunocompromised.
- Both *Mycobacterium intracellulare avium* and *Mycobacterium tuberculosis* can be isolated from stool and blood.
- A patient from Africa with pneumonia should be admitted to a side room until TB has been excluded.
- The risk of TB developing in those infected (i.e. disease reactivation) in HIV increases when CD count is <200.

Progress. This patient was started on anti-tuberculous therapy. She was taken over by the HIV team and had continued care from the Respiratory team for follow-up and contact tracing.

Treatment — drug therapy in TB

- Rifampicin: if body weight <50 kg, 450 mg daily; if body weight ≥50 kg, 600 mg daily.
- Isoniazid: 300 mg daily.
- Pyrazinamide: if body weight <50 kg, 1.5 g daily; if body weight ≥ 50 kg, 2 g daily.
- Ethambutol: 15 mg/kg (test visual acuity before treatment).
- Give all drugs together once daily with breakfast.
- All four drugs for 2 months followed by rifampicin and isoniazid for 4 months (having checked the sensitivities).
- Tuberculous meningitis: recommended duration 12 months:
  - Four drugs for 3 months; rifampicin + isoniazid for 9 months.
  - Corticosteroids are indicated in tuberculous meningitis, pericarditis and spinal tuberculosis with neurological compression.
  N.B. This patient may have multi-resistant TB (MRTB).

Monitor therapy

- Liver biochemistry.
- Patient compliance with medication.

PLEURAL EFFUSION

This is an excessive accumulation of fluid in the pleural space. It can be detected on X-ray when ≥ 300 mL of fluid is present, and clinically when ≥ 500 mL or more is present. The CXR appearances range from obliteration of the costophrenic angle to dense homogeneous shadows occupying part or all of the hemithorax. Fluid below the lung (a sub-pulmonary effusion) can simulate a raised hemidiaphragm. Fluid in the fissures may resemble an intrapulmonary mass.

Case history (1)

A 63-year-old man presented with a 2-month history of increasing breathlessness and could only walk at a slow pace on the level.

On examination, he showed:

- Reduced chest movement on the left

- Reduced tactile vocal fremitus
- Stony dullness to percussion
- Reduced breath sounds
- Apex beat in anterior axillary line (see Fig. 11.2).

Extra signs to look for

- Clubbing: suggests malignancy.
- Glands in neck.
- Wasting.
- Enlarged liver.

What do you do next?

The patient was admitted to the MAU. A diagnostic aspiration was performed after the procedure was explained to the patient and consent obtained.

A syringe with a 21 G needle was used to obtain 20 mL of fluid. This was sent to the laboratory for:

- Protein/LDH
- Cell count
- Culture, including TB
- Cytology for malignant cells.

Result

- Fluid is blood-stained.
- Fluid protein is >30 g/L, which indicates an exudate.
- Few white cells and mesothelial cells.
- Cultures sterile.
- Malignant cells: probably squamous origin.

  Diagnosis. Malignant pleural effusion. There is an underlying squamous cell carcinoma of the bronchus.

  If the diagnosis had not been obtained on the aspirate, a pleural biopsy and a larger volume of pleural fluid with cytological examination of the spun cellular debris could have been performed.

  If there is still no diagnosis, refer to a respiratory physician.

What next?

- The patient has inoperable lung cancer (malignant cells in fluid).
- Treatment should be discussed at an MDT meeting, concentrating on relieving symptoms and possible chemotherapy.

  Drain the effusion (following explanation and consent) with an intercostal drain, ideally placed over the top of the diaphragm.

  An ultrasound to guide placement is useful. A small-bore (10–14 F) intercostal drain should be the initial choice. Clamp intermittently and limit flow to 1 L in the first hour to reduce the risk of re-expansion pulmonary oedema or discomfort from mediastinal shift. Re-expansion pulmonary oedema occurs much more commonly following re-expansion of the collapsed lung associated with a pneumothorax. It relates to endothelial dysfunction and is therefore not hydrostatic. Diuretics are not helpful and may exacerbate any tendency to hypovolaemic hypotension.

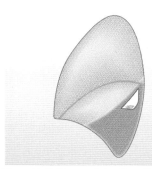

PA aspect –
Homogeneous shadow
rising into the axilla
Fluid level indicates
air/fluid interface =
gas-forming organisms
in the pleural space

Left lateral view –
This is an empyema –
pus in the pleural space.
You cannot aspirate this
with a 'fine' needle!

Figure 11.12 Diagram of chest X-ray (PA and left lateral) of an empyema.

Progress. This man's breathlessness improved after drainage of the effusion and he was discharged with an appointment to see the Palliative Care team.

Case history (2)

A 43-year-old woman developed increasing breathlessness and malaise after being treated for pneumonia with oral cefalexin 2 weeks previously. She was febrile with a temperature of 39°C, flushed and anorexic with signs of a **left pleural effusion**. A pleural tap produced cloudy, infected fluid (an empyema). A diagram of the CXR appearances is shown in Fig. 11.12.

What should you do?

- Drain the fluid by placing an intercostal drain.
- Start antibiotics (after taking blood and fluid cultures). This should cover both aerobic and anaerobic organisms: cefuroxime 1 g IV 6-hourly and metronidazole 500 mg IV 8-hourly for 5 days, followed by oral cefaclor and metronidazole for 2–4 weeks.

- Consult a chest physician/surgeon early if drainage is incomplete. Decortication of the lung or a rib resection and wide-bore drain might be needed.
- Bronchoscopy should be performed to exclude bronchial obstruction. CT scanning is helpful to assess the presence of an underlying lung abscess.

Causes

- Malignancy.
- Mesothelioma.
- Metastatic cancer: breast, bowel.
- Lymphoma.
- Pneumonia.
- Tuberculosis.
- Heart failure.
- Nephrotic syndrome.
- In association with intra-abdominal sepsis or pancreatitis.

Remember

If in doubt:
- Consult a more senior colleague
- Learn under supervision.

Progress. This patient had an **empyema**. She was in hospital for 10 days, as her recovery was slow. She required two further drainages of her empyema but surgery was not necessary. When seen 4 weeks later, she was well.

PULMONARY EMBOLISM (AND DEEP VEIN THROMBOSIS)

Pulmonary embolism (PE) is due to thrombus formed in the systemic veins (rarely, the right side of the heart), which breaks off and embolises in the pulmonary artery. The clinical scenarios depend on whether the emboli block small/medium arteries or the pulmonary artery itself, causing right ventricular obstruction.

The diagnosis of pulmonary embolism can be difficult for a number of reasons:
- It is often not present when thought of.
- It is present when not thought of.
- Presumptive treatment is not without risk.
- Proving the diagnosis may be difficult.

Case history (1)

A 24-year-old woman had been getting breathless for 3 months when referred. Asthma seemed unlikely (peak flow from the referring doctor was 460 L/min) and the CXR was normal. A short pulmonary early diastolic murmur was noted and a Cardiology opinion sought. Spirometry was normal but CO gas transfer was reduced (TL_{CO} 60% predicted). The echocardiographic appearances were normal.

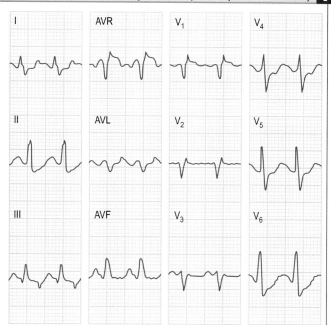

Figure 11.13 Acute pulmonary embolism shown on a 12-lead ECG. (From Feather A, Randall D, Waterhouse M, eds. *Kumar and Clark's Clinical Medicine*, 10th edn. Edinburgh: Elsevier, 2020; Fig. 29.1.)

About 2 weeks later she was admitted in shock. The ECG (Fig. 11.13) showed acute right heart strain (S1, Q3, T3 with dominant R waves in V_1–V_3, and the pulmonary artery diastolic pressure with the right atrial pressure was calculated to be 25 cmH$_2$O (by Doppler echocardiography of the tricuspid regurgitant wave), which is very high.

Diagnosis. This is a **massive pulmonary embolism**.

She was managed on the CCU with alteplase 10 mg IV over 1–2 min, followed by IV infusion of 90 mg over 2 h, and the Doppler echocardiogram used to monitor response. She was anticoagulated with LMW heparin and warfarin.

She responded well to treatment and was returned to the ward.

Progress. A subsequent V̇/Q̇ scan revealed the typical multiple patchy perfusion abnormalities of recurrent minor PE, which explains her 3-month history of breathlessness. The scan has remained abnormal and she has continued to be breathless. Leiden factor V deficiency was discovered and the oral contraceptive stopped. She has been advised to remain on long-term warfarin, although the benefits are disputed.

Other common clinical scenarios caused by pulmonary embolisms

- Acute minor pulmonary infarction producing pleuritic chest pain and possibly haemoptysis.
- Episodic non-specific symptoms in the postoperative patient (such as palpitations and anxiety attacks), possibly followed by a cardiac arrest when at toilet.
- Chronic minor thromboembolism leading to established pulmonary hypertension.

Information

Ninety per cent of patients with a PE have chest pain and/or breathlessness as the major complaint.

The source of dislodged thrombus is most commonly the pelvic or femoral veins, with the classical triad of stasis, hypercoagulopathy or trauma being present in most patients. In some circumstances, air, amniotic fluid, infected clot and even sheared-off IV catheter material may be causal.

Venous thrombosis occurs in 10% of hospitalised patients and was much more common on surgical wards before routine prophylaxis was introduced. Patients with malignancy, advanced cardiorespiratory disease or a past history of venous thrombosis are most at risk.

All medical patients expected to be in bed for more than 3 days should be given DVT prophylaxis. Risk calculation should now guide prophylaxis, which should include pressure stockings as well as heparin (LMW).

Simple investigations

These are usually helpful only when the diagnosis is clinically obvious.
- Plasma D-dimers are very useful; if negative, they rule out PE.
- The ECG or CXR might, however, reveal evidence of alternative causes such as myocardial infarction, pneumothorax or aortic dissection.

Information

An undetectable plasma D-dimer level (reflecting fibrin activation) essentially excludes significant thromboembolism but a raised value is non-specific.

Invasive investigations

CT

Contrast-enhanced, multi-detector CT angiograms (CTAs) have a sensitivity of 83% and specificity of 96%, with a positive predictive value of 92% (higher with 64-multislice scanners).

Radionuclide ventilation/perfusion scanning ($\dot{V}/\dot{Q}$ scan)

This is a good test after measurement of D-dimers. It demonstrates ventilation/perfusion defects, i.e. areas of ventilated lung with perfusion defects. Pulmonary ^{99m}technetium scintigraphy demonstrates the under-perfused areas, while a scintigram, performed after inhalation of radioactive xenon, shows no ventilatory defect. A matched defect may, however, arise with a PE that causes an infarct, or with emphysematous bullae. This test is therefore conventionally reported as a probability (low, medium or high) of PE and should be interpreted in the context of the history, examination and other investigations.

MRI

This gives similar results to CT and is used if CTA is contraindicated.

Echo

The echocardiogram can be very useful in the diagnosis of massive PEs but is of limited value otherwise:

- It might show RV dilatation with paradoxical septal wall movement; pulmonary artery pressure may also be estimated.
- It might exclude or confirm an alternative diagnosis, e.g. cardiac tamponade, LVF.
- RV clot is occasionally imaged and is an adverse prognostic sign, with 10% mortality risk.

Look for DVT. Doppler ultrasound and B-mode venous compression ultrasonography of the legs have largely replaced contrast venography, having sensitivities of 90% and 70%, respectively, for proximal thrombus. They can detect clots in the pelvic or ilio-femoral veins.

Treatment

Supportive therapy with oxygen and analgesia should be given.

In the original trials of IV heparin in patients with obvious clinical venous thrombosis and PE, treatment with heparin reduced mortality from 40% to 7%:

- LMW heparin is licensed for use in DVT and patients with minor PE, e.g. pulmonary infarction, can be treated without admission if the necessary organisation is available in the community. Use unfractionated heparin if rapid reversal is required.
- These treatments only prevent further clot formation.
- Warfarin is started and heparin discontinued once the INR is therapeutic (INR 2–3).
- Six months' warfarin is adequate therapy and 6 weeks might be sufficient in patients with surgery as the provoking factor and no underlying coagulopathy. Anti-thrombin agents, e.g. dabigatran, are being used in place of heparin and warfarin.
- Thrombolytic therapy is used for clot lysis in major PE. There is increasing experience of thrombolytic therapy. Although good evidence of reduced mortality is lacking, there is faster and more complete resolution of echocardiographic abnormalities or $\dot{V}/\dot{Q}$ defects.

Information

Thrombolysis should be used in all patients with cardiogenic shock due to massive PE. You should discuss this with your consultant before treating.

- Emergency embolectomy is rarely a possibility – it can be performed only in cardiothoracic centres.
- Transvenous placement of venocaval filters is used for *recurrent* PE, even though the patient is adequately anti-coagulated.

PNEUMOTHORAX

Case history (1)

A 23-year-old man presented to the A&E department with sudden onset of right-sided chest pain, worse on deep inspiration and associated with acute breathlessness. This started at rest and was not associated with cough. There were no pre-existing medical problems and no other symptoms.

On examination, he was a healthy young man:
- Afebrile, not cyanosed, no signs of DVT
- Pulse rate 100 bpm; respiratory rate 30/min
- Trachea central
- Chest movement reduced right side
- Percussion note hyper-resonant right side
- Breath sounds reduced right side
- Key investigation: CXR (Fig. 11.14), which demonstrated pneumothorax = 1/2 hemithorax.

Key points

Common causes of pleuritic chest pain and dyspnoea are pneumothorax, PE and pneumonia with pleurisy.

Diagnosis

Right-sided spontaneous pneumothorax.

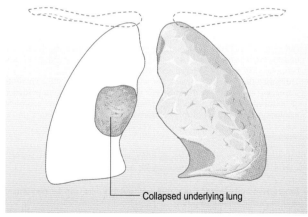

Collapsed underlying lung

Figure 11.14 Diagram of chest X-ray showing collapsed right lung (pneumothorax).

Management of pneumothorax

- If <2 cm: discharge and review next day.
- If there is shortness of breath $\pm$ >2 cm rim on CXR: aspirate.
- If still unsuccessful: insert intercostal drain.

  This man was symptomatic and had a moderate-sized pneumothorax. Aspiration is the first choice. Explain and obtain consent:

Technique for simple aspiration

- Infiltrate with local anaesthetic down to pleura in second intercostal space in mid-clavicular line using 16 FG cannula (or less) at least 3 cm long.
- Once in pleural space, remove needle.
- Connect cannula via three-way tap to chest, 50 mL syringe.
- Stop aspirating when resistance felt, or patient coughs or complains of discomfort, or when 2.5 L aspirated.

  The patient was X-rayed again and the lung was seen to have partially re-expanded.

Further management

The patient was:

- Discharged home after observation and some resolution on CXR, taking his discharge X-ray with him
- Instructed not to fly for 6 weeks or go deep-sea diving
- Given a follow-up appointment in the Chest clinic for 1 week
- Instructed to re-attend (bringing the X-ray) if he became breathless.

  Progress. This man's follow-up X-ray was normal and he has had no further problems.

Case history (2)

A 69-year-old man with long-standing COPD and an exercise tolerance of 100 m on the flat became acutely breathless at rest.

  On examination, he was distressed and cyanosed:

- Using accessory muscles of respiration
- Respiratory rate 40/min
- Pulse 120; BP 100/60
- Barrel-shaped chest with poor expansion
- Hyper-resonant chest with almost inaudible breath sounds.

Main differential diagnoses

- Acute exacerbation of COPD but no obvious infection and symptoms very acute.
- PE.
- Pneumothorax.
- Acute myocardial infarction with LVF.

Action

Urgent CXR and ABGs.

Diagnosis

Life-threatening **tension pneumothorax**: emphysematous lungs with mediastinal shift to the right and complete left pneumothorax.

Management

- Controlled oxygen as per blood gases.
- Urgent insertion of cannula, followed by insertion of intercostal tube.

MANAGEMENT OF INTERCOSTAL TUBE
Insertion of tube

- Explain and reassure patient throughout; obtain consent
- Pre-medicate with opiate and atropine to prevent reflex bradycardia, particularly if patients are anxious, in those with pre-existing lung disease
- Double-check site of pneumothorax
- Site: 4th–6th intercostal space in anterior axillary line — mark with pen and position patient supine with head at 30° and arm abducted to 90°
- Wear sterile gloves
- Drain 10–14 FG (adult). Check assembly and tight connection, and make sure that underwater seal is ready
- Local anaesthetic:
  - Intradermal bleb in appropriate intercostal space
  - Infiltrate deeper with blue then green needle to parietal pleura at upper surface of rib; N.B. neurovascular bundle runs along lower surface
  - Use 5–10 mL 1% lidocaine
  - Check intermittently if in pleural space (air aspirated into syringe).

Insertion of drain

- Make 1–2 cm incision in skin and subcutaneous fat
- Insert two horizontal sutures across incision (leave loose for subsequent sealing of wound on drain site)
- Make wide tract through intercostal muscles down to and through pleura by blunt dissection with forceps (not sharp trocar)
- Insert tube using Seldinger technique and drain assembly without force
- Withdraw metal needle 5 cm and advance tube in apical direction
- Remove metal needle and connect tube to underwater seal
- Secure tube firmly with one or two sutures (1 loop through skin and 4 times round tube); purse string suturing no longer advised as it leaves unsightly scarring
- Loop tube and secure to skin with plaster (*Note:* no kinks)
- Prescribe adequate oral/IM analgesia.

Removal of tube

- Leave tube draining until no further bubbling and then X-ray again (X-ray earlier if in doubt about site or efficacy of tube). *Note:* if level is not swinging, tube is blocked. Clear or replace if lung is not re-expanded
- Some patients need pre-medication for tube removal
- Remove holding suture and withdraw while patient breath-holds in expiration
- Seal wound with one of original sutures
- Observe overnight and if no recurrence of pneumothorax (clinical and X-ray) discharge with Chest clinic appointment in 7–10 days. Patient keeps last X-ray to bring to appointment or to A&E in emergency.

Progress. A CXR at the Chest clinic at 10 days showed full expansion of the lungs. The patient was asymptomatic but apprehensive about having a recurrence. He was reassured that this was unlikely.

CARCINOMA OF THE BRONCHUS

Case history

A 53-year-old male presents with a history of coughing up blood a few hours ago. He has been smoking 20 cigarettes a day for the past 30 years.

On examination, there are diminished breath sounds at the right upper chest anteriorly.

What is the most likely diagnosis and why?

Carcinoma of the bronchus:
* Cigarette smoking is the most common risk factor.
* It is a common cause of haemoptysis in smokers >40 years of age.
* Physical sign of diminished breath sounds suggests bronchial obstruction.

Information

CARCINOMA OF THE BRONCHUS
* Most common form of cancer in both sexes
* Non-small-cell:
  * Squamous cell carcinoma (39%)
  * Large cell carcinoma (10–15%)
  * Adenocarcinoma (25%)
  * Alveolar cell carcinoma (2%)
* Small-cell (20–30%)

What are the diagnostic investigations?

* CXR.
* Sputum cytology.
* Bronchoscopy for histological diagnosis.
* CT.

If histological diagnosis is not made on bronchoscopy, CT-guided percutaneous needle biopsy should be performed.

Radiological manifestations of lung cancer

Screening for lung cancer has been shown in many studies to be ineffective in reducing the mortality rate. CXR is the first diagnostic screening investigation for lung cancer. Evidence on CXR depends on:
* Location of the tumour
* Its effect on neighbouring tissues:
  * Central lung shadow: about 70% of cancers, mostly small-cell and squamous cell, arise centrally and present as a shadow in the hilar region and/or in the mediastinum due to involvement of lymph nodes (Fig. 11.15).

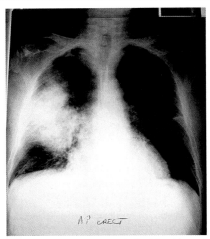

Figure 11.15 Chest X-ray showing a shadow in the right mid-zone (note the area of consolidation with irregular margins).

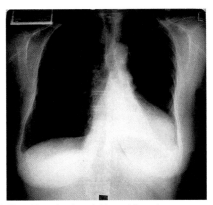

Figure 11.16 Chest X-ray showing a left lower lobe collapse.

- Peripheral lung shadow: some tumours, especially adenocarcinoma, appear as a rounded shadow in the periphery.
- Collapse of lung parenchyma: centrally located tumours often result in collapse of a lobe by obstruction of the bronchus (Figs. 11.16 and 11.17).

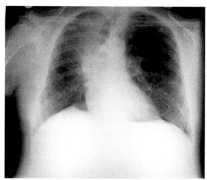

Figure 11.17 X-ray showing right upper lobe collapse.

- Collapsed whole left lung (Fig. 11.18). *N.B.* Collapse of whole lung is also seen postoperatively due to retained sputum.
- Pleural effusion: a large pleural effusion is almost always due to invasion of pleura by malignant cells and its presence is a contraindication to surgical resection. A small pleural effusion might occur without invasion of malignant cells and hence surgical resection may still be considered.
- Rib erosion: the classic presentation is erosion of the first rib seen with an apical neoplasm (Pancoast tumour), often associated with Horner's syndrome. Rib erosion itself is not a contraindication to surgical resection.

Low-dose CT screening has been shown to reduce mortality.

Other presentations are:

- Cachexia or metastatic disease
- Raised hemidiaphragm due to phrenic nerve palsy.

Differential diagnosis

Pneumonia

The possibility of lung cancer should be considered in a smoker with shadow on CXR diagnosed as due to pneumonia:

- Presence of lobar collapse on CXR
- Irregular margins of the lung shadow representing consolidation
- Absence of constitutional symptoms associated with pneumonia
- Symptoms such as haemoptysis and weight loss prior to the development of pneumonia, especially in a middle-aged or elderly smoker.

The patient should be investigated for lung cancer if:

- He/she does not respond to treatment, especially if there are risk factors such as smoking and susceptible age group
- Satisfactory radiological resolution has not occurred 6 weeks following treatment for pneumonia resulting in clinical response.

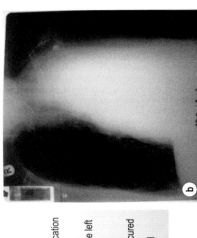

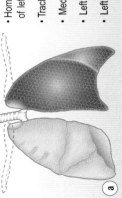

- Homogeneous opacification of left hemithorax
- Trachea deviated to the left
- Mediastinal shift
- Left heart border obscured
- Left diaphragm raised

Figure 11.18 Diagram (a) and chest X-ray (b) showing a complete collapse of the left lung. Note that the mediastinum has been shifted to the left.

Tuberculosis

- TB is more often seen in the young age group.
- Constitutional symptoms such as low-grade pyrexia and night sweats are often present in TB.
- Cavitation is uncommon in lung cancer but may occur in the squamous cell type. The wall of the cavity is thick and irregular in lung cancer.

Management

For practical purposes, carcinoma of the bronchus can be divided into:
- Small-cell lung cancer (SCLC): this is rarely operable.
- Non-small-cell lung cancer (NSCLC).

Management of major complications

Hypercalcaemia (see p. 424)

- IV fluids: 3–4 L.
- Diuretic: furosemide 40 mg IV (ensure adequately rehydrated).
- IV pamidronate: treatment of choice.

Weakness of legs

This suggests spinal cord compression and is a medical emergency, especially with bladder or bowel dysfunction:
- Start dexamethasone 4 mg × 3 daily
- MRI scan of the spine and referral for radiotherapy / surgery.

Stridor

This is due to obstruction above the level of the carina (demonstrated in a flow volume loop):
- Start dexamethasone 4 mg × 3 daily
- Urgent bronchoscopy followed by CT scan of the chest / neck
- Intraluminal growth: referral for laser therapy / stenting
- Extrinsic compression: referral for radiotherapy / stenting.

Superior venocaval obstruction

- Start on dexamethasone 4 mg × 3 daily.
- Refer for radiotherapy.
- Consider heparin or thrombolysis.

What treatments can be offered to a patient?

All patients should be referred to an MDT for discussion of management, which is then discussed fully with the patient before decisions are made.

Progress. This man was found to have non-small-cell carcinoma of the bronchus, squamous cell type. The MDT consensus was that surgery was not an option. He was given radiotherapy followed by chemotherapy. Follow-up at 6 months showed deterioration of his condition and he was referred to the Palliative Care team.

Small-cell lung cancer

Prognostic factors. The staging of SCLC is divided into limited and extensive disease. Systemic therapy is the primary therapeutic modality because of the usually disseminated nature of the disease.

SCLC

- Limited disease: tumour confined to one hemithorax and ipsilateral supraclavicular node
- Extensive disease: involvement of any site outside the hemithorax

Treatment. *Limited disease* is present in approximately 30% of patients. It is best treated with concurrent chemo- and radiotherapy using a combination of cisplatin and etoposide or irinotecan, which increases the survival at 5 years from 15% to 25% compared with radiotherapy alone. A similar degree of improvement can also be achieved with hyperfractionated radiotherapy. Prophylactic whole-brain radiation to prevent cerebral metastases can reduce symptomatic CNS disease and improve overall survival by 5%.

Extensive disease can be palliated with the combination of carboplatin and etoposide or irinotecan; when compared with best supportive care, this can increase median survival from 6 months to 9–13 months and 2-year survival to 20%.

- Severe pain: potent analgesics, e.g. opiates, including fentanyl.
- Bone pain:
  - NSAIDs
  - Local radiotherapy.
- Nerve root pain:
  - Amitriptyline
  - Carbamazepine.

Management of patients with neutropenia following chemotherapy

- Blood (preferably two samples from two different sites) and urine cultures
- CXR
- Culture from any suspected site of infection, e.g. cannula exit site, sputum

Indications for antibiotic therapy
- Absolute neutrophil count <1.0/total WCC <2.5.
- Pyrexia.

Recommended antibiotic regimens
- IV gentamicin 3–5 mg/kg IV once a day (monitor trough levels) and a ureidopenicillin (piperacillin with tazobactam 4.5 g every 6 h).
- In the presence of severe renal insufficiency, replace gentamicin with IV ceftazidime 1–2 g × 3 daily or ciprofloxacin 400 mg × 2 daily.
- Continue antibiotics for 5 days or until WCCs are in normal range and symptoms have remitted.

If no improvement after 48–72 h of antibiotic therapy
- Repeat blood and urine cultures and CXR.
- Consider the following infections:
  - Fungus: blood and urine cultures. Start fluconazole and/or amphotericin

- Protozoa: broncho-alveolar lavage
- Virus: viral serology
- Resistant staphylococcus: more common with central venous catheter; treat with vancomycin.

Indications for filgrastim (recombinant human granulocyte-colony stimulating factor, rhG-CSF)

This is for specialist use only:
- Absolute neutrophil count: 0.2
- Persistent neutropenia (<1.0 for >48 h)
- Stop therapy when absolute neutrophil count is ≥1.5.

SARCOIDOSIS

Sarcoidosis is a multi-system granulomatous disorder of unknown aetiology. It commonly presents with bilateral lymphadenopathy, pulmonary infiltration, and skin and eye lesions.

Case history (1)

You are phoned by a primary care physician who has a 28-year-old woman in the clinic with tender, bluish lumps on the front of her legs. She also complains of stiffness of the ankles and a temperature. The doctor thinks that this is erythema nodosum (EN) but would like another opinion.

Is this EN?

From the description this sounds very likely and you ask the doctor to send the patient up to outpatients, where you will arrange for a CXR to be performed (Fig. 11.19).

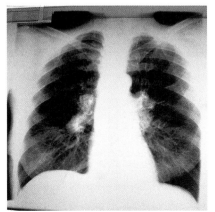

Figure 11.19 Bilateral hilar lymph node enlargement in sarcoidosis.

EN with lymphadenopathy on CXR is a characteristic presentation of **sarcoidosis**. When it presents along with arthritis and fever, it is called Löfgren's syndrome.

In outpatients, the patient poses several questions on hearing her diagnosis.

What is sarcoidosis?

You explain that this is a well-recognised disorder for which no cause is known. You emphasise, however, that in her case the skin rash (EN) will subside within 2 months but the CXR might take up to a year to revert to normal. No treatment is required other than pain relief. The chances of further trouble are negligible.

You discuss this later with your consultant, who reminds you of the extrapulmonary manifestations that can be troublesome (**skin and ocular lesions** are most common):

- **Skin lesions:** 10% of cases. Apart from EN, a chilblain-like lesion (lupus pernio) and nodules are seen.
- **Eye involvement:** 5% of cases. Anterior uveitis (misting of vision, pain, red eye) is common. Posterior uveitis may present with a progressive loss of vision. Conjunctivitis and retinal lesions are seen. Asymptomatic uveitis may be found in 25% of patients.
- **Metabolic hypercalcaemia:** found in 10% but rarely severe.
- **CNS involvement:** rare (2%) but can lead to severe neurological disease.
- **Bone and joint involvement:** arthralgia without EN is seen in 5% of cases.
- **Cardiac involvement:** rare (3%) clinically, although seen in 20% of post-mortems. Ventricular arrhythmias, conduction defects and cardiomyopathy with congestive cardiac failure are seen. The serum ACE is insensitive in cardiac sarcoid and echocardiography should be performed in chronic sarcoidosis.

Your consultant does say that the above list is comprehensive but fortunately the conditions are rare.

Progress. The patient made a good recovery and her EN settled after 2 weeks. A follow-up CXR at 6 months was normal.

Case history (2)

You are contacted by the ENT registrar because he has seen a 48-year-old patient with nasal stuffiness and a blocked nose. He had also noted some blood-stained nasal discharge. An X-ray of the patient's sinuses shows destruction of the nasal bones. He wants you to see the patient because he found out that this man has had long-standing **pulmonary sarcoidosis**. As you walk to the ENT ward, you go over your knowledge of sarcoidosis, remembering that patients with upper respiratory tract involvement usually have pulmonary disease.

On arrival on the wards you retake the history: the patient has been breathless for years and tells you that all his numerous CXRs show that his lungs are 'full of sarcoid'. He has not been on steroids because of their lack of efficacy and side-effects, which have made him non-compliant.

On examination, he is noticeably breathless and cyanosed. Chest examination shows widespread crackles.

You arrange to give the patient oxygen by ordinary face mask (4 L/min).

Investigations are as follows:

- CXR
- FBC:
  - A mild normochromic normocytic anaemia
  - Low lymphocyte count $\pm$ low neutrophils
  - Thrombocytopenia
- Blood gases: PO_2 6.8 kPa, pCO_2 4.3 kPa.

The next morning you return with your consultant, having obtained the patient's old notes.

You note multiple CXRs showing widespread pulmonary infiltration with no hilar lymphadenopathy. The latest CXR also shows a rounded opacity in the right apex — thought to be an aspergilloma.

Fibre-optic bronchoscopy with transbronchial biopsies was performed 10 years ago. This showed epithelial and giant cell granulomas (this test has a 90% sensitivity with pulmonary infiltration).

Lung function tests showed:

- Reduced total lung capacity (restrictive ventilatory capacity)
- Impaired gas transfer (TLCO)
- Low compliance
- Raised serum ACE level: done a few years ago.

Review of his past treatment shows that he has been given steroids on many occasions and azathioprine and methotrexate as steroid-sparing agents.

Your consultant congratulates you on your review of the notes, which is crucial for the future management of this case. In a patient with such severe disease, he suggests you start high-dose steroids and then a trial of azathioprine and infliximab, for which there is some evidence of efficiency.

Progressive respiratory failure is well recognised in sarcoidosis. Unfortunately, recurrence in the transplanted lung (as well as limited availability of organs) has led many centres not to consider transplantation for end-stage pulmonary fibrosis. Lung transplantation may be indicated if this patient fails to improve.

Progress. This man's chest condition remained static, despite a further trial of steroids and azathioprine. He continues to be breathless but is coping, for the moment. He has been referred to the Transplant team for assessment in view of his young age.

Further reading

Breathlessness and wheeze

British Thoracic Society/Scottish Intercollegiate Guidelines Network. British Guideline on the Management of Asthma. 2019. https://www.brit-thoracic.org.uk/quality-improvement/guidelines/.

Respiratory failure

British Thoracic Society/Intensive Care Society. Guidelines for the Respiratory Management of Acute Hypercapnic Respiratory Failure in Adults. 2016. https://www.brit-thoracic.org.uk/quality-improvement/guidelines/.

Roberts CM, Brown JL, Reinhardt AK, et al. Non-invasive ventilation in COPD: management of acute type 2 respiratory failure. *Clinical Medicine* 2008; **8**: 517–521.

COPD – acute exacerbation

British Thoracic Society/NICE. Guideline – COPD in Over-16s. 2019. https://www.brit-thoracic.org.uk/quality-improvement/guidelines/copd/.

Tuberculosis

Bloom BR. A neglected epidemic. *New England Journal of Medicine* 2018; **378**: 291–293.

WHO Global tuberculosis report 2019. https://www.who.int/tb/publications/global_report/en/.

Pleural effusion

British Thoracic Society Pleural Disease Guideline Group. BTS Pleural Disease Guideline 2010. *Thorax* 2010; 65 (Suppl II). Available at https://thorax.bmj.com/content/65/Suppl_2#BTSPleuralDiseaseGuideline2010.

Feller-Kopman D, Light R. Pleural disease. *New England Journal of Medicine* 2018; **378**: 740–751.

Pulmonary embolism (and deep vein thrombosis)

Agnelli G. Current concepts: acute pulmonary embolism. *New England Journal of Medicine* 2010; **363**: 266–284.

Millar CM, Laffan MD. Drug therapy in anticoagulation: which drug for which patient? *Clinical Medicine* 2017; **3**: 233–244.

Pneumothorax

MacDuff A, Arnold A, Harvey J. Management of spontaneous pneumothorax: British Thoracic Society Pleural Disease Guideline 2010. *Thorax* 2010; ii18–ii31. Available at https://thorax.bmj.com/content/65/Suppl_2#BTSPleuralDiseaseGuideline2010.

Carcinoma of the bronchus

Goldstraw P, Ball D, Jett JR, et al. Non-small-cell lung cancer. *Lancet* 2011; **378**: 1727–1740.

National Institute of Health and Care Excellence (NICE). Lung cancer: diagnosis and management. NICE guideline 122. 2019. http://www.nice.org.uk/guidance/ng122.

Van Meerbeeck JP, Fennell DA, De Ruysscher DK. Small-cell lung cancer. *Lancet* 2011; **378**: 1741–1755.

British Thoracic Society guidelines. www.brit-thoracic.org.uk/guidelines.

Royal College of Radiologists: Guidelines on the Non-Surgical Management of Lung Cancer. www.rcr.ac.uk.

SHOCK

Case history (1)

A 60-year-old bank manager presents with crushing central chest pain. This started 45 min ago and has remained constant ever since.

On examination, he is pale and clammy. His pulse is 100/min and poor-volume, and his BP is 90/60.

Diagnosis. Shock – **cardiogenic**; the ECG shows evidence of anterior myocardial infarction (MI).

Case history (2)

A 50-year-old man who works in a bar has been brought to hospital, vomiting a large amount of blood. He gave no history of upper abdominal pain but did admit to drinking a bottle of whisky a day and occasional beers as well.

He also reveals a previous hospital admission with abdominal swelling, which was due to alcoholic liver disease. He was told that his liver disease was bad and that he must stop drinking and take propranolol regularly, as he had varices on endoscopy. He had not stopped drinking, nor was he taking his propranolol.

On examination, he is sweating profusely with visible shaking of his extremities. His pulse rate is 120/min with a BP of 90/60.

Diagnosis. Shock – **hypovolaemia** due to blood loss, probably from oesophageal varices.

Remember

- Shock is a life-threatening condition in which the patient is suffering global hypoxic injury.
- Establish a clear airway.
- Oxygen must be given immediately to all haemodynamically unstable patients.

Physiology (Fig. 12.1)

Shock is 'inadequate tissue oxygenation' where there is failure of the circulatory system due to:

- Failure of the heart to maintain an adequate cardiac output, e.g. MI
- Reduction in the volume of blood within the circulation, e.g. haemorrhage
- Loss of vascular tone within the circulatory system, e.g. sepsis
- Obstruction to the circulation, e.g. pulmonary embolism.

Causes of shock

- Cardiogenic: MI, tamponade, aortic dissection, pulmonary embolism.
- Sepsis: infective causes, e.g. pneumonia, urinary tract infection, meningococcal septicaemia or 'systemic inflammation', resulting from trauma, surgery or anaphylaxis.

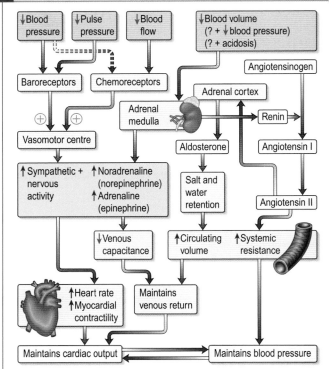

Figure 12.1 The sympatho-adrenal response to shock, showing the effect of increased catecholamines on the left of the diagram and the release of angiotensin and aldosterone on the right. Both mechanisms result in maintaining the BP and cardiac output in shock.

- Hypovolaemia: profound dehydration, haemorrhage.
- Distributive shock: anaphylactic shock
  - Signs of profound vasodilatation: warm peripheries, low BP, tachycardia
  - Erythema, urticaria, angio-oedema, pallor, cyanosis
  - Bronchospasm, rhinitis
  - Oedema of the face, pharynx and larynx
  - Pulmonary oedema
  - Hypovolaemia due to vascular leak
  - Nausea, vomiting, abdominal cramps, diarrhoea.

Ideally, 10 mL of clotted blood should be taken within 45–60 min of the reaction for confirmation of the diagnosis: e.g. by measurement of the mast cell tryptase. Serum should be separated and stored at -20°C. Follow-up of these patients is essential.

Distributive shock: sepsis, severe sepsis and septic shock (see p. 3)

Definition of sepsis (adapted from 3rd International Consensus: Sepsis-3)

- Sepsis is defined as life-threatening organ dysfunction caused by a dysregulated host response to infection.
- Organ dysfunction (severe sepsis) can be identified as an acute change in total SOFA (Sequential Organ Failure Assessment) score of >2 points consequent to the infection:

  The baseline SOFA score can be assumed to be 0 in patients not known to have pre-existing organ dysfunction.

  A SOFA score of >2 reflects an overall mortality risk of approximately 10% in a general hospital population with suspected infection. Patients presenting with modest dysfunction can deteriorate further.
- Patients with suspected infection who are likely to have a prolonged ICU stay or to die in the hospital can be promptly identified at the bedside with qSOFA (quick SOFA), i.e. alteration in mental status, systolic BP ≤ 100 mmHg or respiratory rate of ≥ 22/min.
- Septic shock is a subset of sepsis, in which underlying circulatory and cellular/metabolic abnormalities are profound enough to increase mortality substantially.
- Patients with septic shock can be identified by a clinical construct of sepsis with persisting hypotension requiring vasopressors to maintain mean arterial pressure (MAP) ≥ 65 mmHg and having a serum lactate level >2 mmol/L (18 mg/dL), despite adequate volume resuscitation. On these criteria, hospital mortality is in excess of 40% (Table 12.1).

Symptoms and signs

- Pyrexia and rigors, or hypothermia (unusual, but more common in the elderly and associated with worse prognosis).
- Nausea, vomiting.
- Vasodilatation, warm peripheries.
- Bounding pulse.
- Rapid capillary refill.
- Hypotension, low diastolic pressure, widened pulse pressure.

Table 12.1 The relationship of lactate level in sepsis to mortality

Lactate (mmol/L)	Mortality
<2	15%
2–4	25%
>4	38%

From Trzeciak S, Dellinger RP, Chansky ME, et al. Serum lactate as a predictor of mortality in patients with infection. *Intensive Care Medicine* 2007; **33**: 970–977.

- Occasionally, signs of cutaneous vasoconstriction.
- Other signs:
  - Jaundice
  - Coma, stupor
  - Bleeding due to coagulopathy
  - Rash and meningism
  - Hyper- or hypoglycaemia.

Remember

A patient might have more than one cause of shock, e.g. Case 2 may have an alcoholic cardiomyopathy (pump failure) as well as haematemesis (decreased blood volume).

Is the shock state in Case 1 due to MI, an obstructed circulation or other shock-inducing factors?

A history in a shocked patient of chest pain associated with ECG evidence of an **MI** makes the diagnosis in this case. However, be careful because ECG changes with tachyarrhythmias and some ST segment changes that look characteristic of myocardial ischaemia can also occur in other types of shock.

Is the shock state in Case 2 due to fluid loss? If so, what fluid and from where?

In this case the blood loss is obvious, i.e. haematemesis. Ask the patient to estimate how much was lost. In other cases, blood loss might be concealed, e.g. pancreatitis.

Clinical examination

In assessing the shocked patient the following indices should be monitored:
- Pulse rate and respiratory rate
- Peripheral venous filling/capillary filling
- Limb temperature
- Arterial BP
- Urinary output
- Mental status.

Investigations

- HB and haematocrit, U&Es, liver biochemistry, troponin estimation
- Serum lactate
- ECG and monitor
- CVP (see p. 208)
  - If the CVP is low (<5 mmHg), fluid replacement is necessary
  - If 10 mmHg or more, fluid replacement is probably not required immediately.

Case 1 has a problem with the circulatory pump and probably needs no extra intra-vascular fluid administration.

Case 2 – the haematemesis patient – has lost circulating volume with a low CVP. His problems are with the plumbing circuit, not the heart pump, but his condition might be compounded by coagulation and biochemical disturbances consequent on hepatic insufficiency.

Other investigations (Fig. 12.2)

- Arterial blood gas analysis: in hypovolaemic shock (as in all shock states): there is a metabolic acidosis with a high hydrogen ion concentration and low bicarbonate concentration. In cases with respiratory complications the PO_2 and PCO_2 values will help indicate the need for ventilatory support.
- Lactate levels: serum lactate levels rise approximately in proportion to the severity of the shock.
- X-rays: these are usually of little value in the acute stages of shock management. A CXR will exclude any treatable pathology, such as a pneumothorax or haemothorax, which often complicate insertion of monitoring lines. A CT scan may be helpful in, for example, a case of trauma.

How would you treat?

Both patients should be admitted to high-dependency nursing units in the first instance:

- NEWS score (see p. 6, Fig. 1.1).
- Sequential Organ Failure Assessment (SOFA)
- qSOFA (outside ICU) bedside test:
  - Respiratory rate $\geq 22/min$
  - Altered mentation (GCS) ↓
  - Systolic BP ≤ 100.

  If the score is >2, to outreach CCU and then admit to CCU

Case 1

In cardiogenic hypotension, the key issues are pain relief, arrhythmia management and treatment of pulmonary oedema. Pain relief with incremental doses of IV opiates will aid reduction in myocardial oxygen consumption. Correcting electrolyte disturbances and hypoxia, and controlling angina pain might assist in arrhythmia management. Temporary transvenous pacing might be required for significant bradycardia. Continuous infusion of vasodilators (e.g. glyceryl trinitrate $10-200 \mu g/min$) plus diuretics (e.g. furosemide 40 mg) is needed for pulmonary oedema. Acute revascularisation (thrombolysis, angioplasty) might also be indicated. In the context of persistent hypotension, infusion of inotropic agents such as dobutamine (e.g. $2.5-10 \mu g/kg$ per min) might be necessary while correctable abnormalities are sought (e.g. acute mitral regurgitation following papillary muscle rupture or the development of an ischaemic ventricular septal defect). Percutaneous insertion of an intra-aortic balloon counterpulsation pump may be necessary for refractory cardiogenic hypotension following transfer to a specialist centre as a prelude to surgical intervention.

Progress. This man initially improved on inotropes, diuretics and vasodilator therapy. However, he remained hypotensive, with a BP <90 and poor output. He was transferred to the Cardiac Centre for insertion of an intra-aortic balloon pump. He did not respond and died 3 days later (mortality is 79% for cardiogenic shock).

Information

Patients at risk of further deterioration will have one or more of the following vital signs, which would indicate transfer to an ITU:

- Heart rate >120 bpm

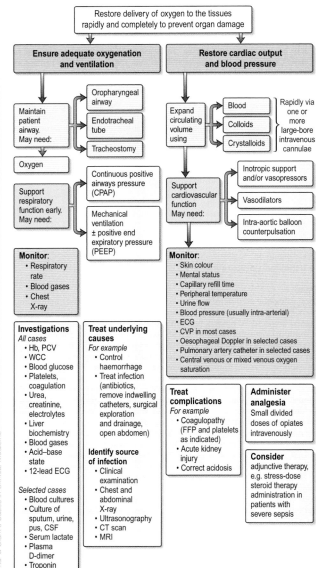

Figure 12.2 Management of shock. Patients require intensive nursing care. FFP, fresh frozen plasma.

- Heart rate <40 bpm
- Systolic blood pressure >200 mmHg
- Systolic blood pressure <80 mmHg
- Respiratory rate >30/min
- Respiratory rate <8/min
- Oxygen saturation <90%
- GCS <8
- Core temperature >39°C
- Core temperature <35°C
- Urine output <0.5 mL/kg per h for 2 consecutive h.

Case 2

In hypovolaemic hypotension the principal issues are reduction in further fluid loss and simultaneous restoration of fluid volumes via wide-bore intravenous cannulae. Infusion of red cells provides sufficient oxygen transport capacity (a target of 70–90 g/L is broadly accepted). Fresh frozen plasma (e.g. to obtain a target INR of <1.5) might be necessary. At the earliest opportunity the patient with haematemesis will require endoscopy to find the bleeding lesion and treat it (see p. 65).

Progress. This man was successfully resuscitated and variceal banding was performed at endoscopy. He left hospital after 7 days and was referred to the local Liver Unit for consideration of liver transplantation (Child Grade C alcoholic liver disease). He did not attend the clinic. He was re-admitted 6 weeks later in hepatic coma and died.

Case history (3)

A 68-year-old man is brought to A&E by ambulance. His wife says that he developed abdominal pain 4 days ago, which has grown progressively worse. He has always suffered from indigestion and pain in the stomach area after food, for which he has taken antacids with some relief.

On this occasion the pains became worse, and she said her husband had refused to get out of bed and appeared to be confused and disorientated. She had called an ambulance, which brought him to hospital.

On examination, he was pyrexial at 39°C. He was pale, unsure of his surroundings and moaning about his abdominal pain. His pulse was 120 bpm with a BP of 90/40, and he had a cold nose. He was breathless and his O_2 saturations were 90%.

Abdominal examination revealed a distended abdomen, tender to the touch, with absent bowel sounds.

What is the cause of shock in this patient?

The patient has septic shock, probably secondary to intra-abdominal sepsis. He will need fluid resuscitation, urgent investigations and probably a laparotomy.

How would you manage this case? (see Fig. 12.2)

Immediate action

- ABCDE.
- Correct hypoxaemia: high-flow O_2 via a face mask.
- Determine cause: examination, CXR and AXR, ECG, arterial blood gases, FBC, U&Es, amylase, blood cultures.

- IV access.
- Initiate treatment: IV fluid resuscitation with 0.9% saline, inotropes if no response to fluid resuscitation.
- Insert a urinary catheter and monitor urinary output.

Shock is a medical emergency. The longer it persists, the lower the chance of recovery because secondary injury, from coexistent hypoxaemia and delayed reperfusion, is now recognised to cause further cytokine activation and the development of multiple organ failure (MOF).

Information

The medical records of many patients admitted to the ICU from the ward show progressive evidence of impending collapse — increasing heart rate, oliguria, tachypnoea or confusion.

Act before shock has become established!

Pathophysiology of septic shock

In sepsis, hypotension primarily results from impaired vascular tone. Sympathetic activation often leads to a high cardiac output with a low systemic vascular resistance. Hypovolaemia can occur from interstitial fluid losses due to widespread endothelial dysfunction and reduced venous tone. In more profound sepsis, myocardial depression also occurs due to circulating cytokines such as tumour necrosis factor (TNF).

Further management

- Early antibiotic therapy, e.g. piperacillin with tazobactam, as it was felt to be an upper GI perforation.
- Attempted early control of the source of infection: seek a surgical opinion for treatment of the abdominal condition.
- Central line for CVP measurement.
- Titration of fluid resuscitation to provide adequate cardiac output with good urine output.
- Inotropic support: give dopexamine, a dopamine analogue which is useful in patients with septic shock, as in this man with a low cardiac output and peripheral vasoconstriction.
- Continuous positive airway pressure (CPAP) or intubation and intermittent positive-pressure ventilation (IPPV).
- Early recourse to stress-dose steroid therapy if requiring vasoconstrictor therapy.
- Control of blood sugar with insulin.

Summary

Timely intervention in patients with sepsis might prevent the progression of shock. Fluid resuscitation and treatment aimed at the primary cause should be instituted rapidly and high-flow oxygen given to limit regional hypoxaemia. Prognosis is dependent on cause and response to treatment. For instance, mortality from urinary sepsis has a better prognosis than a similar clinical situation resulting from peritonitis.

Progress. This man had peritonitis secondary to a perforated ulcer. He was resuscitated and admitted to the ITU. He later had a laparotomy (a laparoscopic surgeon was unavailable) with washout of the peritoneum and oversewing of the ulcer, and an omental patch. He remained in the ITU, needing inotropic support and ventilation for 4 days, and was then transferred to the ward. He eventually made a good recovery. *Helicobacter pylori* eradication was given.

ACUTE RESPIRATORY DISTRESS SYNDROME (ARDS)

Case history

You are called urgently to A&E when on take. A 35-year-old known drug user has been sent urgently to the hospital, having been found unconscious. The GCS is 5 and BP 100/60, with a respiratory rate of 20/min; SaO_2 on high-flow O_2 therapy is 85%.

What are the possible causes of depressed consciousness and what are your immediate actions?

- You need to consider intoxication, hypoglycaemia, respiratory failure, head injury or a post-ictal state.

  On examination, look for evidence of focal neurological signs, pinpoint pupils, trauma to the head or evidence of seizures such as tongue laceration or incontinence.

- Ensure the airway is not obstructed, establish IV access, and take blood gases, blood glucose, and blood and urine for toxicology.

  Arterial blood gas analysis reveals pH 7.2, PaO_2 6.4, $PaCO_2$ 2.5 and lactate 4.1 mmol/L.

What do these results indicate?

Acute type 1 **respiratory failure** with a metabolic (lactic) acidosis.

There is vomitus around the patient's mouth and on his clothing. The CXR shows patchy shadowing at the right base.

Following naloxone administration, he becomes agitated, moving all limbs, but does not respond purposely to command.

What is the immediate management?

Respiratory failure is probably related to aspiration of vomitus. Intubation and IPPV are indicated. CPAP or non-invasive ventilation are contraindicated because of the danger of further vomiting and lack of cooperation.

The man was transferred to the ICU. On the post-take ward round next morning, ventilatory pressures are high for standard tidal volumes and he remains hypoxic on F_iO_2 100%. Your consultant suggests that you make a short presentation on ARDS to the students at the lunch-time meeting.

Key features of ARDS (Berlin definition)

See Fig. 12.3:
- Pulmonary infiltrates: due to an increase in lung interstitial fluid not related to heart failure; by definition, pulmonary artery occlusion pressure <18 mmHg.
- A reduction in pulmonary compliance: i.e. stiff lungs, resulting in high inflation pressures.
- Profound gas exchange abnormalities defined as $PaO_2 : F_iO_2$ ratio (Table 12.2), all with positive end-expiratory pressure (PEEP) ≥ 5 cm H_2O.

Causes

- Severe sepsis, e.g. peritonitis, septicaemia.
- Pulmonary aspiration (as in this case).

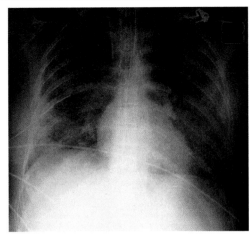

Figure 12.3 CXR appearances in acute respiratory distress syndrome (ARDS). Bilateral diffuse alveolar shadowing with air bronchograms and no cardiac enlargement. (From Feather A, Randall D, Waterhouse M, eds. *Kumar and Clark's Clinical Medicine*, 10th edn. Elsevier, 2021; Fig. 10.30.)

Table 12.2 Berlin definition of ARDS		
Severity	**PaO$_2$: F$_i$O$_2$ ratio**	**Mortality**
Mild	40–26.6 kPa 300–200 mmHg	27%
Moderate	26.6–13.3 kPa 200–100 mmHg	32%
Severe	13.3 kPa < 100 mmHg	45%

From ARDS Definition Task Force. Acute respiratory distress syndrome: the Berlin definition. *Journal of the American Medical Association* 2012; **307:** 2526–2533.

- Multiple trauma and massive transfusion.
- Post-cardiac bypass syndrome.
- Pancreatitis.
- Toxic fume exposure, including smoke inhalation.
- Cerebral injury, e.g. subarachnoid haemorrhage.

Pathophysiology

Profound hypoxaemia results from venous admixture or shunting of deoxygenated blood through poorly ventilated or unventilated lung units. This arises because:

- Endothelial dysfunction leads to widespread interstitial oedema and impaired alveolar capillary perfusion.
- The stiff (low-compliance) lungs result in reduced tidal volume and reduced end-expiratory lung volume; this then causes small airway collapse. Once the airways are collapsed, Laplace's law explains why it is difficult to re-expand them (consider the difficulty in initially blowing up a balloon).
- Additional small airway pathology is present, particularly with direct lung injury, e.g. smoke inhalation.
- The lung can be likened to a wet sponge: the dependent sponge is waterlogged and the air spaces collapsed. Only the non-dependent areas of the lung might be contributing to gas exchange. The additional component of airway inflammation in some causes of ARDS explains the high mortality associated with direct lung injury ($>60\%$).

Management

The high mortality of ARDS is critically dependent on resolution of the primary cause. Treatment of the lung is essentially supportive. Further injury must be avoided by tolerating relative hypoxaemia (aiming to limit oxygen toxicity by F_iO_2 <70%) and allowing permissive hypercapnia (limiting tidal volume to avoid barotrauma — over-distension of functioning lung and risk of pneumothorax). Ventilatory techniques include:

- Deep sedation and neuromuscular paralysis to increase chest wall compliance; a semi-recumbent bed position unless contraindicated
- Small tidal volumes (6 mL/kg of predicted body weight) and prolonged inspiratory time to limit airway pressure
- Use of a minimum amount of PEEP to recruit lung units
- Prone positioning to improve $\dot{V}/\dot{Q}$ matching and clearance of lung secretions.

Experimental methods

- Inhaled nitric oxide to overcome hypoxic pulmonary vasoconstriction, improve $\dot{V}/\dot{Q}$ matching and reduce pulmonary hypertension.
- Rescue therapy with steroids to limit the proliferative fibrotic process of lung repair.
- High-frequency ventilation.
- Extra-corporeal membrane oxygenation.

Outlook

Mortality from ARDS remains high (overall 30–40%). Lung remodelling might, however, result in considerable eventual recovery. Progress of the underlying disease, hospital-acquired infection or the development of cardiogenic shock secondary to RV failure is critical in determining survival.

Progress. The patient developed MOF with impaired hepatic synthesis, including coagulopathy, cholestatic jaundice and acute tubular necrosis requiring haemofiltration. Antibiotic therapy initially was IV cefuroxime infusion 1.5 g 6-hourly and metronidazole 500 mg IV 8-hourly, but subsequently *Pseudomonas* was cultured from respiratory secretions and IV piperacillin was started. A week later a tracheostomy was performed and ventilatory support was progressively weaned over the next 3 weeks. He was discharged from hospital 6 weeks after admission.

Further reading

Faculty of Intensive Care Medicine. Guidelines on the management of ARDS. 2018. https://www.ficm.ac.uk/news-events-education/news/guidelines-management-ards

Herridge MS, Tansey CM, Matte A, et al. Functional disability 5 years after acute respiratory distress syndrome. *New England Journal of Medicine* 2011; **364**: 1293–1304.

Taylor Thompson B, Chambers RC, Liu KD. Acute respiratory distress syndrome. *New England Journal of Medicine* 2017; **377**: 562–572.

SELF-POISONING

Poisoning is a major health problem worldwide. WHO estimates that a million people a year die of self-harm. Chemicals are a major cause, for example copper sulphate used in agriculture, and yellow oleander, with 370,000 deaths every year; approximately 25% are in low/mid income countries.

General points

- 80% of patients seen in A&E will be conscious.
- There is poor correlation between history of amount, type and timing of poisons consumed, and blood toxicology.
- Frequently, more than one drug will have been consumed.
- Alcohol is the most commonly consumed second agent.
- Carefully assess suicide risk, be sympathetic and admit to the MAU.

What particular points do you need to assess on physical examination?

- Assess and record conscious level using the GCS (see p. 463).
- Document respiratory rate and cyanosis (use pulse oximetry).
- Measure BP and pulse.
- Record pupillary size (small with opiates) and reactivity to light.
- Measure temperature: rectally if unconscious.
- If consciousness is depressed, check for coexistent head injury.
- Look for needle tracks or signs of drug use.

Case history (1)

A 25-year-old woman is admitted semi-conscious, smelling of alcohol, having taken an indeterminate amount of an unknown drug at some point earlier that evening.

On examination, she has depressed consciousness (GCS 11), respiratory rate of 12/min, BP of 95/70 and small, reactive pupils.

What should you do?

- Baseline: FBC, urea U&Es, liver biochemistry.
- Paracetamol and salicylate levels at 4 h or thereafter post overdose.
- Blood and urine samples for toxicology: particularly useful in seriously ill patients with altered consciousness.
- O_2 saturation, arterial blood gases if depressed respiration.
- Admit the patient to the MAU.

Information

SELF-POISONING

Take advice from the 24-h National Poisons Information Service (see end of chapter) in all serious overdoses: there might have been recent advances in management of the specific poisoning you are dealing with.

Some common drugs used for overdose exhibit delayed action, e.g. aspirin, paracetamol, tricyclic anti-depressants, iron (more common in children), co-phenotrope, paraquat and all modified-release preparations.

General management

- Nurse in left lateral position.
- Clear mouth of vomitus, debris, obstructing objects.
- Catheterisation of bladder: usually unnecessary, as gentle suprapubic pressure can empty bladder.
- IV cannula.
- Nursing care of mouth and pressure areas.

Respiratory support

- Protect airway because vomiting is a risk: vomiting is particularly associated with opiates, benzodiazepines, alcohol and tricyclic anti-depressants.
- Respiratory depression might occur with opiates, benzodiazepines, alcohol, tricyclic anti-depressants.
- Monitor with pulse oximetry.
- Give oxygen: start with 60% humidified O_2.
- Loss of gag or cough reflex is the prime indication for intubation.

Cardiovascular support

- Watch for hypotension (systolic BP <80 mmHg):
  - Mild: raise end of bed.
  - Severe: use IV volume expanders, e.g. Plasma-Lyte.
  - Very severe: insert CVP line to monitor fluid replacement.
  - Measure urine output: aim for 0.5 mL/kg per h. Urine output is a useful guide to adequacy of the circulation.
- Monitor ECG for arrhythmias.

What other problems might occur?

Blood pressure
- Watch for hypotension (see earlier).
- Avoid vasopressor drugs because these might interact adversely with the poison.
- Less commonly, transient hypertension might be seen with amfetamine and cocaine.

Arrhythmias
- Might arise from hypoxia or metabolic acidosis.
- Bradycardia might occur with beta-blockers, digoxin and organophosphorus compounds.
- Ventricular and supraventricular tachycardias occur due to theophyllines, tricyclic anti-depressants/phenothiazines (due to prolonged QT interval) cocaine, Ecstasy and amfetamine.

Hypothermia
- Can occur due to unconsciousness, especially with phenothiazines and barbiturates.
- Measure temperature rectally.

- Nurse under space blanket with warming, if needed, using water bottles.

Hyperthermia

- Can occur with amfetamines, Ecstasy and cocaine, selective serotonin re-uptake inhibitors (SSRIs), salicylates and tricyclic anti-depressants.

What specific management procedures are there for overdoses?

Reducing absorption

- Gastric lavage: should only be used for life-threatening overdoses and only within the first hour for significant recovery of poison. Avoid lavage if corrosives, paraffin or petrol have been taken because of the risk of inhalation. Always intubate if the patient is unconscious.
- Induced emesis: should not be used because it is ineffective at removal of poison and delays the use of activated charcoal.
- Activated charcoal: binds drugs in the intestine and is valuable for adsorbing most poisons, but is most effective for aspirin, tricyclic anti-depressants and theophyllines. For most drugs, do not use more than 1 h post ingestion of poison or with an oral antidote (see also Active elimination, next section).

Active elimination

- Repeated doses of charcoal might enhance elimination for selected drugs even after the drug has been absorbed. This works for aspirin, barbiturates, quinine, theophylline and carbamazepine.
- Whole-bowel irrigation using non-absorbable polyethylene glycol solution (not to be confused with ethylene glycol or anti-freeze) causes loose stool and forces bowel contents through, rapidly reducing absorption. This is not routinely used.
- Forced diuresis for salicylate poisoning is dangerous and should not be used.
- Urine alkalinisation is mainly used for salicylate overdose (see p. 384).
- Haemodialysis helps in severe salicylate poisoning, barbiturates, ethylene glycol, alcohol and lithium poisoning.
- Haemoperfusion involves passing heparinised blood across absorbents such as charcoal. Works for barbiturates and theophylline.

Antagonising the influences of poisons

- Acetylcysteine or methionine replenishes cellular glutathione stores in paracetamol poisoning.
- Ethanol is a competitive inhibitor of alcohol dehydrogenase and is given in ethylene glycol (anti-freeze) poisoning. Fomepizole is also useful when ethanol is contraindicated, e.g. previous excess alcohol user or liver disease.
- Naloxone and opiates compete at the same receptor.

Progress. The partner of this 25-year-old patient came to the MAU shortly after admission. He had found two empty boxes of diazepam, which she had been taking for acute anxiety over the last few months. He said that her drug misuse might be related to her being made redundant a week ago. She did not require ventilation and woke up gradually. She was very tearful

Kumar & Clark's Cases in Clinical Medicine

Box 13.1 Benzodiazepine overdose

Benzodiazepines account for 40% of all overdoses.

Clinical features
- Drowsiness, ataxia, slurred speech, coma
- Respiratory depression and hypotension might occur

Management – the problems

Respiratory depression or – in combination with alcohol – vomiting and aspiration

Treatment – supportive
- Protect airway and neurological observations
- Gastric lavage is not required
- Flumazenil is a benzodiazepine antagonist that can be used in severe overdose with marked respiratory depression only
- Beware: seizures have followed flumazenil administration
- Patients are usually fit to be discharged at 24 h

---

and apologetic, and did not require psychiatric referral after counselling (Box 13.1).

PARACETAMOL (ACETAMINOPHEN) POISONING

Remember

- Paracetamol is consumed in 45% of overdoses in the UK.
- As little as 7.5–15 g (15–30 tablets) can cause severe hepatic necrosis.

Case history (2)

A young woman, aged 18, was brought into A&E by her boyfriend, who had found her drowsy. A tablet packet – possibly containing paracetamol tablets – and half a bottle of wine were found near her. They had argued the previous night and she had threatened suicide. He thought that she had taken the tablets 6 h ago. A past history of an eating disorder was elicited.

On examination, she was very thin and had a GCS of 10. There were no other physical signs.

Investigations

- Baseline U&Es
- Liver biochemistry (including INR)
- Paracetamol and salicylate levels

This patient's paracetamol level was 140 mg/L and her salicylate level was <10 mg at 6 h post overdose. She was admitted to the MAU.

Points to remember

- Nausea and vomiting are extremely common in the first 24 h.
- Abdominal pain 24 h plus.
- Persistent nausea with subcostal pain usually indicates significant hepatic necrosis.
- Chronic alcohol excess or other enzyme-inducing drugs increase metabolism of drugs.
- Hypoglycaemia may occur.

Remember

Paracetamol is a constituent (with an opiate) of co-proxamol or co-dydramol.

Physical examination (Fig. 13.1)

- Check respiratory rate in case a compound preparation has been consumed.
- Haematuria, proteinuria and loin pain after the first 24 h might indicate acute kidney injury (AKI).
- Later: liver flap and altered consciousness might develop 3 days plus.

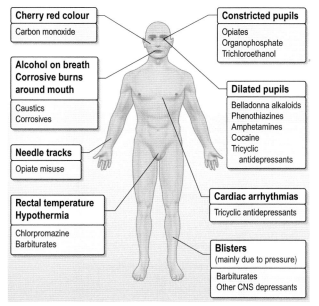

Figure 13.1 Physical signs of poisoning.

Kumar & Clark's Cases in Clinical Medicine

Management — the problems

Paracetamol can cause hepatic necrosis, with maximum damage sustained 72–96 h after ingestion. Renal damage occurs even without major liver damage.

Information

IMPORTANT POINTS
- Severe liver or renal damage: seek specialist advice.
- Contact liver unit if INR >3.0 or alanine aminotransferase >1000 U/L, or there is evidence of acidosis, encephalopathy or hypotension with systolic BP <60 mmHg.
- Hypoglycaemia might develop in first 48 h.
- Alert renal physicians if serum creatinine rises.
- There is evidence that administration of acetylcysteine, even in patients with established hepatic encephalopathy, might improve the prognosis.

How should you manage this patient?

For general management, see page 378.

Treatment nomogram (Fig. 13.2)
- There are two lines on the nomogram: the normal and the high-risk treatment lines.
- The high-risk treatment line should be used for patients who are likely to be glutathione-deplete, e.g. malnourished or HIV-positive patients.
- Alcohol-dependent patients or those on enzyme inducers, e.g. phenytoin, rifampicin or carbamazepine, are also at high risk from lower levels of paracetamol.

This patient's prior eating disorder and low body weight indicate that the high-risk treatment line should be used to interpret the paracetamol levels.

Information

PARACETAMOL OVERDOSE
- The National Poisons Information Service has received reports that the nomogram has not predicted paracetamol toxicity for some patients.
- Investigation indicates that this relates to inaccurate history of timings, quantities and frequency of paracetamol overdose.

Antidotes — regime for treatment

Acetylcysteine by infusion
- Acetylcysteine 150 mg/kg in 200 mL 5% glucose over 15 min.
- Then 50 mg/kg in 500 mL 5% glucose over 4 h, followed by 100 mg/kg in 1 L over 16 h. Total dose 300 mg/kg over 20–25 h.

What are the adverse reactions to acetylcysteine?
- Local itching and rashes at infusion sites.
- Systemic effects include nausea, flushing, angio-oedema, bronchospasm and hypotension. Treatment is with discontinuation of the infusion and an anti-histamine.

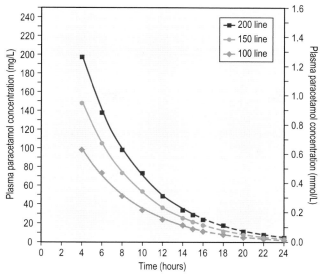

Figure 13.2 Nomogram for treatment of paracetamol poisoning. Note that the treatment lines are uncertain if the patient presents 15 h or more after ingestion, or has taken a modified-release preparation of paracetamol. Although these lines are often extended to 24 h (dotted lines), the concentrations are not based on clinical trial data. (From Feather A, Randall D, Waterhouse M, eds. *Kumar and Clark's Clinical Medicine*, 10th edn. Elsevier, 2021; Fig. 12.2.)

Once these effects have been resolved, the acetylcysteine infusion can be resumed at 100 mg/kg in 1 L over 16 h.

With a GCS of 10, opiates were suspected in this patient, and naloxone 0.8–2 mg IV was also given. As she responded to this, a naloxone infusion was started at a dose of 2 mg diluted in 500 mL with the rate adjusted to clinical response, as a single IV naloxone dose lasts only 30 min, as well as the acetylcysteine.

Intubation and ventilation were not required; pulse oximetry showed no impaired oxygenation.

Summary: how would you treat a paracetamol overdose?

If a patient presents within 8 h (as in this case)

- Gastric lavage or emesis up to 4 h post ingestion.
- Use treatment nomogram at 4 h or later to guide use of acetylcysteine (see Fig. 13.2).
- If there is doubt about the timing, or if more than 12 g has been ingested, treat with acetylcysteine immediately.
- If the 4-h paracetamol level is below the treatment line, discontinue acetylcysteine *except* in patients who are at high risk (see Fig. 13.2).

- If methionine or acetylcysteine is started within 8 h, the prognosis is good and patients can be considered for discharge at the end of the infusion if blood tests are normal.
- Prior to discharge, check that INR and plasma creatinine are normal.
- Advise the patient to return if vomiting ensues.
- Ensure liaison with Psychiatric services.

If a patient presents at 8–24 h post ingestion

- Patients presenting more than 8 h post ingestion are at greater risk of hepatotoxicity; the efficacy of treatment with acetylcysteine declines *but still give it*.
- Individual response to paracetamol overdose can be variable and the validity of the treatment line beyond 15 h post ingestion is not clear.
- If there is doubt about the timing of overdose, or if more than 12 g has been consumed, then treat with acetylcysteine immediately.
- At the end of the infusion, check that the INR and plasma creatinine are normal. If so, the risk of damage is negligible and discharge can be planned.
- If INR or creatinine is abnormal, or the patient develops symptoms, continue to monitor these blood tests till normal.

If a patient presents 24 h plus post ingestion

- The treatment remains controversial but there is evidence of benefits of acetylcysteine in those who develop hepatic encephalopathy.
- All should have INR, creatinine, BM Stix glucose and arterial pH monitored.

Progress. This woman was given acetylcysteine and her INR was monitored within the normal range. She was discharged after being seen by the duty Psychiatrist with an urgent referral to Mental Health Services.

SALICYLATE AND TRICYCLIC ANTI-DEPRESSANT OVERDOSE

Case history

A 16-year-old girl was brought to A&E by her parents after an episode of nausea, followed by severe vomiting. Her parents then found packs of aspirin tablets in her bedroom, which she said she had taken because of difficulties with friends at school. She also complained of tinnitus and deafness. The parents think the aspirin ingestion occurred about 4 h ago.

On examination, she is hyperventilating with peripheral vasodilatation, profuse sweating and tachycardia, suggesting a moderate/severe **salicylate overdose.** She was transferred to the MAU.

- Aspirin is rapidly absorbed: usually peaks at 4 h.
- <150 mg/kg body weight causes mild toxicity
- 150–130 mg/kg body weight causes moderate toxicity
- 300–500 mg/kg body weight causes severe toxicity.
- Beware modified-release formulations: these can prolong absorption.
- Aspirin itself might delay gastric emptying.

Clinical features
- Early features include nausea, vomiting, tinnitus or deafness (severe overdose), sweating and hyperventilation.
- Later features include Kussmaul's respiration, confusion, coma, fits and renal impairment.

Investigations
- Blood gases reveal a respiratory alkalosis.
- Plasma salicylate measured after 4 h.

Management – the problems
- Aspirin delays gastric emptying.
- People who appear well might have very high levels.
- Early hypokalaemia and respiratory alkalosis may be replaced after 4–6 h by metabolic acidosis due to salicylate.
- Hypo-prothrombinaemia might occur (increased prothrombin time/INR).

Treatment
- Gastric lavage was not attempted, as tablets taken 4 h previously.
- Repeated doses of charcoal enhance elimination.
- IV fluids with potassium supplements were given to correct dehydration and hypokalaemia, and to improve urine flow.
- Forced alkaline diuresis should not be used.
- Urine alkalinisation was used when plasma salicylate levels were found to be 620 mg/L: 8.4% bicarbonate (~225 mL) in 1 h with careful monitoring.
- Haemodialysis should be used only when the salicylate level is >700 mg/L.

Progress. This young girl was kept in hospital for 3 days, during which time she fully recovered and her blood gases and electrolytes returned to normal. She was seen with her parents by the Psychiatric department but further counselling was not thought to be necessary.

Information

RISK FACTORS FOR DEATH FROM SALICYLATES
- Age >70 years
- CNS features
- Metabolic acidosis
- Hyperpyrexia
- Late presentation
- Pulmonary oedema
- Salicylate concentrations >700 mg/L (5.07 mmol/L)

Tricyclic anti-depressant overdose

These have become less common since the (much safer) SSRIs became available. Features of overdose are mainly due to anti-muscarinic and alpha-blocking adverse effects. Arrhythmias occur due to prolongation of the QT interval.

Kumar & Clark's Cases in Clinical Medicine

Clinical features

- Drowsiness, confusion but rarely unconsciousness.
- Blurred vision due to fixed dilated pupils.
- Sinus tachycardia with long QT interval.
- Ventricular arrhythmias.
- Hypotension.
- Hypothermia.
- Hyper-reflexia and extensor plantars.
- Agitation, visual and auditory hallucinations: common during recovery.
- Seizures: in <5%.

Treatment – supportive

- Gastric lavage up to 4 h post ingestion for life-threatening amount of drug.
- Activated charcoal: reduces absorption of tricyclics; anti-cholinergic action delays gastric emptying.
- Cardiac monitor and watch for hypotension.
- Neurological observations.
- Seizures: might require IV diazepam 10 mg.
- Ventricular arrhythmias due to prolonged QT interval: should not be treated with anti-arrhythmics but with under-drive or over-drive temporary pacing.
- Rarely, heart block and electrical mechanical dissociation have occurred.
- Occasionally, metabolic acidosis ensues – if pH ≤7.0 develops, this should be corrected with 1.4% sodium bicarbonate.

COCAINE AND ECSTASY

Cocaine (Fig. 13.3) can be inhaled (snorted), injected or swallowed, or separated from its hydrochloride base and melted as crack. Binges with cocaine can last 24–96 h.

Case history

A 32-year-old man is brought to A&E by his friends, who were all at a party together. A large amount of alcohol was drunk and some drugs had been used, mainly cannabis and Ecstasy. The patient had been found semi-conscious, and when his friends tried to move him he seemed to have no movement in the left side of his body.

On examination, he has a GCS of 9. He has signs of a left hemiparesis.

Remember

If a young person presents with a stroke or myocardial infarction, cocaine overdose should always be looked for.

Clinical features of cocaine toxicity

- Euphoria, slurred speech, dilated pupils.
- Pyrexia, sinus tachycardia and hallucinations (auditory, tactile and olfactory).
- Hypertension (may be severe), rarely causing haemorrhagic stroke, hyperventilation.
- Myocardial infarction may occur in 6% of those with chest pain.
- Ventricular arrhythmias, seizures.
- Later kidney injury, disseminated intravascular coagulation (DIC).

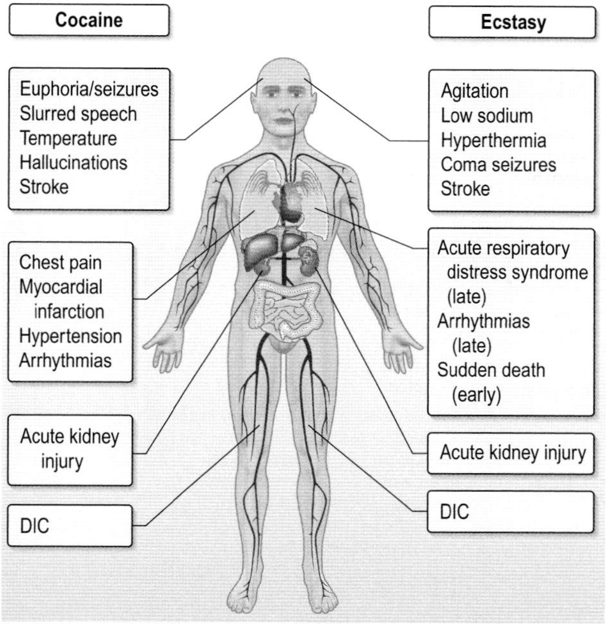

Figure 13.3 Features of cocaine and Ecstasy misuse. DIC, disseminated intravascular coagulation.

Immediate plan

- ABCDE.
- Admit to HDU.
- Blood tests (Hb, WCC, U&Es, glucose, INR).
- Arrange urgent CT scan.

  In this patient, the CT provided evidence of cerebral haemorrhage, so any further active treatment is not required. He was transferred to the Stroke Unit (see p. 159).

  Progress. This young man continued to deteriorate and died 33 h after admission. It was later found that he tried smoking cocaine for the first time.

Ecstasy (see Fig. 13.3)

Ecstasy is an amfetamine derivative known as MDMA, which stimulates the sympathetic nervous system, and prevents neuronal re-uptake of catecholamines, dopamine and serotonin (5-HT).

Clinical features

- There may be agitation, profound dehydration, low sodium due to excess water consumption or anti-diuretic hormone.

- Early arrhythmias (supraventricular or ventricular) occur and can cause sudden death.
- Nausea, vomiting, muscle pain, sinus tachycardia and visual hallucinations.
- Hypertension (might be severe), rarely causing haemorrhagic stroke, chest pain, hyperventilation.
- Hyperthermia, coma, seizures, rhabdomyolysis, rarely fulminant hepatic failure.
- Later: AKI, DIC, acute respiratory distress syndrome (ARDS).

Investigations

- Baseline: FBC, U&Es, glucose, liver biochemistry
- 12-lead ECG
- Paracetamol and salicylate levels at 4 h or thereafter if coexistent overdose suspected
- Urine screen for drugs of misuse
- Imaging, e.g. brain CT

Treatment – supportive

- Activated charcoal reduces absorption within 1 h.
- Early hyponatraemia due to excessive water consumption by Ecstasy users should be looked for before rehydration.
- Cardiac monitor and watch for hypertension.
- Treat agitation or seizures with IV diazepam 10 mg.
- Hyperthermia >39°C can be reduced by 1 L of cold saline. If temperature does not respond, IV dantrolene might help.
- Ventricular arrhythmias should be treated with anti-arrhythmics.

GAMMAHYDROXYBUTYRIC ACID (GHB)

GHB has been used for bodybuilding and for weight reduction. It was sold as a salt, which forms a colourless liquid in water, but is no longer available legally. The seaweed-like taste can be impossible to detect when added to an alcoholic drink. GHB has been used to facilitate 'date rape'. Street names includes 'scoop', 'easylay' and 'liquid X'.

Clinical features

- History might indicate no intent or knowledge of consumption of any drug.
- Initial euphoria, disinhibition, agitation, confusion, nausea and diarrhoea progressing within 1 h to drowsiness and unconsciousness (potentiated by alcohol).
- Nausea, vomiting, muscle pain, sinus tachycardia, and rarely seizures.
- Bradycardia, respiratory depression and even Cheyne–Stokes respiration might rarely occur.
- Be alert to the possibility that such patients might have suffered sexual assault.

Investigations

FOR GHB CONSUMPTION
- Baseline FBC, U&Es (may reveal hypernatraemia and hypokalaemia), blood glucose and liver biochemistry
- Blood gases if patient is unconscious or there is respiratory depression (metabolic acidosis may occur)

Treatment of GHB consumption – supportive

- Activated charcoal reduces absorption within 1 h: observe for a minimum of 2 h, even if apparently much improved clinically.
- Monitor BP, heart rate and pulse oximetry.
- Treat seizures with IV diazepam 10 mg.
- Bradycardia associated with hypotension should be treated with IV atropine.

INSECT STINGS AND BITES

Case history

A 24-year-old had been cleaning a pond in the summer when she was stung by a wasp. A few minutes later she felt unwell and had to lie down, as she felt faint. She then noticed some difficulty in breathing and felt a 'tightening' of her face. After 45 min her symptoms improved.

Diagnosis. Mild anaphylactic reaction to wasp sting. She made a complete recovery.

Information

ANAPHYLACTIC REACTIONS CAN BE FATAL
- Reactions to penicillin: 1 death in every 7.5 million injections
- Bee and wasp stings: severe reactions in 1 : 200 stings
  (USA 60–80 deaths per year)
  (UK 5–10 deaths per year)

ANAPHYLACTIC SHOCK

Typically follows a second or third challenge.

History

- Exposure to insect bite, bee or wasp sting, seafood, nuts, drugs (e.g. penicillin, NSAIDs) or contrast media.
- Dizziness, wheeze and facial swelling.
- Past history of allergy.

Examination

- Facial oedema.
- Tachycardia, hypotension.
- Stridor due to laryngeal oedema.
- Bronchospasm.

Immediate management

- Ensure clear airway and establish large-bore venous access.
- Give oxygen 35% unless hypoxic.
- If there is serious hypoxia and stridor, tracheostomy might be required.
- Lay the patient flat and elevate legs.
- Perform cardiovascular observations.
- Administer 0.5 mg adrenaline (epinephrine) IM (not IV) to create depot support for the circulation.
- Repeat after 5 min if still hypotensive.

- Follow with anti-histamine: chlorphenamine 10 mg IV.
- Then give hydrocortisone 100 mg IV.

Further management

- If persistent hypotension, infuse plasma expander, e.g. 1 L of Haemaccel.
- Salbutamol 2.5–5 mg nebulised or IV for bronchospasm or continued shock.
- An aminophylline infusion for continuing bronchospasm.
- Always identify precipitant.
- Advise on Medic-Alert bracelet.
- Provide the patient with adrenaline (epinephrine) Minijet 0.3 mg and tuition to inject in the thigh in the event of exposure to allergen. This treatment should be carried with the patient at all times.

Prevention

- This is the best.
- Avoid triggering factor, e.g. food, stings.
- Patient education is vital.
- Self-administered adrenaline (epinephrine). Patients should always carry pre-loaded syringes.

Significant websites

https://www.toxbase.co.uk *Toxbase — database of UK National Poisons Information Service*

https://www.toxinz.com *Database of the New Zealand Poisons Centre*

https://www.nlm.nih.gov/enviro/index.html *Environmental health, toxicology and chemical information from the National Library of Medicine*

https://www.who.int/ipcs/poisons/centre/directory/en *Contact details of all poisons centres worldwide*

https://www.wikitox.org *Home of the Clinical Toxicology Teaching Resource Project*

Endocrinology and Diabetes 14

DIABETES MELLITUS

Diabetes mellitus is a syndrome of chronic hyperglycaemia due to relative insulin deficiency or resistance or both.

Case history (1)

You are phoned by a GP who has seen a 50-year-old man in his surgery, complaining of thirst and polyuria. His venous blood glucose is 24 mmol/L. He is tired but otherwise well.
  What are the key decisions in this case?
- Does this patient need admission?
- Does he need insulin?
- What is the immediate management?

Diagnosis. The likelihood is that this patient has **type 2 diabetes** (Table 14.1). The risk of ketoacidosis is small and he will not need admission unless he is either ketotic (ketonuria + + +) or is very dehydrated.

This patient should be advised to avoid sweet drinks (especially sweetened canned drinks) and an appointment arranged for him to attend a diabetic outpatient clinic. Contact the Diabetic Liaison Nurse in your hospital and arrange for the patient to be seen urgently.

Indications for admission

- Severe dehydration (may have hyperosmolality).
- Intercurrent illness such as pneumonia or urinary tract infection (UTI).
- + + + ketonuria.
- Tachycardia or tachypnoea.

Information

DIAGNOSTIC CRITERIA FOR DIABETES MELLITUS
- Fasting venous plasma glucose >7.0 mmol/L (126 mg/dL) after 8 h fast*
- Random venous plasma glucose >11.1 mmol/L (200 mg/dL)*
- HbA1c of >6.5% (48 mmol/mol) (Table 14.2)
  *Two readings are required for asymptomatic individuals. Note also:
- Impaired fasting glucose: 5.6—6.9 mmol/L
- Impaired glucose tolerance: >7.8 and <11.1 mmol/L; 2 h after 75 g oral glucose tolerance test (GTT).
  An oral GTT is required only for borderline cases.

Progress. At the Diabetic Clinic the Diabetic Nurse explained lifestyle changes that are an essential part of treatment, i.e. stopping smoking, and losing weight via diet and exercise. The nurse arranges for an appointment for this patient to be checked by the doctor and for eye testing. He was also started on metformin 500 mg daily, increasing to 1.5 g daily.

Table 14.1 The spectrum of diabetes: a comparison of type 1 and type 2 diabetes mellitus

	Type 1	Type 2
Epidemiology	Younger (usually <30 years of age)	Older (usually >30 years of age)
	Usually lean	Often overweight
	Increased in those of Northern European ancestry	All racial groups. Increased in peoples of Asian, African, Polynesian and American Indian ancestry
	Seasonal incidence	
Heredity	HLA-DR3 or DR4 in >90%	No HLA links
	30–50% concordance in identical twins	~ 50% concordance in identical twins
Pathogenesis	Auto-immune disease	No immune disturbance
	Islet cell autoantibodies	Insulin resistance
	Insulitis	
	Association with other auto-immune diseases	
	Immunosuppression after diagnosis delays beta-cell destruction	
Clinical	Insulin deficiency	Partial insulin deficiency initially
	May develop ketoacidosis	May develop hyperosmolar state
	Always need insulin	Many come to need insulin when beta-cells fail over time
Biochemical	Eventual disappearance of C-peptide	C-peptide persists

HLA, human leukocyte antigen. *Note:* there is a significant rise in the incidence of young patients with type 2 diabetes mellitus, especially in the obese and in Asian populations.

Table 14.2 HBA1c – conversion of percentage values to mmol/mol

Diabetes Control and Complication Trial (HbA1c %)	International Federation of Clinical Chemistry (HbA1c mmol/mol)
4.0	20
5.0	31
6.0	42
6.5	48
7.0	53
7.5	59
8.0	64
9.0	75
10.0	96

Case history (2)

You are telephoned by a GP who has seen a 17-year-old man in his surgery, complaining of thirst and polyuria. He has recently lost 8 kg in weight. His blood glucose is 31 mmol/L.

The key decisions are again:

- Does this patient need admission?
- Does he need insulin?
- What is the immediate management?

This patient is much more likely to be presenting with early **type 1 diabetes** and might not be ketotic yet because he could still have a degree of residual beta cell function (the 'honeymoon' phase). Again, assessment of ketosis, acidosis and dehydration must be made to determine whether he needs admission. He should be seen within 24 h either by the Diabetic Liaison Nurse or in hospital to commence insulin. If there is any doubt, the patient should be seen in A&E immediately.

Progress. At the Diabetic Clinic the patient was found to be dehydrated with mild ketosis. He was admitted to the MAU to commence insulin therapy.

DIABETIC KETOACIDOSIS (DKA)

Case history

A 21-year-old woman presents to A&E, having been generally unwell for 2 weeks and having been treated for a UTI by her doctor.

On examination, severe dehydration, a tachycardia of 120 bpm and a BP of 90/50 mmHg are noted. The nurses have checked the patient's finger-prick blood glucose (BM Stix) and found it to be 30 mmol/L.

Diagnosis. Diabetic ketoacidosis.

How do patients present with ketoacidosis?

- Unwell ± intercurrent illness (e.g. bacterial or viral infection).
- Polyuria and polydipsia.
- Hyperventilation or dyspnoea.
- Vomiting ± abdominal pain.
- Impaired conscious level.

Patients known to have type 1 diabetes mellitus most commonly develop ketoacidosis when insulin is omitted because of missed meals during an intercurrent illness (e.g. gastroenteritis). Patients become rapidly dehydrated (Fig. 14.1) and acidotic (over hours). Tachypnoea or Kussmaul respiration (a deep, sighing respiration) is prominent, with the smell of ketones on the breath. It is the fall in pH that causes coma.

The blood glucose might not be particularly high and severe acidosis may be present, with glucose values as low as 10 mmol/L. This might be due to recent self-administration of insulin, which is insufficient alone to correct the acidosis in the presence of dehydration.

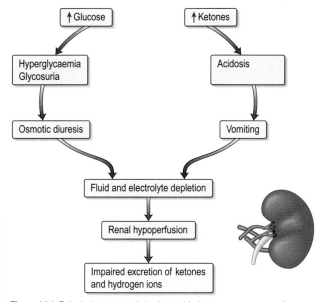

Figure 14.1 Dehydration occurs during ketoacidosis as a consequence of two parallel processes. Hyperglycaemia results in osmotic diuresis, and hyperketonaemia results in acidosis and vomiting. Renal hypoperfusion then occurs and a vicious circle is established as the kidney becomes less able to compensate for the acidosis.

Assessment of severity

Poor prognostic features include:
- Impaired conscious level (indication for urgent intubation)
- pH <7.0
- Oliguria
- Low serum potassium at presentation.

Investigations

- Blood glucose
- ABGs and pH
- U&Es — bicarbonate in venous blood <12 mmol/L — severe acidosis
- Urinalysis (ketones strongly positive + + +)
- Plasma ketones — test with Ketostix
- FBC
- Blood ± urine cultures
- CXR
- ECG and cardiac enzymes

Management

General measures

- Admission to HDU.
- A central line in patients with a history of cardiac disease/renal impairment/autonomic neuropathy, or in the elderly.
- An arterial line to monitor ABGs and plasma potassium.
- Nil by mouth for at least 6 h.
- Nasogastric tube: if there is an impaired conscious level, to prevent vomiting and aspiration.
- Urinary catheter: if there is no urine for 2 h or serum creatinine is high.
- Low molecular weight (LMW) heparin: enoxaparin 40 mg SC daily or thrombin inhibitors.

Remember

Management of DKA requires fluid, insulin, potassium and *care*.

Fluid replacement

Severely shocked patients may require colloid to restore circulating plasma volume. Table 14.3 shows examples of blood values in severe ketoacidosis and compares these with the values seen in the hyperosmolar, hyperglycaemic state (see p. 396).

The guidelines for fluid replacement are shown in Table 14.4. These are applicable to young patients.
- When blood glucose falls to <12 mmol/L, convert to a 5% glucose infusion. This will enable the insulin infusion to be continued. Continued insulin is required to inhibit ketone production.
- Continue with IV fluids 1 L every 4–6 h until the patient is rehydrated and ketosis resolves (~24 h).

Table 14.3 Examples of blood values

	Severe ketoacidosis	Hyperosmolar, hyperglycaemic state
Na^+ (mmol/L)	140	155
K^+ (mmol/L)	5	5
Cl^- (mmol/L)	100	110
HCO_3^- (mmol/L)	5	25
Urea (mmol/L)	8	15
Glucose (mmol/L)	30	50
Arterial pH	7.0 (H^+ >100 nmol/L)	7.35

The normal range of osmolality is 285–300 mOsmol/kg. It can be measured directly, or can be calculated approximately from the formula:

$$Osmolality = 2(Na^+ + K^+) + glucose + urea$$

For example, in the patient with severe ketoacidosis described above:

$$Osmolality = 2(140 + 5) + 30 + 8 = 328 \text{ mOsmol/kg}$$

In the example of non-ketotic hyperosmolar coma:

$$Osmolality = 2(155 + 5) + 50 + 15 = 385 \text{ mOsmol/kg}$$

The normal anion gap is <17. It is calculated as $(Na^+ + K^+) - (Cl^- + HCO_3^-)$.

In the example of ketoacidosis, the anion gap is 40.

In the example of non-ketotic hyperosmolar coma the anion gap is 20.

Mild hyperchloraemic acidosis may develop in the course of therapy. This will be shown by a rising plasma chloride and persistence of a low bicarbonate, even though the anion gap has returned to normal.

Table 14.4 Guidelines for average fluid replacement in young patients

Volume	Duration/timing
1 L 0.9% saline + 20 mmol/KCl	Over the first 30 min
1 L 0.9% saline + 20 mmol/KCl	Over next 1 h
1 L 0.9% saline + 20 mmol/KCl	Over next 2 h
1 L 0.9% saline + 20 mmol/KCl	Over next 4–6 h

Table 14.5 Potassium replacement in patients with diabetic ketoacidosis

Serum potassium (mmol/L)	Amount of KCl (mmol/h)
<3	40
3–4	30
4–5	20
5–6	10
>6	Stop KCl

Insulin regimen

- Add 50 units of soluble insulin to 50 mL 0.9% saline and administer by IV infusion; this equates to 1 U/mL.
- Commence at 6 U/h and continue at 3 U/h after venous glucose falls to <11.5 mmol/L.
- Glucose must then be administered to prevent hypoglycaemia (see earlier).
- Continue IV insulin infusion until ketosis resolves and the patient is eating, and for 2–4 h after the first SC dose of soluble insulin.

Potassium replacement (Table 14.5)

Total body potassium can be depleted by approximately 1000 mmol, and the plasma potassium falls rapidly as potassium shifts into the cells under the action of insulin. Use less potassium in patients with renal impairment or oliguria.

- Monitor serum [K⁺] every 2 h initially, then every 4 h until stable.
- Use pre-mixed potassium-containing infusions wherever possible.

Acidosis

- If the pH is <7.0: isotonic (1.26%) sodium bicarbonate given at a rate of 500 mL over 4 h is safe.
- If the pH is >7.0, bicarbonate need not be given.

Assessment during treatment

- Remember that the role of insulin is primarily to suppress ketogenesis rather than to lower blood glucose.
- Blood glucose (BM Stix every hour, laboratory blood glucose 4-hourly).
- Plasma potassium every 4 h; the main risk is hypokalaemia.
- Repeat ABGs after 2 h. A calculated anion gap (needs chloride estimation) may be adequate for monitoring.

Remember

CAUSES OF DEATH IN DKA
- Hyperkalaemia
- Aspiration due to gastric stasis

- Cerebral oedema due to acidosis $\pm$ over-hydration
- Hypokalaemic respiratory arrest

Progress. This patient started eating and receiving treatment with SC insulin after 48 h. She was shown a video on diabetes and its self-management. She was helped with her insulin injections and discharged on the sixth day with support from the Community Diabetic Nurse.

HYPEROSMOLAR HYPERGLYCAEMIC STATE

Case history

A 60-year-old woman is referred to A&E following a collapse. She has been generally unwell for the last year. Her husband confirms that she has had polyuria and polydipsia with nocturia of 3—4 times every night. Over the last month, she has started using sugar drinks to build herself up because she has been losing weight.

Examination reveals an extremely dehydrated woman with increased tissue turgor. Pulse 100 regular; BP 100/60; JVP not visible; GCS 12.

Investigations revealed:

Na$^+$ 165; K$^+$ 5.9; U 24.7; Cr 170; bicarbonate 20; glucose 64 mmol/L; pH 7.31; pCO$_2$ 4.7 kPa; pO$_2$ 11.2 kPa; plasma osmolality $2 \times (165+ 5.9) + 64 + 24.7 = 429.7$ mOsmol/kg.

Diagnosis. These findings are typical of **hyperosmolar hyperglycaemic state** (see Table 14.3).

Information

CALCULATION OF OSMOLALITY

$2 \times (Na^+ + K^+)$ + glucose (normal range 285—300 mOsmol/kg)

How should this patient be managed?

Hyperosmolar hyperglycaemic state occurs in older patients with type 2 diabetes. It is characterised by a very high glucose, a relatively normal acid—base balance and high plasma osmolality. These patients are also at increased risk of venous and arterial thromboses. The mortality is higher than for DKA. This patient's biochemistry has been slowly getting worse over many weeks, so normalisation must be equally slow.

Remember

Ketones can be found in the urine in any starved person.

How do patients present?

- Middle-aged or elderly patient.
- Insidious onset of polyuria and polydipsia.
- Severe dehydration.
- Altered conscious level.
- Most middle-aged or elderly patients have not previously been diagnosed with diabetes.
- Respiration is usually normal.

- Presentation is usually precipitated by infection, stroke or myocardial infarction.

Diagnosis and investigations

- Plasma glucose: usually >40 mmol/L.
- U&Es: significant hypernatraemia occurs but this is masked by the high glucose. The Na^+ usually increases as the venous glucose, and therefore the extracellular colloid osmotic pressure, fall, and water moves into the intracellular space.
- ABGs: relatively normal.
- Plasma osmolality: typically >350 mOsmol/kg.
- Estimated corrected sodium: to evaluate water loss as a result of hyperglycaemia (see Information box).
- FBC: may show polycythaemia, dehydration or a leucocytosis from infection.
- Creatine kinase: cardiac ischaemia or rhabdomyolysis.
- Troponins.
- ECG: for myocardial infarction or ischaemia.
- CXR: for signs of infection.
- Urine: for urinalysis, microscopy and culture.

Information

CALCULATION OF CORRECTED SODIUM CONCENTRATION

Add 2.0 mmol/L to the measured serum sodium for every 5 mmol/L increase in glucose concentration. Thus a fall in glucose from 50 to 25 mmol/L will be accompanied by a rise in Na^+ of 10 mmol/L.

Remember

The principal cause of death and morbidity in hyperosmolar hyperglycaemic state is arterial and venous thrombosis due to the hyperosmolar state.

Assessment of severity

- The degree of consciousness correlates most closely with plasma osmolality. Coma is usually associated with an osmolality of >400 mOsmol/kg.
- A coexistent lactic acidosis considerably worsens the prognosis.

How would you manage this patient?

General treatment measures

- Aim to correct the high osmolality with fluid and insulin over 48–72 h. Avoid fluid overload and insert a central venous line if there are cardiac problems.
- Manage as for DKA, except:
  - 0.9% saline is the standard fluid for replacement given slowly
  - If Na^+ is >150 mmol/L, use 5% glucose
  - Ensure slow correction of serum sodium (see p. 213)
  - Start insulin at 3 U/h as patients are often sensitive to insulin
  - Anti-coagulate with SC enoxaparin 40 mg daily or a thrombin inhibitor unless contraindicated

Kumar & Clark's Cases in Clinical Medicine

- Insert a urinary catheter if oliguria is present or serum creatinine is high.
- When blood glucose is <10 mmol/L, commence a 5% glucose infusion.
- Once stable, stop insulin therapy and commence oral hypoglycaemic agents or manage by diet alone.

Progress. This patient was discharged on metformin 1 g daily and instructed on lifestyle changes, e.g. controlling weight; an urgent appointment was made with the Community Diabetic Nurse.

HYPOGLYCAEMIC COMA

Case history

A 25-year-old man is brought to A&E by the police, having been found behaving abnormally. He is aggressive and irrational, and attempts to punch the staff. He is restrained and a MedicAlert bracelet is found under his shirt, indicating that he has diabetes. A finger-prick glucose reads 'low'.

Diagnosis. Hypoglycaemia.

Always consider hypoglycaemia in confused patients and check a blood glucose using a glucostix (or BM Stix), confirming with a laboratory determination wherever possible. The most common cause of coma in a patient with diabetes is hypoglycaemia due to drugs. The long-acting sulphonylureas, such as glibenclamide, or long-acting insulins, such as isophane, are prone to do this. Patients who are *not* known to have diabetes but who are hypoglycaemic should have a laboratory-determined blood glucose test, and blood saved (serum) for determination of insulin and C-peptide, the fragment of pro-insulin that is found in endogenous insulin (to diagnose insulinoma or factitious drug administration).

How do patients present? (Box 14.1)

Patients with tightly controlled diabetes can have frequent episodes of hypoglycaemia and can become desensitised to sympathetic activation. These

> **Box 14.1** Presentation of patients with hypoglycaemic coma
>
> Sympathetic over-activity (glucose <3.5 mmol/L)
>
> - Tachycardia
> - Palpitations
> - Sweating
> - Anxiety
> - Pallor
> - Tremor
> - Cold extremities
>
> Neuroglycopenia (glucose <2.6 mmol/L)
>
> - Confusion
> - Slurred speech
> - Localised neurological impairment
> - Coma

patients can develop neuroglycopenia before sympathetic activation and complain of 'loss of warning'. Use of beta-blockers can also minimise the warning signs of hypoglycaemia by blocking the features of an activated sympathetic nervous system.

Conversely, patients with poorly controlled diabetes develop sympathetic signs early and avoid these by running a high blood glucose. They complain of 'being hypo' when their blood sugar is normal or high. They do not require glucose.

Information

Patients with type 2 diabetes who are managed by diet alone or metformin (but no insulin or sulphonylureas) *cannot* become hypoglycaemic.

Assessment of severity

- Hypoglycaemia in a patient with diabetes is defined as <3.5 mmol/L.
- A 'mild' episode requires intervention by the patient.
- A 'severe' episode might lead to coma and requires treatment by a third party.

Investigations

PATIENTS WITH DIABETES WHO HAVE FREQUENT HYPOGLYCAEMIC ATTACKS

- U&Es: hypoglycaemia is more common in diabetic nephropathy because the kidney is one of the sites of insulin metabolism
- TFTs: hypothyroidism is associated with type 1 diabetes mellitus and impairs counter-regulation
- 09:00 cortisol ± short adrenocorticotrophic hormone (ACTH; tetracosactide) stimulation test: hypoadrenalism reduces hepatic glycogen stores (see p. 271)
- Take an alcohol history
- Consider deliberate self-harm

How would you manage hypoglycaemia?

Conscious patient

- Treat with 15–20 g carbohydrate, i.e. four glucose tablets, or glucose drink.

Unconscious patient

- Take blood sample.
- Give:
  - 75 mL 20% glucose IV or
  - 1 mg glucagon IM.
- Do not use 50% glucose in peripheral veins.
- Once recovered, give 1–2 slices of bread or 2–4 biscuits.
- Admit the patient if the cause is a long-acting sulphonylurea or a long-acting insulin, and give a continuous infusion of 10% glucose (e.g. 1 L 8-hourly) and check glucose hourly or 2-hourly.
- Patients should regain consciousness or become coherent within 10 min, although complete cognitive recovery might lag by 30–45 min. Do not give further boluses of IV glucose without repeating the blood glucose. If

the patient does not wake up after 10 min or more, repeat the blood glucose and consider another cause of coma — stroke or a head injury during their confused state.

Hypoglycaemia in the non-diabetic patient

Hypoglycaemia in patients without diabetes is rare and always needs investigation — usually as an inpatient. Always:

- Confirm the hypoglycaemia with a laboratory sample before treatment.
- Take a simultaneous serum sample for insulin and C-peptide, and send it urgently to the laboratory for centrifugation and separation.

Causes of hypoglycaemia

- Drugs:
  - Surreptitious insulin or sulphonylurea ingestion
  - Ethanol
  - Quinine
  - Pentamidine
  - Disopyramide
  - Prescription errors, e.g. chlorpropamide for chlorpromazine (ask for all drugs to be brought in).
- Tumours:
  - Insulinoma
  - Retroperitoneal sarcomas and other malignancies.
- Liver failure.
- Hypopituitarism, causing ACTH, growth hormone (GH) and thyroid stimulating hormone (TSH) deficiency.

Progress. This patient responded to IV glucose and quickly returned to normal. He explained that he was out with friends last night and forgot to eat, but continued to drink alcohol. He thinks he may have given himself the wrong amount of insulin, as he overslept and was late for work.

THE SICK DIABETIC PATIENT

Case history

A 40-year-old man with a 15-year history of type 1 diabetes mellitus and previously documented proteinuria is referred from A&E with vomiting and a feeling of being generally unwell. Glucose was 20 mmol/L, electrolytes were normal and blood gases did not support diabetic ketoacidosis (pH 7.4; bicarbonate 20 mmol/L). An ECG shows evidence of evolving anterior myocardial infarction (MI). This is the typical presentation of a 'silent MI'. Chest pain is frequently atypical or absent in diabetes due to small-fibre neuropathy. The other major cause of this type of non-specific presentation is occult infection and often further investigations are required.

Investigations

- FBC
- U&Es
- ABGs
- CXR
- MSU
- ECG

- Blood cultures
  Other investigations to consider later if occult infection is suspected:
- Abdominal ultrasound or abdominal CT scan
- Tc bone scanning
- Labelled white cell scan

Treatment and progress

This patient has a diagnosis of ST elevation myocardial infarction (STEMI) and requires immediate therapy with aspirin 300 mg chewed and clopidogrel 300 mg oral gel. He was immediately transferred to the Coronary Care Unit for further assessment and possible percutaneous coronary intervention, which is instantly available (see p. 268). His diabetes was initially controlled on insulin infusion because he was kept nil by mouth for the cardiac procedures (Table 14.6). The infusion was continued until the patient was eating and drinking. Insulin treatment has been proven to improve outcome in patients with diabetes in the immediate period after MI.

Once eating and drinking, the patient can be converted back to his/her usual insulin regimen or, if tight glycaemic control is essential, on to × 4 daily insulin (see later), which gives greater ease of adjustment.

Remember

Always inspect the feet carefully in unwell diabetic patients — infected ulcers are common and may be painless.

Protocol for converting diabetics from IV to SC insulin

- Calculate total dose over last 24 h.
- Give 25% of total as soluble insulin 30 min before each meal (i.e. × 3 daily).
- Give 25% of total dose as intermediate-acting isophane insulin at 22:00.

Table 14.6 IV infusion insulin management of type 1 diabetes mellitus in hospital

Level of blood glucose (measured hourly)	Insulin infusion (units/h)
<4.0 mmol/L	0.5
4.0–7.0 mmol/L	1
7.1–9.0 mmol/L	2
9.1–11.0 mmol/L	3
11.1–14.0 mmol/L	4
14.1–17.0 mmol/L	5
17.1–28 mmol/L	6
>28 mmol/L	8

Note: this is only a guide and insulin doses should be adjusted upwards if the patient is known to have a high insulin requirement, and always reviewed regularly to see if the doses are appropriate. The aim is to keep blood glucose in the 7–9 region.

- Monitor blood glucose fasting and 2 h after meals (post-prandial) — each finger-prick glucose measures the adequacy of the previous dose.
- Aim for glucose <10 mmol/L post-prandial and <8 mmol/L fasting.
- Don't discontinue IV insulin until 1–2 h *after* the first SC insulin dose is administered because IV insulin has a half-life of only 3 min.

MANAGEMENT OF NEW TYPE 2 DIABETICS PRESENTING FOR SURGERY

Case history

You are asked to see a 50-year-old man with no previous history of diabetes, who is admitted for coronary artery bypass graft (CABG) surgery and found to have a blood glucose of 13 mmol/L. This patient has suffered from angina for 5 years and still has symptoms on maximal medical therapy. He has had coronary angiography, which shows triple-vessel disease, and his Cardiologist has recommended surgery rather than percutaneous coronary intervention.

How would you manage this patient?

- Ask about symptoms of diabetes, e.g. thirst, polyuria, lack of energy.
- Check that a laboratory glucose has been sent to confirm the diagnosis of diabetes (random glucose 13.4 mmol/L).
- Discuss the patient's angina symptoms and the urgency of CABG surgery with the Cardiologist.
- It is agreed by all, including the patient, that his diabetes should be treated and blood sugar controlled before surgery is performed.
- He is referred to the Diabetic Liaison Nurse for assessment and discussion of treatment as an outpatient.

Remember

Always bring diabetes under control before patients undergo surgery, unless this is an emergency.

Information

ASSESSMENT OF NEW PATIENTS WITH DIABETES
- Carry out a biochemical assessment of long-term glycaemic control (e.g. HbA1c)
- Measure body weight
- Measure blood pressure
- Measure plasma lipids
- Measure visual acuity
- Examine the retina through dilated fundi (ophthalmoscope initially, followed by retinal photo)
- Test urine for protein
- Test blood for renal function (creatinine and eGFR)
- Check general condition of the feet, peripheral pulses and sensation
- Review cardiovascular risk factors
- Introduce self-monitoring and injection techniques if insulin is required
- Review dietary knowledge

Progress. This patient was managed with lifestyle changes and metformin, initially 500 mg daily. He will undertake surgery when his HbA1c is <7% (53 mmol/mol).

Management for surgery

Non-insulin-treated patients should stop medication 2 days before the procedure. Patients with mild hyperglycaemia (fasting blood glucose <8 mmol/L) can be treated as non-diabetic. Those with higher levels are treated with soluble insulin prior to the procedure/surgery, and with glucose, insulin and potassium infusion during and after the procedure (see p. 405). Be careful of hypoglycaemia due to the additive effect of medications taken previously. Postoperatively, patients should return to their normal management regimen when they begin eating and drinking.

Who needs insulin perioperatively?

- All patients who usually use insulin.
- All acute surgical emergencies (type 1 and type 2 diabetes).
- All patients undergoing major surgery (type 1 and type 2 diabetes).

In other words, all diabetic patients should receive insulin, except type 2 diabetic individuals undergoing minor surgery. For patients on insulin, give the usual evening and/or night-time insulin, and commence glucose and insulin as described at 06:00.

Urgent surgery in patients with diabetes

Surgery requires patients to fast for several hours. In addition, a general anaesthetic and surgery themselves place significant stresses on an individual. The hormonal response to stress involves a significant rise in counter-regulatory hormones to insulin, in particular cortisol and adrenaline (epinephrine). For this reason, patients with diabetes undergoing surgery will require an increased dose of insulin, despite their fasting state. Long-acting hypoglycaemic agents must be stopped the night before surgery because hypoglycaemia might otherwise occur. In the case of an emergency operation where the patient has taken a long-acting insulin, an infusion of 10% glucose can be used (usually with potassium), together with a controlled infusion of insulin.

The procedure for **insulin-treated patients** is simple:

In patients whose diabetic control is poor and who are not undergoing emergency surgery, diabetic control should be reassessed and therapy adjusted to achieve an HbA1c <8.5% (70 mmol/mol), if possible preoperatively.

Preoperative glucose levels should be in the range of 7–11 mmol/L.

The patient's usual insulin is given the night before the operation and, whenever possible, diabetic patients should be first on the morning procedure/operating list.

An infusion of glucose, insulin and potassium is given during the procedure/surgery. The insulin can be mixed into the glucose solution or administered separately by syringe pump. A standard combination is 16 U of soluble insulin with 10 mmol of KCl in 1 L of 5–10% glucose, infused at 125 mL/h. The insulin dose is adjusted:

- Blood glucose <4 mmol/L – 8 U/L
- Blood glucose 4–15 mmol/L – 16 U/L
- Blood glucose 15–20 mmol/L – 32 U/L.

Postoperatively, the infusion is maintained until the patient is able to eat. Other fluids needed in the perioperative period must be given through a separate IV line and must not interrupt the glucose/insulin/potassium infusion. Glucose levels are checked every 2–4 h and potassium levels are monitored. The amount of insulin and potassium in each infusion bag is adjusted either upwards or downwards, according to the results of regular monitoring of the blood glucose and serum potassium concentrations.

The same approach is used in the emergency situation, with the exception that a separate variable-rate insulin infusion may be needed to bring blood glucose under control before surgery.

THE DIABETIC FOOT

Case history

The chiropodist in the Diabetic Clinic asks you to review an 84-year-old woman who is complaining of severe pain in her big toe. She had attempted to cut a toe nail a week ago and the toe had become painful and infected. She is known to have type 2 diabetes, for which she takes glibenclamide 10 mg daily. She does not have regular supervision of her diabetes.

On examination, she has a 2 cm ulcer on the medial side of her big toe with swelling and erythema.

Remember

- Many foot problems are avoidable. Older diabetic patients must be taught good foot care and should not cut their own toe nails.
- Diabetic foot problems can occur in patients with type 1 and type 2 diabetes.

What further points would be helpful in the history?

- Is there a previous history of foot problems?
- Does she regularly inspect and wash her feet? Is she careful about buying shoes of the correct size?
- How good is her sight?
- Does she live alone? Does she have any help?
- Is there any suggestion of peripheral vascular disease, e.g. intermittent claudication?
- Is there any suggestion of peripheral sensory problems? Does she complain of numbness or burning in her feet?

Remember

Fifty per cent of patients have no previous history of neuropathy or peripheral vascular disease.

What particular points do you look for on examination?

- Inspect the lesion. Take a swab for culture.
- Look for signs of neuropathy:
  - Dry skin
  - Evidence of sensory loss to pin-prick/light touch/vibration

- Check ankle jerks — absent knee and ankle jerks and sensory loss indicate a neuropathy.
- Look for signs of vascular insufficiency:
  - Check peripheral pulses
  - Are the toes cold?

Pathogenesis of foot ulcers

- Most ulcers occur as a result of trauma.
- Neuropathy causes:
  - Reduced sensitivity
  - Altered proprioception with 'high pressure' on parts of the foot
  - Autonomic dysfunction, leading to dry skin with cracks and fissures.
- Peripheral vascular disease:
  - Very common
  - Leads to ischaemic ulcers (pure ischaemic ulcers in 10%). Ninety per cent of ulcers are due to neuropathy alone, or a combination of neuropathy and ischaemia.

Information

DIABETES IN INDIA
- There are 50 million people with diabetes mellitus.
- Foot problems are very common: these are due to neuropathic and infective causes rather than vascular ones.

Management

- Admit the patient to an MAU.
- Take swabs for microbiology.
- Arrange an urgent X-ray to look for foreign bodies, gas and osteomyelitis.
- Early effective antibiotic treatment is essential:
  - Use broad-spectrum antibiotic cover until cultures are available, e.g. flucloxacillin, amoxicillin and metronidazole
  - Discuss with a microbiologist.
- Control the diabetes with insulin until the foot is healed, when oral treatment can be restarted.
- Establish the presence of other diabetic complications (see earlier).
- Ask the Diabetic team to carry out a full assessment and arrange for future follow-up care.

Information

MEGGITT—WAGNER CLASSIFICATION OF DIABETIC FOOT ULCERS
- Grade 0: high-risk foot with no ulcers
- Grade 1: superficial ulcer
- Grade 2: deeper ulcer infection/cellulitis; no bone involvement
- Grade 3: osteomyelitis and foot ulceration
- Grade 4: localised gangrene (toes, forefoot or heel)
- Grade 5: gangrene of entire foot

Progress. This woman was admitted to the MAU and seen by the Tissue Viability Nurse for daily dressing of her foot ulcer. The inflammation settled and she was discharged after 6 days with full nursing care at her own home. She was continued on glibenclamide and metformin. Note that 40% of patients have a recurrence within 1 year after ulcer healing.

DIABETES IN PREGNANCY

Case history (1)

You are asked to see a 28-year-old woman who is 18 weeks pregnant and has been found to have a blood glucose of 10 mmol/L. She is asymptomatic and gives no history of diabetes.

Diagnosis. Gestational diabetes.

How should this patient be managed?

Meticulous glycaemic control is of paramount importance in pregnancy. The patient should initially be taught to monitor her blood glucose levels and be advised on lifestyle changes, including diet. Blood glucose levels should be measured 1 h after each meal. If blood glucose is <7 mmol/L, then insulin is not required. Oral hypoglycaemic agents are avoided in pregnancy because they cross the placental barrier (although there is evidence that glibenclamide is safe), so that if glucose levels are >7 mmol/L, insulin therapy is required. High levels of glucose are associated with risk of neonatal macrosomia, fetal death and postnatal hypoglycaemia. Thus the patient should be commenced on soluble insulin with each meal and a long-acting insulin at night if glucose is not controlled to <7 mmol/L.

Information

- Normal women have lower blood glucose during pregnancy.
- Thresholds vary between diabetic units but a fasting glucose >6 mmol/L or a random/post-prandial glucose >7.8 mmol/L is an indication for home blood glucose monitoring.
- Diet should be healthy but not restricted.
- Pregnant women have a low threshold to start insulin.

Progress. This patient required insulin therapy, which was continued until she delivered at normal term.

Case history (2)

You are called to the labour ward to see a patient who is on insulin. She has been on soluble insulin 12 U three times daily and isophane insulin 18 U last thing at night, with very good control of her blood sugar. She is now in labour and is nil by mouth.

What is your immediate management of this patient?

An infusion of 5% glucose containing 10 mmol of KCl and 16 U of insulin in 1 L is commenced at an initial rate of 125 mL/h.

The dose of insulin is adjusted with hourly glucose assessment (see p. 402), with a target blood glucose of 4–9 mmol/L. The infusion is maintained until the patient is able to eat and drink.

It is essential to determine whether the patient had type 1 diabetes before pregnancy (in which case, insulin should never be stopped) or whether she has gestational diabetes, when insulin therapy can be stopped after delivery. The placental hormones cause insulin resistance and, after the third stage of labour, gestational diabetes can disappear.

Progress. This mother has type 1 diabetes, so she was commenced on her pre-pregnancy dose of insulin when she started eating. IV insulin must be continued until 4 h after the first dose of SC insulin. She is followed up at her doctor's Diabetic Clinic.

CUSHING'S SYNDROME

Cortisol is the principal endogenous glucocorticoid secreted from the adrenal glands; the amount is controlled by the level of plasma ACTH.

Cushing's syndrome is caused by excess glucocorticoids for the reasons shown in the Information box, of which exogenous corticosteroid administration is the commonest.

Patients have undiagnosed Cushing's syndrome for some time, and present because of metabolic decompensation due to either hypokalaemia (which can be severe), or hyperglycaemia and resultant dehydration.

Other complications follow, including secondary infection, bruising and bleeding, uncontrollable hypertension and osteoporotic fractures (Fig. 14.2).

Information

CAUSES OF CUSHING'S SYNDROME
(Percentages in brackets refer to incidence of the primary cause)
- Excess corticosteroid administration
- Pituitary-dependent Cushing's disease (85%)
- Adrenal adenoma (10%)
- Ectopic ACTH protection (5%)

Case history

A 55-year-old woman presents with a 2-year history of atypical depression and 3 weeks of confusion, altered behaviour and an inability to climb stairs due to muscular weakness. Her weight has increased marginally but she has lost muscle bulk from the arms and legs.

On examination, she was obese and plethoric, with a moon face and buffalo hump. Her skin was thin with multiple striae over breasts, abdomen and thighs.

Diagnosis. Cushing's syndrome.

The patient was dehydrated and was found to have glycosuria, with a blood glucose of 30 mmol/L.

ABGs reveal:
- pH 7.60
- pO_2 12.0 kPa
- pCO_2 5.4 kPa.

This patient has a metabolic alkalosis due to the chronic hypokalaemia found in Cushing's. Electrolytes came back from the laboratory, confirming your suspicions:
- Na^+ 145 mmol/L
- K^+ 2.5 mmol/L
- Urea 15.0 mmol/L

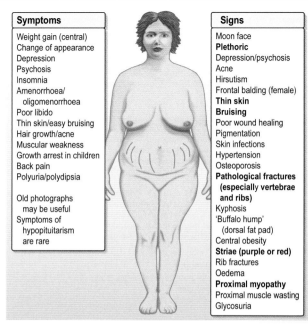

Symptoms		Signs
Weight gain (central)		Moon face
Change of appearance		**Plethoric**
Depression		Depression/psychosis
Psychosis		Acne
Insomnia		Hirsutism
Amenorrhoea/		Frontal balding (female)
oligomenorrhoea		**Thin skin**
Poor libido		**Bruising**
Thin skin/easy bruising		Poor wound healing
Hair growth/acne		Pigmentation
Muscular weakness		Skin infections
Growth arrest in children		Hypertension
Back pain		Osteoporosis
Polyuria/polydipsia		**Pathological fractures**
		(especially vertebrae
Old photographs		**and ribs)**
may be useful		Kyphosis
Symptoms of		'Buffalo hump'
hypopituitarism		(dorsal fat pad)
are rare		Central obesity
		Striae (purple or red)
		Rib fractures
		Oedema
		Proximal myopathy
		Proximal muscle wasting
		Glycosuria

Figure 14.2 Symptoms and signs of Cushing's syndrome. Bold type indicates the signs of most value in discriminating Cushing's syndrome from simple obesity and hirsutism.

- Creatinine 120 μmol/L
- Bicarbonate 37 mmol/L
- Glucose 27 mmol/L.

How would you manage this patient?

The hypokalaemia and hyperglycaemia need prompt treatment. Total body potassium is likely to be extremely low, and as potassium is replaced, the initial effect will be to reduce the bicarbonate rather than to increase the extracellular (serum) potassium.

- Start potassium replacement both orally and IV (not more than 20 mmol in any 3 h) to provide at least 200 mmol per day.
- Rehydrate the patient with 0.9% saline + potassium chloride (40 mmol/L) added to each bag (see p. 405) with 2-hourly K^+ monitoring.
- Start an IV infusion of insulin at 4 U/h. This might exacerbate the fall in serum potassium.
- After 48 h the patient was rehydrated with a serum K^+ of 4.5 mmol/L.

- *Confirm the diagnosis of Cushing's syndrome.*
  - Collect 24 h urine for urinary free cortisol (normal <700 nmol in 24 h).
  - Measure midnight cortisol (normal <50 nmol/L).
  - Give 8 h low-dose dexamethasone suppression (0.5 mg 6-hourly for 48 h at 09:00, 15:00, 21:00, 03:00 followed by 09:00 cortisol).

Progress. Cushing's is confirmed and the patient is referred for specialist investigation. These investigations will include determination of ACTH dependence, pituitary and adrenal CT scanning, and localisation procedures.

HYPERTHYROIDISM

Case history (1)

A 65-year-old woman is brought to A&E with acute breathlessness and cough, producing frothy, blood-tinged sputum.

On examination, she had profuse sweating with rapid severe breathlessness. She has atrial fibrillation (AF), and auscultation reveals wheezes and crackles throughout the chest. Your diagnosis of **pulmonary oedema** is confirmed by the CXR, which shows bilateral perihilar shadowing and Kerley B lines of interstitial oedema.

The ECG shows fast AF (160/min) but there is no evidence of cardiac ischaemia or other abnormality (Fig. 14.3).

What should you do?

- Admit the patient to the HDU and start treatment of acute heart failure, oxygen, IV furosemide 50 mg and vasodilatation therapy with glyceryl trinitrate infusion 100−200 μg/min.

  She responds well but still has fast AF.
- *Urgent.* TFTs reveal a free T4 of 45 pmol/L (normal range 9.0−23) with a suppressed TSH.

  Diagnosis. Hyperthyroidism.

Treatment

- Control the heart rate using beta-blockers (propranolol 40 mg every 8 h), and digoxin if required.
- Avoid amiodarone, as this will potentially interfere with investigation and management.
- Anti-coagulate the patient (heparin and warfarin, or thrombin inhibitors, e.g. rivaroxaban).

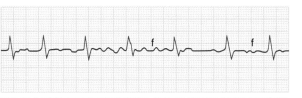

Figure 14.3 ECG showing atrial fibrillation. Note the absolute rhythm irregularity and baseline undulations (*f* waves). (From Kumar P, Clark M, eds. *Kumar and Clark's Clinical Medicine*, 9th edn. Edinburgh: Elsevier, 2017; Fig 23.46A.)

- Start anti-thyroid medication, e.g. carbimazole 40 mg daily (or methimazole).
- Determine the cause of the hyperthyroidism (see later).

Beta-adrenoreceptors are sensitised to normal circulating catecholamines by high levels of thyroxine and beta-blockade is useful in achieving symptom control in hyperthyroidism; it is also helpful in treating high-output heart failure and achieving rate control. Propranolol is used in high doses (40 mg every 8 h) because, being lipid-soluble, it crosses the blood−brain barrier.

Remember

- TSH is invariably suppressed in hyperthyroidism (except for the exceptionally rare TSH-secreting pituitary adenoma).
- Hyperthyroidism often presents in the elderly with AF and few other features.

Investigations

- Thyroid anti-microsomal auto-antibodies and anti-thyroglobulin antibodies (in the serum): positive in up to 90% of patients with Graves' disease
- Thyroid technetium scan to distinguish a 'hot nodule' (focal uptake) from Graves' disease (uniform uptake) and from viral thyroiditis (zero uptake)

Progress. This woman was confirmed as having Graves' disease. She was followed up for her hyperthyroidism with reduction of her carbimazole dosage. A Cardiologist advised her to stay on digoxin and warfarin, and she remained in AF at 6 months.

Case history (2)

A 75-year-old woman is referred with weight loss, general malaise and apathy.
  Clinical examination is unremarkable, except for a mild tachycardia of 100 bpm.
  Routine investigations (remembering to include TFTs) (Table 14.7) have now been phoned through by the Biochemist with the following results:
- Free T_4: 56 pmol/L (normal range 9−23 pmol/L)
- TSH <0.1 mU/L (normal range 0.3−5.5 mU/L)

Elderly patients can have atypical presenting features of hyperthyroidism, which may be dominated by weight loss, apathy and fatigue.

Remember

Weight loss without obvious cause always requires a TSH measurement.

Information

HYPERTHYROIDISM IN THE ELDERLY
- Weight loss
- Atrial fibrillation
- Lethargy
- Proximal myopathy

Causes of hyperthyroidism

Common causes
- Graves' disease.

Table 14.7 Characteristics of TFTs in common thyroid disorders[a]

	TSH (0.3–3.5 mU/L)	Free T$_4$ (10–25 pmol/L)	Free T$_3$ (3.5–7.5 pmol/L)
Thyrotoxicosis	**Suppressed (<0.05 mU/L)**	**Increased**	**Increased**
Primary hypothyroidism	**Increased (>10 mU/L)**	Low/ low–normal	Normal or low
TSH deficiency	Low–normal or subnormal	**Low/ low–normal**	Normal or low
T3 toxicosis	Suppressed (<0.05 mU/L)	Normal	**Increased**
Compensated euthyroidism	**Slightly increased (5–10 mU/L)**	**Normal**	Normal

[a]The clinically most informative tests in each situation are shown in bold.

- Multinodular goitre.
- Toxic solitary nodule.
- Viral thyroiditis.
- Amiodarone.

Rare causes
- TSH-secreting pituitary adenoma.
- Choriocarcinoma.
- Factitious (self-medication).

Tests in patients with goitres

- **Thyroid function tests:** TSH plus free T$_4$ or T$_3$.
- **Thyroid antibodies:** to exclude auto-immune aetiology.
- **Ultrasound:** ultrasound with high resolution is a sensitive method for delineating nodules and can demonstrate whether they are cystic or solid. In addition, a multinodular goitre may be demonstrated when only a single nodule is palpable. Unfortunately, even cystic lesions can be malignant and thyroid tumours may arise within a multinodular goitre; therefore fine-needle aspiration (see next point) is often required, and is performed under ultrasound control at the same time as the scan.
- **Fine-needle aspiration (FNA):** In patients with a solitary nodule or a dominant nodule in a multinodular goitre, there is a 5% chance of malignancy; in view of this, FNA should be performed. This can be done in the outpatient clinic. Cytology in expert hands can usually differentiate the suspicious or definitely malignant nodule. FNA reduces the necessity for surgery, but there is a 5% false-negative rate, which must be borne in mind (and the patient appropriately counselled). Continued observation is required when an isolated thyroid nodule is assumed to be benign without excision.

- **Thyroid scan** (99^m technetium): This can be useful to distinguish between functioning (hot) or non-functioning (cold) nodules. A hot nodule is only rarely malignant; however, a cold nodule is malignant in only 10% of cases and FNA has largely replaced 99^m technetium scans in the diagnosis of thyroid nodules.

Drug treatment in hyperthyroidism

- Rapid symptomatic treatment (if necessary): propranolol 40–80 mg 8-hourly.
- Control thyroid over-activity:
  - Carbimazole 40 mg once daily *or*
  - Propylthiouracil (PTU) 200 mg × 3 daily.

The last two drugs inhibit the formation of thyroid hormones (Fig. 14.4). Carbimazole and PTU will induce hypothyroidism after 4–8 weeks at these doses, and either treatment should be titrated down to a maintenance level (e.g. carbimazole 10 mg daily) or thyroxine should be added back at a dose of 100–150 μg in a 'block and replace' regimen. Patients are typically treated for 6–18 months with anti-thyroid drugs. All patients commencing anti-thyroid drugs should be warned about possible rashes, which are common and usually self-limiting without discontinuation, and severe sore throats or mouth ulcers, which may indicate a dangerous fall in neutrophils.

Treatment with radio-iodine is frequently employed if patients relapse after medical treatment but may also be used as primary treatment, particularly in multinodular goitres or toxic adenoma. Surgery is reserved for large goitres or for patient preference after relapse.

Remember

Agranulocytosis occurs in 1 : 1000 patients on anti-thyroid drugs. All patients prescribed anti-thyroid drugs should be warned to report severe mouth ulcers or sore throats immediately, and should have an urgent FBC if symptoms are experienced.

Information

INVESTIGATION OF A SOLITARY NODULE

- All solitary nodules >1 cm should be evaluated, as should 'dominant' nodules in nodular goitres.
- Fine-needle aspiration cytology is the first-line investigation to identify a papillary carcinoma or follicular neoplasm.
- Ultrasound is used to diagnose multinodular goitre.
- Isotope scanning might identify a toxic 'hot' solitary nodule; these are almost always benign.

Progress. This patient was treated with carbimazole and at 3 months was euthyroid.

Case history (3)

You have been phoned by a doctor who has received the results of some TFTs on one of his patients. The blood test report showed a high free T4: 45 pmol/L (normal range 10–25) with a suppressed TSH (<0.1 mU/L). On further questioning, it transpires that the test was performed in a patient who was unwell with a painful neck. You recommend a thyroid technetium uptake scan, which shows minimal uptake, and arrange for the patient to come to outpatients in 2 weeks.

When you see the patient he is better but still clinically hyperthyroid. Repeat TFTs are as follows: free T4 7.0 pmol/L; TSH 25 mU/L.

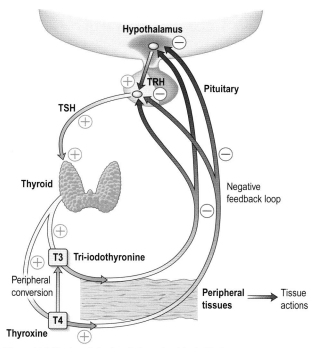

Figure 14.4 The hypothalamic–pituitary–thyroid axis. Pituitary thyroid stimulating hormone (TSH) is secreted in response to hypothalamic thyrotropin releasing hormone (TRH) and stimulates secretion of T4 and T3 from the thyroid. T4 and T3 have actions in peripheral tissues and exert negative feedback on pituitary and hypothalamus.

This patient is now biochemically hypothyroid, although the initial biochemistry demonstrated hyperthyroidism.

This presentation is strongly suggestive of **viral thyroiditis (de Quervain's)**. Thyroid hormones are released in the early stage (when the patient is thyrotoxic) and patients typically become biochemically, and later clinically, hypothyroid. The tissue effects of high levels of thyroxine last longer than their serum levels and symptoms often lag behind the biochemical changes.

Progress. Viral thyroiditis does not usually require treatment; hypothyroidism is often transient, although a short course of thyroxine (3–6 months) should be used if high TSH persists. Autoantibodies might be positive because of the viral damage and do not necessarily predict long-term thyroid dysfunction. TFTs at 6–12 months were normal in this patient.

Features of viral (de Quervain's) thyroiditis

- Neck discomfort or pain on swallowing; a short course of prednisolone is used if pain is severe.
- History of viral illness.
- Hyperthyroidism (usually 1–3 weeks), followed by hypothyroidism, and then resolution.
- Disparity between clinical features and biochemistry.
- High ESR.
- Reduced uptake on technetium uptake scan.
- Weakly positive anti-thyroid antibodies.

Case history (4)

A 42-year-old woman was brought to A&E as an emergency with a 24 h history of vomiting, diarrhoea and two seizures. She had become confused and was now very drowsy.

She was accompanied by her partner, who explains that she has been unwell for 6 months with a thyroid problem, for which she takes tablets. Following a severe cold 7 days ago, he thinks that she has stopped her therapy.

On examination, she has a GCS of 8 with the following findings:

- Tachycardia >145—bpm, ? atrial fibrillation
- Hyperpyrexia >41°C
- Heart failure
- Jaundice
- Psychosis.

Patients who have two or more of the above have a high mortality. Symptoms can also include vomiting, diarrhoea, seizures and coma.

Thyroid storm

This is defined as being present in a patient with biochemical hyperthyroidism and any two of the above features. It is a rare medical emergency because thyrotoxicosis is now easy to diagnose biochemically and can be treated earlier than formerly.

It can be precipitated by thyroid surgery, the administration of radioiodine, the withdrawal of or non-compliance with anti-thyroid medication and by acute illness.

Treatment

- Cooling of the patient with tepid sponging and a fan. Do not use aspirin, which is contraindicated in thyroid storm (it displaces thyroxine from its binding globulin and increases the free T4).
- Beta-blockers (propranolol 5 mg IV then 40–80 mg 8-hourly orally) unless contraindicated by asthma. (*Note:* heart failure is not a contraindication to beta-blockers.)
- Fluid replacement. This needs careful assessment with central venous monitoring. Heart failure will rapidly come under control once the patient's heart rate is lowered.
- Hydrocortisone 100 mg IV 6-hourly. This blocks T4 to T3 conversion.
- Propylthiouracil 250 mg 4-hourly.

- Potassium iodide 60 mg 8-hourly, as iodine blocks thyroxine synthesis and release. This should be given at least 1 h after the propylthiouracil, which blocks iodine incorporation but not uptake.

Progress. This woman responded to her emergency treatment and was referred back to the Endocrine team, who have now recommended radioactive thyroid treatment.

AMIODARONE AND THYROID FUNCTION

Case history

A 45-year-old woman presents in A&E with increased breathlessness over the last few days. On direct questioning she says that she has been losing weight (8 kg) for 4 months. She gives a past history of heart problems, for which she is under the care of a Cardiologist. She is unsure of the exact problem but says that she does take tablets for an irregular pulse and has brought them with her. She is on amiodarone and also takes warfarin and a diuretic.

On examination, she has an irregular pulse 120/min, and a raised JVP with crackles at both bases.

You diagnose **mild heart failure with atrial fibrillation**, which is confirmed by ECG.

Treatment

You increase her diuretic to furosemide 80 mg daily and start her on enalapril at a small initial dose of 2.5 mg daily.

Progress. On post-take ward round your consultant is pleased with your summary of the woman's condition and your initial management. He asks you about the weight loss, which you have noted but so far have no explanation for.

Fortunately, you have done many blood tests, including TFTs, the results of which are now available. These show a free T4 30.7 pmol/L and a TSH <0.1 mU/L.

How should you proceed?

- Confirm how long the patient has been on amiodarone and check the clinical record to establish whether there are any previous TFT results, particularly those before amiodarone therapy was commenced.
- Amiodarone can cause hypo- or hyperthyroidism. In patients who have nodular thyroid disease the synthesis of thyroxine may be autonomous and is limited only by iodine availability: thyrotoxicosis may be precipitated. In others, the Wolff–Chaikoff effect may result in hypothyroidism. Amiodarone also blocks T4 to T3 conversion, causing a high T4 and normal T3.
- Examine the patient for clinical evidence of hyperthyroidism.
- The patient is clinically as well as biochemically thyrotoxic, so start carbimazole 40 mg daily and ask the patient's Cardiologist to discontinue amiodarone and use other therapy for her atrial fibrillation. Amiodarone-induced thyrotoxicosis can require high doses of carbimazole and sometimes prednisolone is helpful in controlling the condition. Because amiodarone contains large amounts of iodine, radioiodine cannot be used.

Amiodarone contains a substantial amount of iodine and has a half-life of about a month. Thus amiodarone behaves like slow-release iodine.

TFTs on amiodarone:

- Normal
- High free T4, normal TSH due to reduced conversion: monitor
- Subclinical thyrotoxicosis, i.e. suppressed TSH: change therapy
- Clinical thyrotoxicosis: change treatment and control over-activity
- Hypothyroidism: titrate thyroxine very gradually starting at 25 µg daily.

Wolff and Chaikoff first noted that excessive iodine suppresses thyroid function and causes short-term atrophy of the thyroid gland. Surgeons use this effect by administration of potassium iodide for 10 days before surgery. This is also why potassium iodide is used in thyroid storm.

Progress. The Cardiologists agreed that this patient should stop amiodarone and start verapamil. They said that two attempts at DC conversion had failed in the past and DC was unlikely to be successful now. The patient became euthyroid after 3 months' carbimazole therapy.

HYPOTHYROIDISM

Case history

A 42-year-old woman is seen in the Well Women's Clinic because she is having irregular periods that are sometimes very heavy. She thinks she has become menopausal and wonders about hormone replacement therapy (HRT). A more detailed history reveals that she has general malaise, weight gain (5 kg in 6 months), constipation and a hoarse voice.

On examination, she is overweight at 68 kg (BMI 30). There is no palpable goitre but she does have swollen, non-pitting oedema of her legs and slow relaxation of her ankle jerks.

***Diagnosis*: Hypothyroidism.**

Investigations show a raised TSH (30 µg/L) and free T4 of 4.2 pmol/L, confirming hypothyroidism. Interpretation of TFTs is shown in Fig. 14.5.

Hypothyroidism is now diagnosed by a multitude of practitioners:

- Lipid clinic: cause of hypercholesterolaemia
- Psychiatrists: organic psychosis or depression
- Neurologists: ataxia
- ENT surgeons: dysphonia or deafness
- Cardiologists: during follow-up of amiodarone treatment
- Dermatologists: dry skin or hair
- Gynaecologists: menorrhagia, oligo- or amenorrhoea, infertility
- Geriatricians: screening test
- Diabetologists: screening test in diabetes.

In primary hypothyroidism, the TSH will *always* be elevated and often very high.

Adult-onset primary hypothyroidism is usually due to auto-immune disease, unless there has been:

- Amiodarone treatment

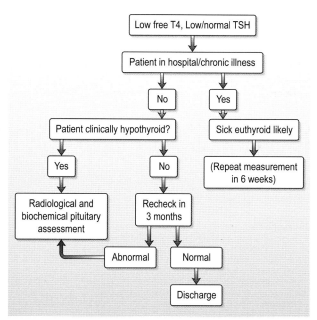

Figure 14.5 Interpretation of thyroid function tests. TSH, thyroid stimulating hormone.

- Previous thyroid surgery
- Previous radio-iodine treatment
- Viral or post-partum thyroiditis.

Treatment

The patient, who is otherwise fit and not at risk of ischaemic heart disease, is started on 100 μg levothyroxine daily.

And then?

It takes about 6 weeks for a steady state to be reached. Aim to increase the levothyroxine dose in 25 μg increments every 6 weeks until the TSH is within or just below the normal range (3–3.5 mU/L). Occasionally, patients require only 50–75 μg daily, although usually 100–150 μg daily is required. Think about associated auto-immune diseases:

- Vitamin B_{12} deficiency
- Myasthenia gravis
- Addison's disease

- Coeliac disease
- Other organ-specific auto-immune diseases.

If the patient has angina, be very careful indeed. Many clinicians start at 25 µg per day (or even alternate days) and increase every 4–6 weeks. With hypothyroidism or when attempting thyroxine replacement with unstable angina, treat the heart disease first.

What is compensated hypothyroidism?

Early in the course of hypothyroidism the TSH is elevated (4–20 mU/L) but T4 and T3 are normal. Opinion differs as to the need for treatment. Most Endocrinologists replace with levothyroxine:

- If autoantibodies are present in high titre
- If the patient has typical symptoms of hypothyroidism
- In the presence of a high cholesterol
- If TSH is >10 mU/L.

Progress. The patient made a complete recovery on levothyroxine therapy and did not require HRT.

ADDISON'S DISEASE

Case history

A 35-year-old teacher has been under the care of a Gynaecologist, whom she consulted for amenorrhoea and menopausal symptoms. She has been increasingly tired and has lost weight over a 6-month period. She presents acutely to A&E with a 2-day history of vomiting and postural hypotension.

On examination, she has a dull, slightly grey/brown pigmentation, easily seen on her palmar creases. Her blood pressure is 80/60 with a postural drop.

Electrolytes:
- Sodium: 127 mmol/L
- Potassium: 5.2 mmol/L
- Urea: 16 mmol/L
- Creatinine: 140 µmol/L.

The clinical presentation and electrolytes indicate **adrenal insufficiency.** Treatment with glucocorticoids (e.g. hydrocortisone) and IV 0.9% saline is life-saving in this situation and should be started immediately after a blood sample is taken for plasma cortisol/ACTH measurements.

Adrenal insufficiency presents gradually – over months – but also, as in this case, with acute haemodynamic collapse, often precipitated by infection, trauma or surgery. Crises can also occur in patients with known Addison's disease during relatively trivial episodes such as a viral infection; for this reason, patients are advised to increase (typically double) the dose of hydrocortisone during illness.

Patients who are on long-term steroids for inflammatory conditions such as asthma also have pituitary adrenal suppression but do not develop the same pattern of electrolyte disturbance and rarely become so unwell because they have preserved mineralocorticoid (i.e. aldosterone) secretion.

Clinical findings in Addison's disease

Acute
- Hypotension (may be severe or postural).

- Nausea and vomiting.
- Diarrhoea.
- Hyponatraemia and hyperkalaemia.
- Metabolic acidosis.
- Hypercalcaemia.
- Mild elevation of TSH.

Chronic
- Weight loss and anorexia.
- Fatigue.
- Generalised weakness.
- Hyperpigmentation.
- Arthralgia and myalgia.
- Depression, apathy and confusion.

Information

COMMON CAUSES OF ADRENAL FAILURE
Primary
- Auto-immune: often associated with other auto-immune disease (e.g. type 1 diabetes mellitus, hypothyroidism, premature ovarian failure)
- Tuberculous adrenalitis: consider in immigrant populations/developing countries
- Drugs (e.g. ketoconazole, metyrapone)

Secondary (i.e. due to ACTH deficiency)
- Long-term glucocorticoid therapy (oral, inhaled, topical or intranasal steroids)
- Hypopituitarism

Immediate management of this patient (Fig. 14.6)

General
- Give IV 0.9% saline.
- Correct hypoglycaemia with 5% glucose.
- Identify and treat a precipitating cause.

Specific
- Take samples for cortisol and ACTH.
- Hydrocortisone (100 mg IM); the intramuscular route gives sustained plasma levels.
- Continue hydrocortisone 50–100 mg IV/IM × 4 daily.

Investigations

FURTHER INVESTIGATIONS
- FBC (anaemia, normochromic normocytic)
- Glucose (hypoglycaemia)
- Serum calcium (might be high)
- ABGs (acidosis)
- CXR (TB, carcinoma)
- Short tetracosactide test (see Information box) if necessary to confirm diagnosis
- Pituitary MRI if hypopituitarism suspected

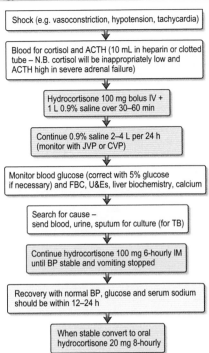

Figure 14.6 Management of acute adrenal failure. (From Kumar P, Clark M, eds. *Kumar and Clark's Medical Management & Therapeutics*. Edinburgh: Elsevier, 2011; Fig. 20.19.)

The initial cortisol in this woman was <100 nmol/L and so Addison's disease is confirmed. In a less clear-cut case, use a tetracosactide test.

Progress. Once the patient had recovered and was eating and drinking, hydrocortisone replacement was rapidly tapered to 20 mg daily, given as 10 mg (06:00) + 5 mg (12:00) + 5 mg (18:00) to try to mimic the physiological circadian rhythm. Fludrocortisone was commenced at 100 μg daily.

Information

SHORT ACTH (TETRACOSACTIDE) TEST
- Omit morning and previous evening dose of hydrocortisone
- Take baseline blood sample for cortisol and ACTH
- Administer tetracosactrin 250 μg IM or IV
- Take further blood samples for cortisol at 30 and 60 min
- 30-min cortisol <500 nmol/L is abnormal (500–600 nmol/L is borderline)

PATIENTS ON STEROIDS FOR SURGERY

Case history

A 50-year-old woman who is known to have chronic asthma and who has been on oral prednisolone between 10 mg and 40 mg for at least the last 10 years is admitted for a right hemicolectomy for a caecal carcinoma. Her asthma has been difficult to control on inhalers alone and she finds that it worsens whenever her dose of oral prednisolone is reduced to 10 mg, which she is on at present.

How should the patient's steroids be continued following surgery?

Patients who have been on prednisolone for more than 3 months are likely to have a suppressed pituitary–adrenal axis (Fig. 14.7). Adrenal mineralocorticoid production will be normal, so that the risks of a typical Addisonian crisis are small, but nevertheless this patient will not be able to mount the

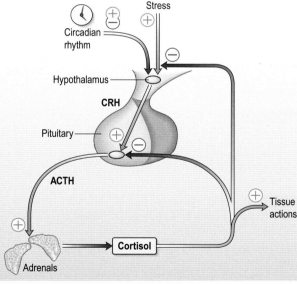

Figure 14.7 Control of the hypothalamic-pituitary-adrenal axis. Pituitary adrenocorticotrophic hormone (ACTH) is secreted in response to hypothalamic corticotrophin-releasing hormone (CRH) triggered by circadian rhythm, stress and other factors, and stimulates secretion of cortisol from the adrenal. Cortisol has multiple actions in peripheral tissues and exerts negative feedback on pituitary and hypothalamus.

normal cortisol response to surgery. Glucocorticoid replacement should be given as follows:

- At induction: hydrocortisone 100 mg IM; *then*
- 50–100 mg IM or IV daily for 3 days.

An IV infusion of hydrocortisone (25–100 mg over 24 h, i.e. 1–4 mg/h) should be given to all patients who will have a prolonged period nil by mouth or who are on the ITU. The pharmacokinetics of hydrocortisone are such that such a continuous infusion of 4 mg will achieve a steady-state plasma cortisol level of >500 nmol/L, similar to patients on the ITU with normal adrenals. A serum cortisol sample after 12 h of infusion can be used to titrate the hydrocortisone infusion down to achieve a cortisol level of 500–750 nmol/L. Hydrocortisone 100 mg every 6 h, when given IM, will also achieve a similar concentration of cortisol.

Note: Oral hydrocortisone has greater bioavailability than IV hydrocortisone.

Information

Once-daily steroids are used in pharmacological doses to treat inflammatory conditions. Such treatment is not appropriate for hydrocortisone replacement in patients with Addison's disease or congenital adrenal hyperplasia (who might not be able to synthesise any adrenal steroids), or following adrenalectomy, when there is a risk of true Addisonian crises. These patients need twice-daily treatment.

Progress. This patient's postoperative period was prolonged due to her asthma and she spent 48 h in the ITU. She eventually made a good recovery but continues to need oral steroids.

HYPERCALCAEMIA

Case history

A 56-year-old female patient who has been found to have fibroids has been admitted for a hysterectomy. She has treated hypertension but no other known illness, and no symptoms other than menorrhagia. A routine biochemical screen has revealed a corrected calcium of 2.75 mmol/L (normal range 2.20–2.60 mmol/L).

Information

An incidental finding of a raised serum calcium is a common presentation of hypercalcaemia and should be evaluated.

What is the appropriate management of this case with mild hypercalcaemia?

In mild to moderate hypercalcaemia with a corrected calcium <3.00 mmol/L:

- Ensure breast examination and CXR are reviewed
- Ensure adequate hydration preoperatively
- Continue IV 0.9% saline (1 L 8-hourly) postoperatively until patient is drinking freely
- U&Es and calcium postoperatively
- Follow-up with full investigation.

- U&Es and eGFR
- Serum parathyroid hormone (PTH)
- ESR
- Serum electrophesis and immunofixation for paraprotein
- Serum free light chain assay
- 24-h urine collection for calcium estimation
- CXR
- TFTs
- Serum angiotensin-converting enzyme (ACE) levels (for sarcoidosis)

Clinical features of moderate/severe hypercalcaemia

- Malaise, tiredness, fatigue.
- Anorexia and weight loss.
- Thirst and polyuria.
- Non-specific musculoskeletal symptoms.
- Renal calculus (stones).
- Osteoporosis ('bones').
- Abdominal pain ('groans').
- Confusion ('psychic moans').

Causes

Information

- Primary hyperparathyroidism is the most common cause of mild to moderate hypercalcaemia.
- Malignancy accounts for 50% of severe hypercalcaemia and is usually apparent with physical examination + CXR and breast examination.

PTH-dependent

- Primary hyperparathyroidism (the most common cause of mild hypercalcaemia).
- Tertiary hyperparathyroidism (in the context of chronic kidney disease).
- Familial hypocalciuric hypercalcaemia (slightly raised PTH).

PTH-independent

- Myeloma.
- Solid tumours: breast, bronchus, kidney, lymphoma.
- Vitamin D excess (especially the 1 alpha analogues of vitamin D).
- Sarcoidosis.
- Thyrotoxicosis.
- Glucocorticoid insufficiency.

Biochemical features of primary hyperparathyroidism

- Elevated PTH in the presence of hypercalcaemia. High normal PTH with hypercalcaemia also suggests hyperparathyroidism because any other cause of hypercalcaemia should suppress the PTH.
- Elevated or high/normal 24 h urinary calcium excretion (normal range 2–8 mmol/24 h).

- Low bicarbonate 15—20 mmol/L (PTH excess causes a mild renal tubular acidosis).
- Moderately elevated ESR.
- Normochromic anaemia.

Familial hypocalciuric hypercalcaemia (FHH) is a benign, familial, autosomal dominant condition caused by a mutation of the calcium-sensing receptor in the kidney and parathyroid gland. It is not associated with renal calculi and is asymptomatic. It can be difficult to distinguish from asymptomatic primary hyperparathyroidism. A low urinary calcium suggests the diagnosis, which is confirmed by examining family members.

Treatment of primary hyperparathyroidism

Patients who are symptomatic or who have complications should all be referred for parathyroid surgery, whatever the serum calcium level.

Most authorities suggest that the majority of asymptomatic patients should also be treated surgically because they are at risk of developing complications, and should certainly be referred for specialist opinion.

Progress. This patient had an uneventful postoperative recovery following her hysterectomy but did not want to consider any further surgery unless it became absolutely necessary. She is being followed with regular serum calcium levels.

SEVERE HYPERCALCAEMIA

Case history

A 72-year-old woman is referred with a diagnosis of 'recurrent hyperparathyroidism'. She had a past history of primary hyperparathyroidism, treated surgically 10 years previously, and had been maintained on a low dose of oral calcium.

Three months prior to admission she had become generally unwell, weak and lethargic. She reported weight loss of 5 kg. The GP had performed blood tests: corrected calcium 3.5 mmol/L; urea 16 mmol/L; creatinine 150 μmol/L. Renal function was previously normal. The patient arrived dehydrated and vomiting. She was found to have a fungating breast carcinoma, which she had kept secret.

- Recurrence of hyperparathyroidism after surgical cure is unusual and suggests a familial cause of hyperparathyroidism (e.g. multiple endocrine neoplasia) or an alternative cause, e.g. breast cancer.
- Hypercalcaemia causes dehydration by creating a secondary type of nephrogenic diabetes insipidus. As calcium clearance is itself dependent on GFR, hypercalcaemia can rapidly decompensate in the presence of fluid depletion.

Management of this patient's severe hypercalcaemia

Information

Severe hypercalcaemia is defined as: corrected calcium >3.5 mmol/L or >3.0 with evidence of dehydration.

- Aggressive rehydration with 0.9% saline 4—6 L over 24 h.
- Central venous pressure monitoring is usually necessary.
  This is usually sufficient to bring calcium down to 3.0 mmol/L.
- Bisphosphonate: treatment of choice for hypercalcaemia of malignancies or of undiagnosed cause; 60—90 mg infusion of disodium pamidronate

via a cannula in a large vein causes normalisation of serum calcium in 80% of patients after 48–72 h.

Other treatments:

- Glucocorticoids (e.g. prednisolone 60 mg daily is used in sarcoidosis or vitamin D toxicity).
- In life-threatening hypercalcaemia, haemodialysis may be necessary.

Progress. This patient's calcium level remained within the normal range for 2 weeks. She was referred to the Oncology department for treatment of the breast cancer and was started on an oral bisphosphonate, as skeletal secondaries were demonstrated.

HYPOCALCAEMIA

Case history

Three days after a total thyroidectomy, a 32-year-old patient develops tingling and numbness around the mouth and in the extremities. She has become emotionally labile.

On examination, tapping the facial nerve (Chvostek's sign) causes her upper lip to twitch. A serum calcium is 1.82 mmol/L corrected. How do you proceed?

Management

The patient's parathyroid glands might have been inadvertently removed. Before the plasma calcium result is available, an urgent assessment of the patient must be made to determine the severity.

Clinical features of hypocalcaemia

- Abnormal neurological sensations and neuromuscular excitability.
- Numbness around the mouth and paraesthesia of the distal limbs.
- Hyper-reflexia.
- Carpal and pedal spasms.
- Tetany contractions (may include laryngospasm).
- Generalised seizures.
- Chvostek's sign is elicited by tapping the facial nerve just anterior to the ear, causing ipsilateral contraction of the facial muscles (positive in 10% of normal people).
- Trousseau's sign is elicited by inflating a BP cuff for 3 min at the level of systolic BP. This causes mild ischaemia, unmasks latent neuromuscular hyper-excitability and enables carpal spasm to be observed.
- ECG: prolonged QT interval.

Information

CAUSES OF TETANY
In the presence of alkalosis

- Hyperventilation
- Excess antacid therapy
- Persistent vomiting
- Hypochloraemic alkalosis, e.g. primary hyperaldosteronism

In the presence of hypocalcaemia

- See later

How do you assess severity?

The symptoms and signs described are a much better guide to prognosis than the absolute value of the plasma calcium. In the presence of a low calcium (corrected calcium <2.0 mmol/L), any of the above features should be taken as evidence that urgent treatment is required.

Treatment of this patient (Table 14.8)

- Administer 10 mL calcium gluconate (10 mL of 10% calcium gluconate [2.20 mmol]) before the plasma calcium result is back.
- Hypocalcaemia is usually transient.

Investigations

- Plasma calcium (and albumin) and phosphate
- Plasma magnesium
- U&Es
- Plasma PTH level (low in hypoparathyroidism, high in vitamin D deficiency
- Vitamin D level
- Skull X-ray (intracranial calcification of chronic hypocalcaemia)

Causes of hypocalcaemia

- Hypoparathyroidism (primary, secondary or, most commonly, post-surgical).
- Renal failure (associated hyperphosphataemia).
- Vitamin D deficiency (giving rickets and osteomalacia).
- Pseudo-hypoparathyroidism (resistance to PTH).
- Severe magnesium deficiency (causes both reduced PTH secretion and resistance to PTH action).
- Acute pancreatitis.
- Rhabdomyolysis.

How do you manage symptomatic hypocalcaemia?

The aim of acute management is not to return the calcium to normal but to ameliorate the acute manifestations of hypocalcaemia (see Table 14.8).

Progress. This patient's serum calcium was normal on the fourth postoperative day and she made an uneventful recovery.

Information

Administration of alfacalcidol (0.5–1.0 μg), together with oral calcium gluconate, is used for chronic hypoparathyroidism with regular calcium monitoring.

PHAEOCHROMOCYTOMA AND PARAGANGLIOMA

Phaeochromocytomas are rare catecholamine-producing tumours derived from neuroendocrine cells, usually involving the adrenal glands (90%) or elsewhere in the sympathetic chain (paragangliomas).

Table 14.8 Management of symptomatic hypocalcaemia

Severity of hypocalcaemia	Recommended action
Emergency	
Spontaneous tetany, laryngospasm, seizures	Give 10 mL calcium gluconate 10% over 5 min IV, then proceed as below
Acute severe hypocalcaemia	
Frequent spasms/distressing symptoms and corrected calcium <2.00 mmol/L *or*	Calcium infusion: calcium gluconate at 15 mg/kg IV over 4 h in 1 L 0.9% saline. This is equivalent to [(weight in kg) × 1.7] mL of 10% calcium gluconate
Mild symptoms and corrected calcium of <1.90 mmol/L	ECG monitoring is essential for patients with arrhythmias
	Check magnesium level and correct if low
Acute mild hypocalcaemia	
Mild symptoms with calcium 1.90–2.20 mmol/L	Oral calcium supplements
	Calcium carbonate (600 mg Ca^{2+} daily) 1–2 tablets 2–3 × daily. Preferably between meals to increase availability of calcium for intestinal absorption
	If hypocalcaemia associated with insufficient vitamin D, give calcium carbonate with colecalciferol 1 tablet 2–3 × daily (Ca^{2+} 600 mg)
Chronic hypocalcaemia	
Symptoms frequently mild unless accompanied by osteomalacia	Oral calcium supplements (as above)
	If due to dietary vitamin D deficiency, use oral calcium as above
	With hypoparathyroidism, either primary, secondary or persisting following thyroid/parathyroid surgery: add alfacalcidol 1 μg daily. This medication requires careful monitoring and usually endocrine follow-up

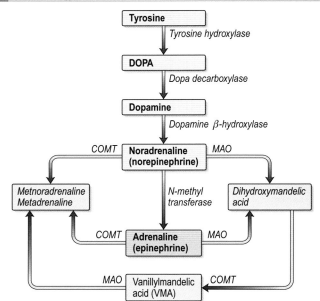

Figure 14.8 The synthesis and metabolism of catecholamines. DOPA, dihydroxyphenylalanine; COMT, catechol-O-methyl transferase; MAO, monoamine oxidase.

Case history

Three hours after a surgical procedure for colonic malignancy, a 62-year-old woman becomes hypertensive with tachycardia, inappropriate lactic acidosis and hyperglycaemia. When you review the notes, you discover that she has a 3 cm adrenal mass seen on a CT scan preoperatively, which was felt to be an incidental finding by the surgical team. On further questioning, you determine that she has had a history of paroxysmal palpitations, flushing, sweating attacks and headaches for years.

This history and CT findings would be compatible with a phaeochromocytoma.

Phaeochromocytoma is known as the 10% tumour (see Information box). It can be diagnosed during routine screening of hypertensive patients (found in only 0.1% of hypertensive subjects), the investigation of unusual episodes or cardiac events of uncertain aetiology. Phaeochromocytomas are usually associated with hypertension, 'attacks' and/or headache. They secrete adrenaline (epinephrine) or noradrenaline (norepinephrine) (Fig. 14.8).

Information

PHAEOCHROMOCYTOMA — THE 10% TUMOUR
• 10% are bilateral

- 10% are extra-adrenal, usually around the sympathetic chain, when they are known as paragangliomas
- 10% are malignant

How do these tumours present?

Symptoms and signs of catecholamine excess include:
- Hypertension (sustained or paroxysmal)
- Anxiety attacks
- Palpitations and tachycardia
- Cold extremities
- Cold sweats, tremor, pallor
- Cardiac arrhythmias, including atrial and ventricular fibrillation
- Hypertensive crises, which may be precipitated by intercurrent illness, surgery or drugs (e.g. beta-blockers, tricyclic anti-depressants, metoclopramide and naloxone)
- Pulmonary oedema with normal LV function
- Unexplained lactic acidosis
- Apparent type 2 diabetes.

Associations

A family history is vital, particularly in young patients, and might reveal the following autosomal dominant conditions:
- Neurofibromatosis type I (neurofibromata, café-au-lait spots, Lisch nodules [iris hamartomas] and axillary freckling)
- von Hippel—Lindau disease (cerebellar haemangioblastomas, retinal haemangiomas and renal cell carcinoma)
- Multiple endocrine neoplasia type 2 (medullary thyroid carcinoma and hyperparathyroidism)
- Hereditary paraganglioma syndromes (phaeochromocytoma, carotid body tumour).

Diagnostic tests

These include:
- U&Es: potassium often low; urea may be high if dehydrated.
- Glucose: hyperglycaemia.
- Urinary catecholamines (adrenaline, noradrenaline and dopamine) are measured by most laboratories. Two sets of normal 24 h urinary catecholamines make a phaeochromocytoma very unlikely.
- Plasma (heparinised) catecholamines (adrenaline, noradrenaline and dopamine) are specific but not sensitive tests. The blood must be taken directly to the laboratory for centrifugation.
- MRI/CT scan of the adrenals should be delayed until biochemical diagnosis but is useful in localising the lesion.
- MIBG (^{131}I-meta-iodobenzylguanidine) scan: MIBG is taken up selectively by adrenal tissue and is useful for localisation of tumour, particularly in extra-adrenal sites.

How would you manage this case?

- Give adequate fluid replacement with 1 L 0.9% saline initially over 1 h, then 1 L 8-hourly, usually with CVP monitoring.

- Initiate oral alpha-blockade: phenoxybenzamine 10 mg × 3 daily, increasing gradually to 40 mg × 3 daily.
- When the BP is controlled with phenoxybenzamine and a reflex tachycardia occurs, add propranolol 10–40 mg × 3 daily. Don't use labetalol.
- Surgery: hypotension commonly occurs intraoperatively when the tumour is removed, and this should be managed with blood, plasma expanders and inotropes as required. Inotropes should be used only when the patient is appropriately fluid-replete. Expansion of intravascular volume 12 h before surgery significantly reduces the frequency and severity of postoperative hypotension.
- In an emergency (hypertensive crisis), IV phentolamine (1–5 mg) should be used, but great care should be taken to rehydrate the patient adequately in order to prevent severe hypotension.

Progress. This patient improved with alpha- and beta-blockade and her BP stabilised. She was referred to the Endocrine department, which, after further investigations, recommended surgical removal of the tumour.

HYPOPITUITARISM

Pathophysiology

Deficiency of hypothalamic releasing hormones or of pituitary trophic hormones can be selective or multiple. Thus isolated deficiencies of GH, luteinising hormone/follicle stimulating hormone (LH/FSH), ACTH, TSH and vasopressin are all seen; some cases are genetic and congenital, while others are sporadic and auto-immune or idiopathic in nature.

Multiple deficiencies usually result from tumour growth or other destructive lesions. There is generally a progressive loss of anterior pituitary function. GH and gonadotrophins are usually first affected. Hyperprolactinaemia, rather than prolactin deficiency, occurs relatively early because of loss of tonic inhibitory control by dopamine. TSH and ACTH are usually last to be affected.

> **Case history**
>
> A 60-year-old man is admitted with a sudden onset of explosive headache and a left IIIrd nerve palsy. A CT scan showed no evidence of an intracranial haemorrhage. A lumbar puncture showed a mild lymphocytosis.
>
> Viral meningitis is suspected but his recovery is slow. He is noted to have small testes and a hypogonadal appearance. Six weeks later, he is re-admitted with weight loss and a chest infection. Endocrine screening shows a low 09:00 serum cortisol and undetectable serum testosterone.

Diagnosis. Hypopituitary coma and apoplexy.

Pituitary apoplexy occurs with infarction or haemorrhage into an undiagnosed pituitary tumour. It produces severe headache with sudden visual field defects or ocular palsy. Axial CT scanning can miss pituitary apoplexy but MRI usually shows the tumour.

Features of pituitary apoplexy

Pituitary infarction can be silent. Apoplexy implies the presence of symptoms:

- Headache occurs in 75% of cases (may be of sudden onset, and very severe or mild)

- Visual disturbance (compression of optic tract, usually causing bitemporal hemianopia)
- Ocular palsy present in 40% of cases: unilateral or bilateral
- Nausea/vomiting
- Meningism
- Hemiparesis.

Clinically, pituitary apoplexy can be very difficult to distinguish from subarachnoid haemorrhage, bacterial meningitis, mid-brain infarction (basilar artery occlusion) and cavernous sinus thrombosis.

Initial investigations

An MRI of the pituitary reveals a tumour mass. *Note:* MRI will often reveal a pituitary tumour, although it cannot distinguish between recent and old haemorrhage (CT might help).

A single clotted blood sample should be taken to measure cortisol, thyroid function, prolactin, GH, testosterone (in men) and the gonadotrophin hormones.

Assessment of severity: pituitary apoplexy

The course of pituitary apoplexy is variable. Headache and mild visual disturbance can develop slowly and persist for several weeks. In the acute form, apoplexy might cause optic nerve compression, haemodynamic instability and coma, and is potentially fatal. Neurosurgical advice should always be sought. Residual endocrine disturbance invariably occurs. Panhypopituitarism is the usual result. Table 14.9 shows the replacement therapy that is required.

Information

- Neurosurgical decompression via a trans-sphenoidal route is the definitive treatment for pituitary apoplexy.
- Obtundation and visual deterioration are absolute indications for neurosurgery.
- Patients without confusion or visual disturbance generally do well without surgery.

Management of this patient's acute hypopituitarism

- Diagnostic samples for cortisol, TFTs and prolactin (single plain venous sample).
- Hydrocortisone 100 mg (preferably IM) should be administered when the diagnosis is suspected.
- Give glucose if the patient is hypoglycaemic.
- Investigate and treat his chest infection.

How do patients with hypopituitarism present?

- Patients present at times of stress (e.g. following a general anaesthetic) with hypoglycaemia due to the combination of a lack of GH, cortisol and thyroxine, all of which have a counter-regulatory effect on insulin.
- Post-partum infarction of the gland occurs following post-partum haemorrhage and vascular collapse during a difficult delivery

Table 14.9 Replacement therapy for hypopituitarism

Axis	Usual replacement therapies
Adrenal	Hydrocortisone 15—40 mg daily (starting dose 10 mg on rising/5 mg lunchtime/5 mg evening)
	(Normally no need for mineralocorticoid replacement)
Thyroid	Levothyroxine 100—150 µg daily
Gonadal	
Male	Testosterone IM, orally, transdermally or implant
Female	Cyclical oestrogen/progestogen orally or as patch
Fertility	HCG plus FSH (purified or recombinant) or pulsatile GnRH to produce testicular development, spermatogenesis or ovulation
Growth	Recombinant human growth hormone used routinely to achieve normal growth in children
	Also advocated for replacement therapy in adults where growth hormone has effects on muscle mass and well-being
Thirst	Desmopressin 10—20 µg 1—3 times daily by nasal spray or orally 100—200 µg 3 times daily
	Carbamazepine, thiazides and chlorpropamide are very occasionally used in mild diabetes insipidus
Breast (prolactin inhibition)	Dopamine agonist (e.g. cabergoline 500 µg weekly)

FSH, follicle-stimulating hormone; GnRH, gonadotrophin-releasing hormone; HCG, human chorionic gonadotrophin.

(Sheehan's syndrome). This diagnosis should be suspected with failure to lactate, amenorrhoea and general ill-health post partum.

- Other features of hypopituitarism are non-specific and include tiredness, weakness, loss of body hair, loss of libido (sexual interest) and features of hypothyroidism.
- Note that patients with ACTH deficiency have no postural BP drop and normal electrolytes, as adrenal mineralocorticoids (aldosterone) are unaffected.

Assessment of severity: acute hypopituitarism

The degree of hypopituitarism bears little relationship to the clinical state of the patient. In the absence of stress, patients with severe hypopituitarism might have few complaints. Examination in males might reveal small testes and women can demonstrate either amenorrhoea or inappropriately low post-menopausal gonadotrophins. Patients with mild hypopituitarism might become profoundly unwell at times of stress, such as during an intercurrent infection.

Causes

- Destruction of the pituitary gland by primary or metastatic tumour.
- Ischaemic necrosis after post-partum haemorrhage.
- Pituitary apoplexy.
- Post-pituitary surgery or radiotherapy.
- Primary empty sella syndrome.

Investigations of anterior pituitary function

- Baseline blood samples must be taken for cortisol, free thyroid hormone levels, testosterone LH, FSH, prolactin and GH levels.
- Dynamic investigation of pituitary function can be deferred and the patient should be treated expectantly with hydrocortisone (e.g. 10 mg × 2 daily once stable).
- Imaging using CT with fine cuts through the pituitary or MRI is indicated to find any space-occupying lesion.

Progress. This patient's hypopituitarism improved without surgery and at 3 months his serum hormone levels were normal. He was evaluated further for possible treatment of his pituitary adenoma.

DIABETES INSIPIDUS

Transient diabetes insipidus (DI) often occurs after pituitary surgery because of vasopressin deficiency, and can also occur acutely following head injury. Consider DI if asked to see a patient with polyuria and polydipsia who has normal blood glucose. DI is also a cause of hypernatraemia.

Case history

You are called to see a patient who had a trans-sphenoidal hypophysectomy the day before for a non-functioning pituitary adenoma. He has made a good recovery from surgery but now complains of severe thirst and is passing large volumes of dilute urine.

Results of his ***investigations:***
- Na^+: 146
- K^+: 4.0
- Urea: 4.7
- Creatinine: 90
- Urine specific gravity (dipstick): 1.001.

Diagnosis. This patient probably has transient **diabetes insipidus.**

How would you manage this patient?

- Ensure adequate access to water or commence IV glucose 5% and 0.18% saline to match urine output if the patient cannot drink enough.
- Make sure an accurate fluid balance chart is being maintained.
- If urine output is >200 mL/h for 2 consecutive hours, check plasma and urine osmolality.
- DI is confirmed by the presence of a high plasma osmolality (>290) in the presence of an inappropriately low urine osmolality (<500 mOsmol/kg).
- Start desmopressin: adult dose 0.5–1.0 μg SC stat followed by 10–40 μg × 3 daily as an intranasal spray.
- If the plasma osmolality is low, the patient might be over-drinking due to a dry mouth, and a low urine osmolality is appropriate. In this

Kumar & Clark's Cases in Clinical Medicine

Box 14.2 Cranial and nephrogenic causes of diabetes insipidus (DI)

Cranial DI
- Hypothalamic tumour
- Basal skull fracture
- Neurosarcoidosis
- Other hypothalamic diseases
- Idiopathic
- Infection
- Inflammatory

Nephrogenic DI
- Drugs:
  - Diuretics
  - Lithium
- Hypercalcaemia
- Hypokalaemia
- Kidney disease, e.g. renal tubular acidosis
- Idiopathic

---

circumstance, administration of desmopressin will cause a further fall in plasma osmolality and can be dangerous.

Other causes of diabetes insipidus

Diabetes insipidus is either cranial (CDI) or nephrogenic (NDI) due to the inability of ADH to act on the kidney (Box 14.2).

Progress. This patient's DI was transient and he improved with IV fluids.

SYNDROME OF INAPPROPRIATE ANTI-DIURETIC HORMONE (SIADH)

Inappropriate secretion of ADH results in retention of water and subsequent hyponatraemia. Mild symptoms of confusion, irritability and nausea occur as sodium levels fall below 125 mmol/L (125 mEq/L); fitting and coma occur as the sodium falls below 115 mmol/L. A diagnosis of SIADH can be made only in a patient who is clinically normovolaemic with normal thyroid and adrenal function.

Case history

A 65-year-old smoker complained of a chronic cough and haemoptysis. A CXR revealed a hilar mass. He was referred to the Chest Clinic for further investigation.

Electrolytes: Na^+ 118; K^+ 4.4; urea 3.3; creatinine 100; glucose 4.9; measured plasma osmolality 255.

In view of the low plasma osmolality, a spot urine was also sent to the Biochemistry department: urinary sodium 30 mmol/L; urinary osmolality 350 mOsmol/kg.

This patient's urinary osmolality is high for his current plasma osmolality. Normally, the kidney can make urine as dilute as 100 mOsmol/kg (urine SG = 1.0001) or as concentrated as 1300 mOsmol/kg in a patient who is dehydrated (urine SG = 1.4000). The current urinary osmolality has to be interpreted with knowledge of the current plasma osmolality.

This patient does indeed have **inappropriate ADH**. He was put on 1 L fluid restriction daily and commenced on demeclocycline.

Mild hypovolaemia is a potent stimulus for vasopressin (ADH) release, and volume-depleted patients given hypotonic fluid will frequently become hyponatraemic. Evaluation of volume status and recent fluid charts is essential in assessing hyponatraemia.

Information

SYNDROME OF INAPPROPRIATE ANTI-DIURETIC HORMONE (SIADH)
- Dilutional hyponatraemia due to excessive water retention
- Low plasma osmolality with higher 'inappropriate' urine osmolality
- Continued urinary sodium excretion >30 mmol/L
- Absence of hypokalaemia (or hypotension)
- Normal renal, adrenal and thyroid function

How would it present?

Most commonly, patients with true SIADH present with incidentally discovered hyponatraemia. Alternatively, they might present with a fit or episodes of confusion.

Causes

- Small-cell lung carcinoma (commonest).
- Drugs (e.g. carbamazepine, selective serotonin re-uptake inhibitors [SSRIs]).
- Pneumonia.
- Tuberculosis.
- Intracranial pathology.
- Other neuroendocrine tumours.

What other causes of hyponatraemia should you think of?

It is essential for other causes of hyponatraemia (in particular, diuretics) to be excluded. The diagnosis of SIADH cannot be made in a patient who is on diuretics. The differential diagnosis of hyponatraemia includes hypothyroidism, adrenal and renal insufficiency, and chronic states such as cirrhosis and congestive cardiac failure.

Investigation of hyponatraemia

- Take a drug history, e.g. diuretics, SSRIs or carbamazepine.
- U&Es and plasma osmolality: hyponatraemia will be seen.
- Urinary electrolytes and osmolality.
- The patient will have a low plasma osmolality (<280) and an inappropriately concentrated urine (>300).
- Free T4 and TSH to exclude hypothyroidism.
- Cortisol and short ACTH test (see p. 422) to exclude Addison's disease.
- CXR and chest CT (tuberculosis, carcinoma).
- CT/MRI brain to exclude intracranial pathology.

Treatment

- Fluid restriction
- Demeclocycline.

Progress. On fluid restriction and demeclocycline, this patient's serum Na$^+$ returned to normal levels. He was referred to the Oncologists for management of his bronchial carcinoma.

Further reading

Diabetic ketoacidosis, hyperosmolar hyperglycaemic state and hypoglycaemic coma

Umpierrez G, Korytkowski M. Diabetic emergencies — ketoacidosis, hyperglycaemic hyperosmolar state and hypoglycaemia. *Nature Reviews: Endocrinology* 2016; **12**: 222–232.

The diabetic foot

Armstrong DG, Boulton ASM, Bus SA. Diabetic foot ulcers and their recurrence. *New England Journal of Medicine* 2017; **376**: 2367–2375.

Cushing's syndrome

Loriaux DL. Diagnosis and differential diagnosis of Cushing's syndrome. *New England Journal of Medicine* 2017; **376**: 1451–1459.

Hyperthyroidism

Franklyn JA, Boelaert K. Thyrotoxicosis. *Lancet* 2012; **379**: 1155–1166.

Addison's disease

Nagarur A, Axelrod L, Dighe AS. A 27-year-old woman with nausea, vomiting, confusion and hyponatraemia. *New England Journal of Medicine* 2017; **376**: 1159–1167.

Hypercalcaemia

Bilezikian JP, Bandeira L, Khan A, et al. Hyperparathyroidism. *Lancet* 2018; **391**: 168–178.

Phaeochromocytoma and paraganglioma

Neumann UPH, Young WF, Eng C. Pheochromocytoma and paraganglioma. *New England Journal of Medicine* 2019; **381**: 552–565.

DIPLOPIA

Diplopia (double vision) occurs when there is an acquired defect of movement of an eye (paralytic squint). It is maximal in the direction of action of the weak muscle.

Case history (1)

A 70-year-old man with type 2 diabetes presents with a 12 h history of double vision. He is taking metformin and glibenclamide for his diabetes.

On examination, there is ptosis in the left eye, which is deviated downwards and laterally (down and out) and fails to elevate or move medially (Fig. 15.1). The pupils both react normally. He is otherwise well. Random blood glucose is 11.5 mmol/L. HbA1c is 8% (64 mmol/mol).

The **diagnosis** is a *mononeuritis* (usually a pupil-sparing IIIrd nerve palsy), a complication of diabetes mellitus.

What immediate action would you take?

- Achieve better diabetic control.
- Put a patch over the eye.
- Reassure the patient that recovery is likely (but not definite) over weeks.

If recovery does not occur, refer the patient to a Neurologist for an MRI scan and investigation of causes of mononeuritis multiplex (see p. 441).

Information

- A **painless IIIrd nerve palsy with preserved pupil reactions** commonly occurs in the setting of diabetes due to nerve infarction.
- If a headache, especially of sudden onset, is present, a posterior communicating artery aneurysm compressing the IIIrd nerve in front of the midbrain is a likely cause. Such a lesion also commonly involves the parasympathetic pupillary constricting fibres so that the pupil is fixed and dilated. MR angiography is indicated in this situation (Fig. 15.2).

Progress. This man's diplopia improved over the next 2 months.

Case history (2)

A 35-year-old woman presents with 3 months of intermittent double vision.

On examination, there is mild restriction of upgaze and lateral gaze of the left eye, and mild restriction of upgaze of the right eye. There is mild bilateral ptosis. Further examination reveals fatigability of the ptosis and of the eye movements.

A *clinical diagnosis* of **myasthenia gravis** was made.

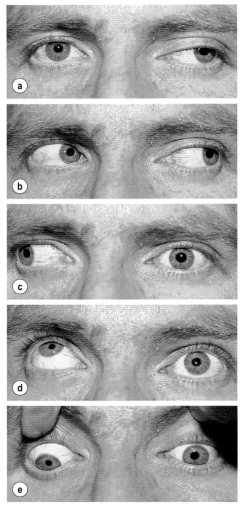

Figure 15.1 Partial left IIIrd nerve palsy with mild ptosis in a man *without diabetes*. (a) Large left pupil; (b) normal left gaze; (c) no adduction of left eye on right gaze; (d) poor elevation; (e) poor depression.

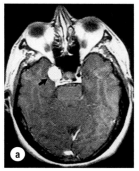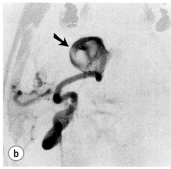

Figure 15.2 (a) MRI showing left cavernous carotid aneurysm (arrow); (b) MR angiogram showing an aneurysm (arrow). (From Albert D, Miller J, Azar D, et al. *Albert and Jakobiec's Principles and Practice of Ophthalmology*, 3rd edn. Saunders/Elsevier, 2008, with permission.)

What action would you take?

Confirm the diagnosis of myasthenia by:

- Measurement of serum acetylcholine receptor antibodies (present in 40% of cases with eye involvement only with 100% specificity)
- EMG studies, including the extra-ocular muscles
- MRI of mediastinum to exclude thymoma.

This patient was diagnosed as having myasthenia gravis and was referred urgently to a Neurologist. Myasthenia gravis is sometimes restricted to the ocular system and can present as a variable gaze palsy that is difficult to interpret in terms of individual muscles or cranial nerves. There is not always a history of fatigability. Some of the many causes of diplopia are listed in Box 15.1.

Treatment

Treatment of myasthenia gravis includes oral anticholinesterases, e.g. neostigmine or pyridostigmine (dosage gradually increased), steroids, immunosuppression and plasmapheresis. Restricted ocular myasthenia carries a better prognosis, as swallowing and the respiratory muscles may be permanently spared.

Thymectomy may be necessary, even in patients without a thymoma.

This woman remains well on pyridostigmine at regular intervals through the day but in view of the high doses required (> 360 mg) she was put on immunosuppressive therapy (azathioprine and steroids). She experienced side-effects of abdominal colic from the pyridostigmine and this was helped by oral propantheline.

Case history (3)

A 30-year-old, 27-weeks pregnant woman complains of 4 weeks of headache, nausea, brief 1 s episodes of visual loss, and horizontal double vision that is worse on distance gaze.

Kumar & Clark's Cases in Clinical Medicine

Box 15.1 Causes of diplopia

Muscle/obstructive

- Orbital masses
- Orbital pseudotumour (ocular myositis)
- Myasthenia
- Latent squint (visible when tired)

Cranial nerves

- Mass lesion in path of IIIrd, IVth or VIth nerves
- Mononeuritis multiplex
- False localising due to raised intracranial pressure

Central

- Brainstem inflammation
- Demyelination
- Brainstem mass lesion
- Infarction
- Haemorrhage

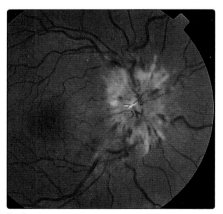

Figure 15.3 Papilloedema.

On examination, she is found to have bilateral papilloedema (Fig. 15.3) and bilateral restriction of lateral gaze consistent with VIth nerve palsy.

What action would you take?

- MRI or CT scan of head.

In this case the ventricles were normal and therefore it was safe to proceed to a lumbar puncture. The opening pressure was recorded at 30 cm (normal pressure <25 cm). A volume of CSF (usually around 20 mL) should be removed, so as approximately to halve the opening pressure.

Diagnosis. This woman has **idiopathic intracranial hypertension (IIH)**. This is most common in overweight females and rare in males.

Precipitating factors

- Pregnancy.
- Weight gain.
- Polycystic ovaries.
- Tetracyclines.
- Vitamin A excess (including retinoids).
- Steroids.

Management

Repeated lumbar puncture and removal of CSF, e.g. every 1–2 weeks, has been widely used but is probably not helpful; conversely, weight reduction is effective. Drugs such as acetazolamide can be of assistance. Treatment is directed primarily at preventing visual loss due to uncorrected papill-oedema, and secondly at relief of headache/diplopia. The visual fields must be checked formally at intervals by screen perimetry to monitor any enlarge-ment of the blind spots. If repeat puncture is unsuccessful in this usually self-limiting condition, optic nerve fenestration or even ventriculoperitoneal shunting may be necessary.

> **Remember**
>
> - There are a number of secondary causes of raised intracranial pressure without dilated ventricles or other space-occupying lesion, e.g. venous sinus thrombosis and meningeal disease.
> - MRI/MR venography and examination of CSF constituents are therefore mandatory.

Progress. This patient's condition improved post partum.

LOSS OF VISION

Case history (1)

A 64-year-old man presents in A&E with visual loss in the right eye for 3 h. He had a pre-vious episode several months earlier. He describes the loss as a horizontal screen des-cending over his vision. You are called by the A&E officer to give an opinion. When you arrive the visual loss has recovered.

What is the most likely diagnosis?

Temporary monocular visual loss with a horizontal defect in this age group is very likely to be **amaurosis fugax**. This is often caused by thromboembo-lism in the ophthalmic artery and is a symptom of carotid stenosis.

Investigations and management

See pages 161 and 163.

What is the differential diagnosis?

Transient ischaemic attacks (TIAs) are usually diagnosed clinically. Other causes of visual loss are shown in Box 15.2.

Kumar & Clark's Cases in Clinical Medicine

> ### Box 15.2 Causes of acute or transient visual disturbance
>
> **Ophthalmological**
> - Glaucoma
> - Amaurosis fugax
> - Giant cell (temporal) arteritis
> - Anterior ischaemic optic neuropathy
> - Central retinal vessel occlusion
> - Vitreous haemorrhage
> - Retinal detachment
> - Uveitis, keratitis
>
> **Neurological**
> - Optic neuritis/demyelination
> - Compressive lesion of the optic nerve, chiasm, tract
> - Transient ischaemic attack/stroke of posterior cerebral circulation
> - Migraine
> - Occipital, temporal, parietal haemorrhage
> - Occipital, temporal, parietal space-occupying lesion
> - Temporal lobe epilepsy
> - Raised intracranial pressure

Remember giant cell arteritis, which causes acute visual loss. It responds to steroids (see p. 194).

Abrupt and progressive visual loss over days is also seen in elderly hypertensives. There is often disc swelling and later disc pallor. This is due to an arteriopathy of the posterior ciliary artery resulting in ischaemia of the optic disc and causing an anterior ischaemic optic neuropathy. Urgent management by a specialist is with heparin infusion and mannitol.

Progress. This patient's carotid Doppler showed a 70% stenosis in the carotid artery and an internal carotid endarterectomy was performed. He has had no further episodes.

Case history (2)

A 24-year-old woman complains of several attacks of loss of vision, lasting up to 1 h, in the right eye, accompanied by a left-sided pounding headache. Closer questioning reveals that the defect is, in fact, in the right visual field of both eyes.

Visual hemifield disturbance, sometimes with shimmering or jagged line scotomata, is a relatively common aura experienced by patients with **migraine**. Occasionally, there is no headache.

If the symptoms are dramatic or atypical, or especially if there are any fixed symptoms or signs, an MRI scan should be performed to check for an underlying vascular lesion such as an arteriovenous malformation or underlying epileptogenic lesion, including occipital tumour.

Treatment

- Paracetamol 1 g, aspirin 900 mg (dispersible formulation) or an NSAID, e.g. ibuprofen 400–600 mg or naproxen 500 mg, is given, as early as possible during an attack. Gastric emptying is reduced during the attack and so dispersible formulations are preferred.

- Anti-emetics (e.g. metoclopramide 10 mg or domperidone 10 mg) is also given.
- If these measures are ineffective, use a 5-hydroxytryptamine $(5HT)_{1B}/_{1D}$ serotonin receptor agonist (triptan). These drugs relieve both the pain and the nausea. Triptans should be avoided in patients with vascular disease or uncontrolled/severe hypertension. They should be given at the onset of the headache (e.g. during the aura phase). There are several triptans available with a spectrum of efficacy, e.g.:
  - Sumatriptan 25–100 mg at onset of headache; repeat if necessary after at least 2 h, maximum 300 mg in 24 h; SC 6 mg sumatriptan has the highest efficacy and produces the most rapid response.
  - Zolmitriptan 2.5 mg at onset; repeat if there is only a partial response after 2 h; 5 mg also available.
  - Rizatriptan 10 mg at onset; repeat after 2 h if there is only a partial response.
  - Oro-dispersible formulations exist for some triptans but absorption is slower.
- If there is no response to an initial dose, do not persist with subsequent doses during the same attack. However, the drug may be effective in subsequent attacks.

Progress. This patient's headache improved with paracetamol and sumatriptan. With subsequent episodes of migraine she was able to self-administer sumatriptan, an anti-emetic and paracetamol at the onset of her headaches. In this regimen her migraine has been manageable.

BELL'S PALSY

Case history

You are called to see a 45-year-old man who woke up this morning with a 'numb' left face, a droopy left eyelid and drooling from the left side of his mouth.

On examination, it is apparent that his 'numbness' represents left facial weakness in the upper and lower distributions. There is no sensory loss and there are no lesions of the skin around or inside the ear (Ramsay Hunt syndrome).

An acute VIIth nerve lesion, **Bell's palsy** (Fig. 15.4) is usually due to a viral infection (often herpes simplex). It involves the VIIth (facial) nerve (motor only), occasionally with a loss of taste on the tongue and hyperacusis. There should be no sensory loss or other cranial nerve involvement.

Management. Treatment is with steroids (60 mg prednisolone for a week, tailing down over the subsequent 1–2 weeks). An anti-viral, e.g. valaciclovir 1000 mg × 3 daily also for 1 week, is recommended by some, although randomized trials are inconclusive. The patient should be reassured and the cornea protected if exposed. Sometimes recovery is incomplete and faulty re-innervation of the facial muscles or of the lacrimal gland may occur. Relapses are seen.

Bilateral or recurrent Bell's palsy, or one that shows no recovery after several weeks, should be investigated with an MRI scan, possibly CSF analysis, and investigations for causes of **mononeuritis multiplex**.

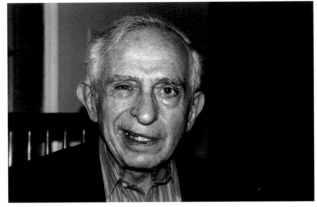

Figure 15.4 Bell's palsy.

Investigations

MONONEURITIS MULTIPLEX
- FBC
- U&Es
- Blood glucose
- Serum auto-antibodies
- Serum anti-cardiolipin antibodies
- Serum anti-neutrophil cytoplasmic antibody (ANCA)
- Treponemal serology
- *Borrelia* serology
- Serum and CSF angiotensin-converting enzyme (ACE)
- Serum electrophoresis and Bence Jones protein
- CXR

Remember

- Sarcoidosis should be suspected in cases of bilateral Bell's palsy.
- Melkersson–Rosenthal syndrome is a rare condition causing bilateral Bell's palsy and tongue swelling with other features.
- Progressive multiple cranial nerve palsies should lead to suspicion of malignant meningitis, or lymphomatous or carcinomatous infiltration.

Progress. This patient was treated with steroids and aciclovir, and the palsy resolved over a few weeks. He has had no further recurrences.

VERTIGO

Vertigo, the definite illusion of movement of the subject or surroundings, typically rotatory, indicates a disturbance of the vestibular nerve, brainstem or, very rarely, cortical function. Deafness and tinnitus accompanying vertigo indicate involvement of the ear or cochlear nerve.

Case history (1)

An 85-year-old woman presented to A&E with a history of severe nausea, vomiting and dizziness, which started on waking one morning 2 weeks previously. She was confused and dehydrated. On rehydration, she was able to give a clear history of true vertigo (the sensation of the environment spinning or rotating about her). The symptoms were precipitated by head movement, especially when she turned her head in bed.

    On examination, she has normal eye movement. The rotational nystagmus in both eyes was brought on by sudden head movements (Hallpike's manoeuvre).

What is the likely diagnosis?

This history is typical of **vestibular neuronitis**, the aetiology of which is uncertain. It occurs at any age. Recovery generally takes place to a large extent over 2–3 weeks, although complete recovery might take several months. Cinnarizine and other vestibular suppressants give symptomatic relief but are best avoided in the long term.

    Peripheral vestibular lesions are characterised by positional vertigo, i.e. influenced – often in a stereotyped way – by head movement. This is manifest in the Hallpike's test (see Information box and Fig. 15.5), which characteristically reveals a rotational nystagmus.

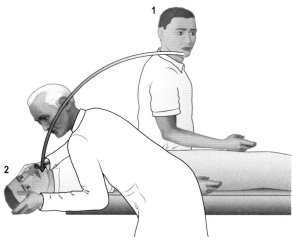

Figure 15.5 Hallpike manoeuvre for diagnosis of benign paroxysmal positional vertigo.

Information

HALLPIKE'S TEST
The patient is sat on a couch with the eyes open and facing the side of the lesion. The examiner swings the patient backwards so that he/she is supine and the head is below the horizontal. Nystagmus following a latent interval of a few seconds is commonly noted if the test is positive.

A **central vestibular lesion** is sometimes also positional but generally fails to habituate (i.e. on Hallpike's testing, continued repetition of the same movement results in no reduction in the unpleasantness or in the nystagmus).

Caloric tests are the definitive investigation to differentiate the two sites and to lateralise the lesion.

Remember

- If there is suspicion of a central lesion, an MRI scan should be performed.
- Always check for associated deafness, tinnitus, cranial nerve lesions or cerebellar disturbance for early identification of a cerebellopontine angle lesion, most commonly an VIIIth nerve schwannoma ('acoustic neuroma').

Main causes of vertigo

Peripheral

- Vestibular neuronitis.
- Benign paroxysmal positional vertigo.
- Ménière's syndrome.
- Lesion of the VIIIth nerve, e.g. schwannoma.
- Inner ear infections, infiltrations.

Central

- Brainstem infarction, inflammation or demyelination.
- Brainstem space-occupying lesion.
- Posterior circulation TIA.
- Migraine.
- Complex partial seizures.

Progress. This patient's vertigo settled after 5 days and has not recurred.

Case history (2)

A rather anxious woman presents to A&E with occasional, very brief blackouts and a long history of dizziness in crowds or when walking past fast-moving traffic. She prefers to avoid any sudden head movements, especially in certain directions and when turning in bed. Hallpike's test is positive.

What is the likely diagnosis?

Benign paroxysmal positional vertigo (BPPV). This is a relatively common disorder presenting with true vertigo, particularly on head movement. There are often vague 'vestibular hypersensitivity' symptoms, especially precipitated when there are conflicting visual inputs such as being stationary in a fast-moving visual field. Occasionally, the vertigo may be so sudden and dramatic as to present as a blackout.

Diagnosis

Largely clinical, although caloric testing may reveal mild dysfunction and MRI helps to exclude other conditions.

Management

Vestibular physiotherapy is given in the form of Cawthorne−Cooksey exercises (repetitive eye and head movements) and vestibular suppressants (e.g. β-histine). In some cases the cause is said to relate to fragments of calcification in the semicircular canals; some specialists perform the Epley manoeuvre, a gentle manipulation and rotation of the head, in an attempt to dislodge these fragments away from the receptors. Some severe cases may be successfully treated by surgical section of the nerve to the ampulla of the posterior semicircular canal.

Progress. The patient has vestibular physiotherapy and was taught to continue the exercises at home. She continues to have dizziness in crowds but is better.

Case history (3)

A 70-year-old man presents with sudden onset of vertigo, vomiting, gait unsteadiness and left facial numbness.

On examination, there is coarse unidirectional nystagmus, a reduced left corneal reflex, a left Horner's syndrome, mild dysphagia and palatal deviation to the right, left-sided ataxia and impaired pin-prick on the right arm and leg.

This is a **partial left lateral medullary syndrome** due to a stroke in the territory of branches of the posterior or anterior inferior cerebellar arteries. The vertigo is usually not positional. Nystagmus of brainstem origin is often coarse, may be in any direction, and is frequently unidirectional and sometimes monocular.

Management

As for stroke − see next section.

STROKE

This is the sudden onset of focal neurological symptoms caused by interruption of the vascular supply to a region of the brain (ischaemic stroke) or intracerebral haemorrhage (haemorrhagic stroke). It is a common cause of mortality and physical disability.

Pathophysiology

Ischaemic stroke (infarction of central nervous tissue) results from cerebral infarction secondary to either arterial thromboembolism or emboli arising from the heart (e.g. in atrial fibrillation, mural thrombus after acute myocardial infarction, or rarely from vegetations in infective endocarditis).

Cerebral haemorrhage is often caused by microaneurysm rupture in small penetrating arteries in hypertensive patients. It can also occur because of rupture of an aneurysm or arteriovenous malformation, or because of amyloid angiopathy in older patients. It accounts for around 15% of strokes.

Other causes of stroke in younger patients include arterial dissection, venous sinus thrombosis, thrombophilia, vasculitis and paradoxical embolisation through a patent foramen ovale.

Case history (1)

A 70-year-old man presents with a two-and-a-half-hour history of right-sided arm, leg and face weakness and loss of speech. He has no headache but is mildly confused. He has a history of ischaemic heart disease.

On examination, he had a global dysphasia, full visual fields, upper motor neurone (UMN) distribution right facial weakness, and dense weakness (UMN distribution) of the right side with absent reflexes and an upgoing plantar response on that side. His pulse was regular.

A clinical diagnosis of **left middle cerebral artery ischaemic stroke** is made.

Information

STROKE DIAGNOSIS

Simple history and examination — FAST:

- *F*ace — sudden weakness of the face
- *A*rm — sudden weakness of one or both arms
- *S*peech — difficulty speaking, slurred speech
- *T*ime — the sooner treatment can be started, the better.

What immediate action would you take in this case (i.e. cerebral infarct)?

- Is thrombolysis to be considered? Yes. However, this stroke occurred less than 180 min ago; therefore, if available, immediate diffuse weighted MRI (more sensitive than CT), should be performed (see Fig. 15.6b). Unfortunately, it was not available for this patient.
- CT will distinguish haemorrhage immediately but infarction cannot be seen early on (see Fig. 15.6a).

An early CT scan is also useful in stroke to check for subarachnoid or intracerebral haemorrhage and to help exclude other conditions that may masquerade as stroke, such as tumour, cerebral abscess and cerebral venous sinus thrombosis.

In this patient the CT showed no evidence of haemorrhage; therefore, **cerebral infarction** was likely.

He was given IV tissue plasminogen activator (tPA) after ruling out contraindications and obtaining patient consent as soon as possible (*minutes count*): total dose 0.9 mg/kg; maximum 90 mg. Give 10% of the total dose over 1 min and the remainder over 60 min by infusion (thrombolytic therapy is recommended by Cochrane reviews).

(If there had been a contraindication to the therapy or if thrombolysis was not available, he would have been given 300 mg aspirin.)

Remember

- If cerebral haemorrhage is shown on CT: *don't* give any therapy that might interfere with clotting, e.g. aspirin or heparin.
- If it is a posterior fossa haemorrhage: refer to the Neurosurgeons for possible emergency clot evacuation.

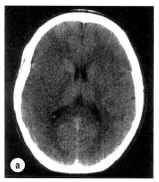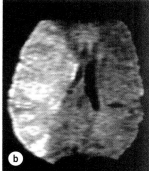

Figure 15.6 (a) CT of a middle cerebral infarct performed in the early stages, showing subtle changes in the right middle cerebral artery territory; (b) MRI of same region done at the same time as the CT, showing the full extent of the damage. (Courtesy of Dr Paul Jarmon.)

Other immediate action

- Give O$_2$ by mask.
- Do blood tests (Hb, WCC, U&Es, glucose, ESR).
- Direct admission to hospital Stroke Unit.
- Check:
  - BP: do not over-correct systemic hypertension in acute phase
  - Swallowing: nil by mouth and IV fluids in any major stroke; assess properly by speech therapist (Speech and Language Therapy [SALT] team)
  - Asymptomatic aspiration: common, and therefore early referral to physiotherapy and other support services should be arranged
  - Any concurrent infection, other illness or electrolyte disturbance: check for and treat.
- If there is evidence of cerebral oedema and risk of coning, give IV mannitol.

Thrombolysis

This significantly increases the chances of having no disability or minimal disability after stroke by reducing infarct size. Recombinant tissue plasminogen activator (rt-PA; alteplase) should be given within 4–5 h. Clot retrieval from a large cerebral artery is being widely used.

Thrombectomy

Clot retrieval is also beneficial after large-vessel occlusions.

Further management

- Start aspirin 75 mg daily (24 h after if tPA has been given).
- Clopidogrel 300 mg loading dose then 75 mg daily.
- Anti-coagulants if in atrial fibrillation.

Kumar & Clark's Cases in Clinical Medicine

• Serum cholesterol: if fasting is >3.5 mmol/L (not in acute situation), give atorvastatin 10 mg daily.

Progress. This patient did not make an early clinical improvement, as can occur after thrombolytic therapy (37%), but by 3 months he was ambulant, with a minor neurological deficit, and had improved speech.

Case history (2)

A 56-year-old man presents with weakness of the left hand and face lasting 3 h and resolving gradually. He had a similar episode 3 months earlier and made a complete recovery. He is a type 2 diabetic and a smoker. A Doppler ultrasound reveals that he has a 90% stenosis at the origin of the right internal carotid artery. This is a transient ischaemic attack (TIA).

Transient ischaemic attack

A TIA is a transient episode of neurological dysfunction caused by focal brain, spinal cord or retinal ischaemia without acute infarction. The previous definition, with its arbitrary 24 h timescale, is no longer used as the end point is now tissue injury.

Examples include:

• Anterior circulation — sudden transient loss of vision in one eye (amaurosis fugax), aphasia, hemiparesis; *or*
• Posterior circulation — diplopia, ataxia, hemisensory loss, dysarthria, transient global amnesia.

TIAs may herald the onset of stroke (one-quarter of patients developing stroke have had a TIA, usually within the previous week). The **ABCD^2 score** can help to stratify stroke risk in the first 2 days (Table 15.1). A score of <4 is associated with a minimal risk, whereas >6 means the patient is at high risk for a stroke within 7 days of a TIA.

Table 15.1 ABCD^2 score

Parameter	Score
Age >60 years	1
BP >140 mmHg systolic and/or >90 mmHg diastolic	1
Clinical features:	
• Unilateral weakness	2
• Isolated speech disturbance	1
• Other	0
Duration of symptoms (min)	
• >60	2
• 10–59	1
• <10	0
Diabetes	
• Present	1
• Absent	0

- If patients are at a high risk of a TIA, i.e. ABCD^2 score >4, or have had two recent TIAs, especially within the same vascular territory, they should be admitted for investigation and treatment (see later).
- *All* patients should be referred to a TIA Clinic and ideally seen within 24 h. Investigation and treatment should be regarded as *urgent* and should be *completed* within 7 days.

Investigations

- Look for the source of the embolus — carotids (Doppler) and cardiac (echo).
- ECG.
- CT brain.
- Further investigation with MRI of the brain and vascular system is often required.

Treatment

- Anti-platelet therapy as for stroke (see pp. 451 and 157).
- Modification of vascular risk factors — smoking, hypertension; give statins as above.
- Early endarterectomy for symptomatic 70–99% carotid artery stenosis (within 1 week if possible).
- Anti-coagulation for atrial fibrillation (see p. 261) (aspirin 300 mg daily for 2 weeks, then anti-coagulate with **heparin** and **warfarin** or **dabigatran**).

Progress. In this patient an endarterectomy was performed. He has made lifestyle changes and has been well over the last 2 years.

Case history (3)

A 40-year-old man presents with a 1-week history of headache followed by loss of speech and a right hemiparesis. His weakness worsens over the next 24 h and he becomes confused. A CT scan is normal at this time. A subsequent MRI scan reveals an infarct in the left frontal lobe with small haemorrhages elsewhere in the hemispheres. His ESR and auto-antibodies are normal. CSF analysis reveals 35 lymphocytes/mm^3 but is otherwise normal. A right frontal brain biopsy reveals **primary cerebral granulomatous angiitis** (a rare necrotising inflammation with granulomatous vasculitis of the brain and meningeal vessels). He is treated with high-dose steroids and cyclophosphamide.

What are the causes of strokes in this young age group?

In the younger age group, there are other causes of stroke, such as vasculitis or structural cardiac lesions. In many of these conditions, specific treatment is indicated. Cerebral vasculitis is difficult to diagnose because systemic inflammatory markers may be normal. The CSF and intra-arterial angiography are sometimes also normal. Even a cerebral/meningeal biopsy may miss involved vessels because the condition is often patchy.

Investigations

ADDITIONAL INVESTIGATIONS IN THE YOUNGER AGE GROUP
- MRI head
- Auto-antibodies, including anti-cardiolipin, ANCA
- Lupus anti-coagulant
- Serum electrophoresis

- Serum lactate/pyruvate
- Urine for protein and casts
- Urine homocysteine
- Echocardiogram
- 24 h ECG
- Consider CSF analysis

Progress. This patient was initially treated with high-dose steroids and cyclophosphamide. The steroids were reduced gradually and oral cyclophosphamide continued for 6 months.

SUBDURAL HAEMORRHAGE

This is caused by venous bleeding in the subdural space from rupture of a vein. It usually follows a head injury, often trivial.

Case history

A 77-year-old woman was admitted 2 weeks previously with failure to manage at home alone. There had been a 2-year history of cognitive decline that seemed to have accelerated to precipitate the admission.

On examination, she was confused and disorientated, unable to repeat a five-digit number, and had an upgoing left plantar response. Her Glasgow Coma Scale score (GCS, see p. 463) was 12.

Diagnosis. A CT scan revealed **bilateral subdural haematomas** (Fig. 15.7).

Subdural haemorrhage can present rather acutely following a fall, with sudden onset of headache and diminished consciousness. The diagnostic challenge lies in identifying other cases that present vaguely without focal

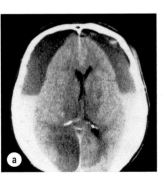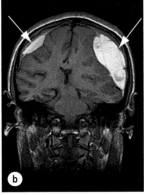

Figure 15.7 Bilateral subdural haematomas (arrows). (a) CT scan; (b) MR (T1) image.

signs and with no history of trauma. A number of factors are associated with increased risk of apparently spontaneous subdural haemorrhage:

- Old age
- Cerebral atrophy, dementia
- Alcohol excess, general debility
- Bleeding diathesis/anticoagulant therapy
- Intracranial lesion such as tumour
- Brain surgery, especially ventricular shunt insertion for normal pressure hydrocephalus.

Management

The management of subdural haematomas depends on their size and the severity of symptoms. Small ones may simply be managed conservatively with follow-up CT scanning. Larger or more acutely symptomatic subdurals should be surgically evacuated.

Progress. This patient had an acute subdural haemorrhage that precipitated her deterioration. This was managed surgically with overall improvement in her cognitive state.

PARKINSON'S DISEASE

Parkinson's disease is a neurodegenerative disorder affecting nigrostriatal dopaminergic cells, as well as other brain cells.

It causes a combination of tremor, rigidity and akinesia, developing slowly over many months or years.

Case history

A 75-year-old man with Parkinson's disease presented with uncontrollable gyrating movements of his arms and legs. On obtaining a detailed history it transpired that he was on levodopa therapy. This had recently been increased to co-careldopa 50/200 (a mixture of carbidopa and levodopa) three tablets × 4 daily.

What is the problem?

This patient has dyskinesia — a common, late side-effect of levodopa (LD) therapy for parkinsonism. About 10% of patients per year of therapy will develop such dyskinesias, involving uncontrollable choreo-athetoid movements and dystonic posturing. At this stage in the illness, the severity of dyskinesia is dose-dependent and so a balance has to be struck between 'off' symptoms of bradykinesia and rigidity and 'on' dyskinetic symptoms. In this case, the co-careldopa was prescribed at too high a dose.

When commencing LD therapy, patients are generally started on co-careldopa 25/100 or co-beneldopa (100 mg/25 mg tablets: a mixture of benserazide hydrochloride and LD in proportions of 1 : 4) × 3 daily. These drugs consist of a combination of LD and a peripheral DOPA decarboxylase inhibitor (DDI) to prevent inappropriate peripheral activation to dopamine. The dose of these drugs can be gradually increased in amount and frequency as the underlying disease worsens.

Alternatively, patients may receive a controlled-release preparation; co-careldopa 50/200 has nearly twice the bioavailable strength of straight careldopa but the co-beneldopa (25/1000) preparation is a more equivalent dose. The controlled-release preparations may be given once at night to help with nocturnal or early morning 'off' symptoms, or may be given 2–3 times

Kumar & Clark's Cases in Clinical Medicine

a day alone or in combination with straight LD in an effort to smoothen fluctuating symptoms.

Occasionally, dyskinesias occur in relation to dramatic fluctuations in LD levels rather than in relation to high peak levels; the solution in this situation is to place the patient on a higher dose of longer-acting medication.

Other treatment available

- Exercise and physiotherapy are useful.
- Initiate pharmacological treatment when there is impairment/disability resulting from symptoms.
- Early treatment with monoamine oxidase B (MAOB) inhibitors (**selegiline** or **rasagiline**) may delay the need for more definitive dopamine replacement therapy by several months.
- **Dopamine agonists (DAs)** are used in patients <70 years. Although they are less effective and less well tolerated than LD, they are also associated with fewer long-term motor complications.
- In older patients (i.e. those more severely affected at diagnosis), start LD + DDI (**co-beneldopa** or **co-careldopa**) because of fewer side-effects.
- Non-ergot DAs (**pramipexole** and **ropinirole** oral 3 times daily, or once daily with slow-release formulations, **rotigotine** via transdermal patch) are used in preference to ergot-derived drugs.
- All patients with Parkinson's disease will eventually require treatment with LD, often in combination with a DA. A typical starting dose is 50 mg of LD (e.g. **co-careldopa** 62.5 mg) 3 times daily, increasing after 1 week to 100 mg 3 times daily.

Progress. This patient was put on a lower dose of co-careldopa and the dyskinesia settled.

MULTIPLE SCLEROSIS (MS)

MS is an autoimmune disease of unknown aetiology. It causes plaques of demyelination throughout the brain and spinal cord. Acute relapses are caused by focal inflammatory demyelination, which causes a conduction block. These plaques can be demonstrated using an MRI scan (Fig. 15.8).

Case history (1)

A 28-year-old man presents with several days of pain and progressive loss of vision in one eye.

Examination showed diminished visual acuity 6/36 and disc swelling (papilloedema). He had previously had an episode of difficulty in walking and urinary incontinence, which had recovered fully after several weeks.

What is the problem with his eyes?

The swelling of the disc, along with diminished visual acuity, suggests optic neuritis, as other causes of papilloedema do not usually give visual disturbance. Optic neuritis is a common early presentation of MS. The previous

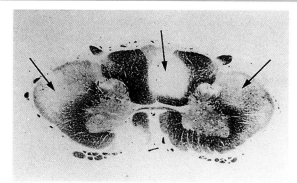

Figure 15.8 Multiple sclerosis — showing plaques in the posterior column and lateral corticospinal tracts (arrows). (Courtesy of the late Dr Ian MacDonald.)

history, suggesting an episode of transverse myelitis (inflammation of the cord), indicates dissociation in space and time, providing strong clinical support for the diagnosis of MS.

What action would you take?

- An **MRI** should be performed to look for the demyelinating lesions of MS.
- **CSF analysis** for oligoclonal bands is usually unnecessary to corroborate the diagnosis further.
- **Visual evoked potentials** are likely to be delayed in the affected eye but may also reveal sub-clinical involvement of the other eye, providing evidence for dissociation in space.
- **Medication**. Recovery after an episode of optic neuritis is aided by IV methylprednisolone, e.g. 1 g/day for 3 days.

Progress. This patient's vision improved following his steroid therapy. However, the MRI showed demyelinating lesions of MS and he is being followed up in the Neurology Clinic.

Case history (2)

A previously well 25-year-old woman develops double vision, vertigo and unsteadiness, as well as speech and swallowing problems, over 2 days. She is admitted to hospital, where she rapidly deteriorates, becoming confused and hypoxic. She requires ventilatory support. An MRI scan reveals a number of small bilateral periventricular white matter lesions, along with lesions in the brainstem and cerebellar peduncles. She is given IV methylprednisolone and recovers well over the next 2 weeks, apart from residual mild vertigo and intermittent diplopia.

Remember

MS may sometimes present dramatically as a brainstem syndrome with central respiratory problems and rapid severe bulbar failure. Early supportive management and steroids are

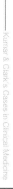

essential in such cases. There may be excellent recovery following the relapse. Patients with known MS who suffer a relapse involving bulbar function or dysarthria should similarly be carefully observed.

Case history (3)

A patient with known MS who has frequent severe relapses, bladder instability and incontinence, and painful leg spasms wonders if anything can be done for her incurable condition.

What would you suggest?

Many forms of treatment are being used; as yet there is no evidence to support one over the other.

- **Acute relapses.** Short courses of steroids, such as IV methylprednisolone 1 g/day for 3 days or high-dose oral steroids, are used widely in relapses and do sometimes reduce severity. They do not influence long-term outcome.
- **Preventing relapse and disability.** Beta-interferon (both IFN β-1b and β-1a) by self-administered injection is used in relapsing and remitting disease. This is defined as at least two attacks of neurological dysfunction over the previous 2 or 3 years followed by a reasonable recovery. IFN β-1b is also used for secondary progressive MS. Interferon certainly reduces the relapse rate in some patients and prevents an increase in lesions seen on MRI. Unwanted effects are flu-like symptoms and irritation at injection sites. Beta-interferons are expensive.
- **Glatiramer acetate**, an immunomodulator, has been shown to reduce relapse frequency in ambulatory patients with relapsing remitting MS – similar to beta-interferon.
- **Natalizumab** is a monoclonal antibody that inhibits migration of leucocytes into the CNS by inhibitory α-4 integrins found on the surface of lymphocytes and monocytes. It is useful in severe, relapsing remitting MS that is unresponsive to other treatments. It is associated with a risk of progressive multifocal leucoencephalopathy (PML), and all patients need close surveillance for this and hypersensitivity reactions.
- **Alemtuzumab**, an anti-CD52 monoclonal antibody that destroys T- and B-cells, reduces disease activity.
- **Mitoxantrone** is used in primary progressive MS in specialist centres. It is potentially cardiotoxic and myelosuppressive.
- **New oral disease-modifying drugs**, e.g. **fingolimod**, a sphingosine-1-phosphate receptor modulator, and **cladribine** (both given orally), an immunomodulator of lymphocytes, have shown benefit in ongoing trials.

Progress. This patient was admitted for re-assessment. She was treated with baclofen for her spasms and spasticity, and gabapentin for neuropathic pain. An anti-muscarinic (oxybutynin) was tried for her urinary problems but eventually she was taught to self-catheterise intermittently. The Physiotherapists, Occupational Therapists and a Social Worker were asked to review her. Disease-modifying therapy was thought to be inappropriate for her advanced condition.

ENCEPHALITIS

This is an inflammation of the brain parenchyma, which is often due to a virus.

Case history (1)

A 45-year-old man presents with a 1-week history of malaise, followed by increasing confusion, headache, meningism and a seizure.

On examination, he was confused, with a GCS of 10. He had fever, neck stiffness and hyper-reflexia of the left arm and leg.

Diagnosis. A tentative diagnosis of **encephalitis** was made.

What action would you take?

- Supportive care: including respiratory support if necessary.
- Treatment of any seizures: ictal and post-ictal states are a reversible element of changes in conscious level.
- CT scan: showed no space-occupying lesion.
- Lumbar puncture: there was a lymphocytosis.
- Serology and PCR: for likely aetiological agents (see later).
- *If there is even a remote possibility that the cause is herpes simplex virus 1 (HSV1), start aciclovir immediately, IV 10 mg/kg × 3 daily.* HSV is treatable; most other causes are not (Box 15.3). Patients have been known to relapse and respond to further treatment.

Box 15.3 Causes of encephalitis/meningoencephalitis

Viral

- Herpes simplex (HSV 1 and 2)
- Measles
- Rubella
- Epstein–Barr virus
- Varicella zoster virus
- Echo
- Coxsackie
- Cytomegalovirus
- Human immunodeficiency virus
- Japanese B (most common worldwide)
- West Nile encephalitis
- Tick-borne encephalitis
- Post-viral: acute disseminated encephalomyelitis (ADEM)

Bacterial

- Legionnaire's
- *Mycoplasma*
- *Listeria*
- Tuberculosis

In immunocompromised people, think of unusual organisms, e.g. fungal.

> **Remember**
>
> • Most cases of viral encephalitis present in the same way, the symptoms being milder than those for a bacterial meningitis. In many cases the viral cause can be worked out from the epidemiological pattern, e.g. from the geographical area where the disease was contracted and the season of the year.
> • The term 'encephalitis' encompasses any acute febrile illness, perhaps with some meningeal involvement, that is accompanied by acute generalised or focal cerebral disturbance. Thus there is considerable overlap with meningitis.

> **Investigations**
>
> **FURTHER INVESTIGATIONS**
> • An MRI scan showed temporal oedema.
> • An EEG excluded generalised or complex partial status epilepticus.
> • If there is a possibility of immunosuppression (as a result of AIDS, lymphoproliferative disorders or iatrogenic), this should be investigated.

Progress. The MRI was highly suggestive of an **HSV1 encephalitis** and this was confirmed by serology and PCR. The patient was treated with IV aciclovir. Although he survived, he was left with a significant residual deficit. He was sent for rehabilitation but had problems with his memory, which is particularly common following HSV1 encephalitis.

> **Remember**
>
> • All cases of encephalitis in developed countries should be given aciclovir.
> • HSV is treatable; most other causes are not.

> **Case history (2)**
>
> A 25-year-old woman has an upper respiratory tract infection. Following recovery, she becomes drowsy over a period of 48 h.
>
> **On examination**, she is apyrexial with a GCS of 9. She has abnormal eye movements and gaze-evoked nystagmus. There is marked spasticity in the limbs.
>
> **Investigations:** CT shows effacement of cerebral sulci but it is safe to do a lumbar puncture. Lumbar puncture reveals 40 lymphocytes/mm³. The patient requires intubation to protect the airway.
>
> A provisional diagnosis of HSV1 encephalitis is made.
>
> **Follow-on:** a subsequent MRI scan reveals diffuse and confluent T2 hyper-intensities in the periventricular white matter and brainstem, and also within cerebral grey matter.

What is the diagnosis?

Acute disseminated encephalomyelitis (ADEM). This is considered to be a post-viral (sometimes post-*Mycoplasma*) inflammatory condition, mainly affecting the white matter, although the distinction from a direct viral encephalitis may be blurred. At the other end of the scale, the distinction from a severe initial attack of MS might also be unclear, although the latter attack is usually milder, more likely to be associated with CSF oligoclonal bands, and characterised in retrospect by repeated attacks. However, treatment of both ADEM and MS attacks is similar, namely with high doses of steroids. Because of the nature of presentation of ADEM, anti-virals are usually also given.

Progress. This patient was treated with IV methylprednisolone, followed by a course of oral steroids, and made a good recovery after several weeks, with some residual pyramidal gait difficulty.

FALLS

Case history (1)

A 70-year-old man presents with recurrent falls. ***On examination***, he has a rigid increase in tone, worse in the trunk than the limbs, marked bradykinesia and extreme mental slowness. He is unable to move his eyes vertically or laterally. He walks with a rather upright gait. He is thought to have Parkinson's disease but has had a poor response to levodopa.

What is the diagnosis?

This man has **progressive supranuclear palsy** (PSP; also known as Steele–Richardson syndrome). Parkinson's disease usually results in falls late on in the disease. Early falls should lead to suspicion of PSP or multi-system atrophy (which does not cause early cognitive problems).

Information

STEELE–RICHARDSON SYNDROME
- Parkinsonism
- Axial rigidity
- Dementia
- Defective upward-and-lateral gaze

Some common causes of falls are listed in Box 15.4. Some simply relate to stance or gait difficulties.

Progress. This patient continued to deteriorate and died of pneumonia 6 months later.

Case history (2)

A 65-year-old woman is worried she has epilepsy. She suffers repeated falls when walking outside. There is no warning before falling; she tends to graze her knees and hands, and recovers immediately in a state of embarrassment. If she loses consciousness at all, it could be for a split second only because she is certainly aware when she hits the ground.
  There is no abnormality on examination.

What is the diagnosis?

The diagnosis is **drop attacks**. These are benign episodes that commonly occur in middle-aged to elderly women. There is no loss of consciousness and they are not considered epileptic (see p. 474). They are due to sudden changes in lower limb tone, presumably brainstem in origin.

Progress. This patient was reassured that she did not have epilepsy and was helped by using a walking stick.

Box 15.4 Causes of falls

Preserved consciousness

- Leg weakness
- Spasticity
- Extrapyramidal syndromes
- Ataxia, periodic ataxia
- Vertigo
- Drop attacks
- Cataplexy
- Epilepsy, myoclonus

Loss of consciousness

- Epilepsy
- Faint
- Syncope (cardiac or vascular insufficiency)
- Vertebrobasilar TIA
- Intermittent hydrocephalus
- Metabolic, e.g. hypoglycaemia
- Toxic encephalopathy
- Other encephalopathies

TRAUMATIC BRAIN INJURY

Case history

A 25-year-old man is knocked unconscious by a blow from a sledgehammer. He regains consciousness after a few minutes and attends A&E. He is nauseated and in pain but reasonably alert, with a GCS (Table 15.2) of 14. A skull X-ray shows a linear skull vault fracture. Although he remains reasonably well for many hours, his conscious level rapidly deteriorates to a GCS of 5. A subsequent CT scan reveals a large extradural blood collection that requires emergency drainage by craniotomy.

Extradural haemorrhage is a serious secondary effect of head injury. These bleeds occur into a tight space, resulting in a rather long lucid interval as the blood slowly accumulates. CT reveals a convex, hyper-dense collection in the acute phase. By contrast, subdural haemorrhages bleed more freely into a more easily opened space so the shape is concave on CT and there is little lucid interval.

Progress. Following his craniotomy and drainage, the patient gradually recovered over the next few days. However, 2–3 weeks later, he was still amnesic and needed constant attention. He is being followed up by the Neurologists.

General Management of Traumatic Injuries

Remember

- Always monitor head injuries carefully and record changes in GCS rather than simply considering one value in isolation.

Table 15.2 Glasgow Coma Scale (GCS)	
Parameter	**Score**
Eye opening (E)	
Spontaneous	4
To speech	3
To pain	2
No response	1
Motor response (M)	
Obeys	6
Localises	5
Withdraws	4
Flexion	3
Extension	2
No response	1
Verbal response (V)	
Orientated	5
Confused conversation	4
Inappropriate words	3
Incomprehensible sounds	2
No response	1

Glasgow Coma Scale = E+ M+ V (GCS minimum = 3; maximum = 15.) (From Feather A, Randall D, Waterhouse M, eds. *Kumar and Clark's Clinical Medicine*, 10th edn. Elsevier, 2021; Box 26.28.)

- The result of secondary swelling by haemorrhage or oedema (the latter is common in children) is raised intracranial pressure (ICP), leading to reduced perfusion pressure and coning.

Effects and complications of traumatic brain injury

Primary effects
- Diffuse axonal injury.
- Contusion.
- Laceration.
- Vascular lesions.

Secondary effects
- Extradural haemorrhage.
- Subdural haemorrhage.
- CSF leak, infection.
- Hydrocephalus.
- Compromised airway, respiration.
- Hypotension.

Late sequelae

- Chronic daily headache.
- Post-traumatic stress disorder: rare.
- Vertigo.
- Cognitive impairment.

Information

Post-traumatic amnesia of >24 h indicates severe brain injury.

What action would you take in a patient with a head injury?

- Attend first to any secondary or concomitant general problems, i.e. resuscitation, hypovolaemic shock, hypotension or compromised airway.
- Assess severity, using circumstances of injury and period of amnesia as a guide.
- Establish whether there is anterograde amnesia: the inability to form memories from the time of injury to the time of continuous normal memory is the most accurate guide.
- Brainstem damage in head injury can affect central respiratory drive, bulbar function and pressor responses.
- Regular GCS measurements; <5 at 24 h implies severe injury and 50% of such patients die.
- Do a CT scan (Box 15.5).

How would you manage the following problems?

- If the patient is deteriorating or has evidence of raised ICP: consider insertion of a bolt, which is simply a tube into the ventricle through which ICP can be recorded.
- If ICP is >20 mmHg: there is a need to treat. Give enough mannitol IV to raise the plasma osmolality to 300 to decrease the ICP, although the benefits of mannitol are still controversial. Mannitol also has poorly understood neuroprotective effects. Hyperventilation with intermittent positive pressure ventilation (IPPV) will also lower the ICP.
- If the patient has haemorrhages: a craniotomy may be indicated.

Box 15.5 NICE guidelines for head injuries: criteria for immediate request for CT scan of the head (adults)

- GCS <13 on initial assessment in the A&E department
- GCS <15 at 2 h after injury on assessment in the A&E department
- Suspected open or depressed skull fracture
- Any sign of basal skull fracture (haemotympanum, 'panda' eyes, CSF leakage from the ear or nose, Battle's sign)
- Post-traumatic seizure
- Focal neurological deficit
- More than one episode of vomiting
- Amnesia for events >30 min before impact

Follow-up

Check for continued improvement in the weeks subsequent to the head injury. At 2–3 weeks post injury, the development of hydrocephalus is a major complication.

Case history

A 30-year-old man falls from a second-storey building and is immediately unconscious. He is admitted comatose, GCS 5, although he is breathing spontaneously. There are no external injuries and a CT scan of the head is normal. He does not regain consciousness.

Diffuse axonal injury is the primary effect of traumatic brain injury and a common cause of vegetative state. There is usually immediate loss of consciousness followed by prolonged coma.

Milder axonal injury is reversible, e.g. in concussion. This damage occurs with brain accelerations or decelerations such as hitting the floor or wall, rather than by a direct blow to the head. The mechanism of damage is due to stretching of axons, causing Ca^{2+} entry and neurofilament damage, and interrupting axonal transport over the next 12 h. Certain areas are particularly vulnerable, such as the parasagittal white matter, internal capsule, cerebellar peduncles, posterior corpus callosum and dorsolateral midbrain.

Progress. This patient was in a coma for a week and never recovered. Consent was obtained for his organs to be used for transplantation.

SEVERE BRAIN INJURY

Case history

Your patient has had a severe hypoxic cerebral episode following a cardiac arrest. He is currently stable from a cardiac point of view but comatose (GCS 5) and requiring ventilatory support on the ITU. He has been given 24 h of induced hypothermia 32–34°. The ITU staff and the patient's relatives want an indication of the likelihood of useful recovery.

What action would you take?

First, check for a remediable cause of coma or any confounding factors worsening the patient's responsiveness (see Investigations box). For example:

- Brain imaging may reveal a potentially treatable but unsuspected condition, possibly additional to the primary pathology, such as subdural or intracerebral haemorrhage or hydrocephalus.
- An EEG may show abnormalities indicative of an unsuspected metabolic encephalopathy or sub-clinical seizure activity.
- The patient may still be under the influence of long-acting anaesthetic agents or other sedative drugs.

Investigations

- Brain imaging
- EEG
- Recent drug history
- Electrolyte imbalance

- Presence of sepsis
- Ongoing low cardiac output

Aspects of examination to assess routinely

- GCS (see Table 15.2).
- Eye movements:
  - Following, roving, conjugate
  - Optokinetic nystagmus (following a moving grid pattern)
  - Vertical and horizontal doll's head movement.
- Pupils.
- Corneal reflexes.
- Bulbar function: is the patient tolerating the ET tube?
- Respiratory function: level of ventilator support.
- Tone and reflexes.
- General examination, e.g. chest, infected pressure sores, abdominal guarding.

What are your prognostic indicators?

There are some prognostic values, depending on the time after the initial cerebral insult. The following criteria indicate **poor outcome**:
- Absent or extensor plantar response 72 h after cerebral insult.
- Absent pupillary or corneal reflexes 72 h after cerebral insult.

In general, every case must be assessed on its merits, especially with regard to the nature of the original insult and whether it was a discrete event or likely to result in ongoing brain injury.

Note: relatives should not be given conflicting or inaccurate information.

Beware

Determination of brain death is made only by the appropriate consultant specialists who assess − on separate occasions − the various brainstem reflexes and responses listed under 'Aspects of examination', earlier. The nature of the insult must be clear and remediable causes must be excluded. Because the criteria for brain death are heavily weighted towards brainstem function and, in the UK, EEG corroboration is not required, the locked-in syndrome (Table 15.3) should be excluded. In this state, a severe pontine lesion prevents access to or from the outside world. The only signs of relatively spared higher-level function may be preserved vertical optokinetic nystagmus or eye following, and preserved vertical doll's eye reflexes.

MENINGITIS

Case history (1)

A 55-year-old man, a heavy alcohol user, is brought to A&E with headache, confusion and a high fever.

On examination, he is found to be photophobic and to have neck stiffness. He is thought by the A&E staff to have meningitis and is immediately given IV benzylpenicillin because they were unclear about the most likely organism. You are called urgently to A&E.

Table 15.3 Differential diagnosis of the vegetative state

Condition	Vegetative state	Minimally conscious state (MCS)	Locked-in syndrome	Coma	Death confirmed by brainstem tests
Awareness	Absent	Present	Present	Absent	Absent
Sleep–wake cycle	Present	Present	Present	Absent	Absent
Response to noxious stimuli	±	Present	Present (in eyes only)	±	Absent
Glasgow Coma Scale score	E4, M1–4, V1–2	E4, M1–5, V1–4	E4, M1, V1	E1–2, M1–4, V1–2	E1, M1–3, V1
Motor function	No purposeful movement	Some consistent verbal or purposeful behaviour	Volitional vertical eye movements or eye blink typically preserved	No purposeful movement	None or only reflex spinal movement
Respiratory function	Typically preserved	Typically preserved	Typically preserved	Variable	Absent
EEG activity	Typically slow wave activity	Insufficient data	Typically normal	Typically slow wave activity	Typically absent

(Continued)

Table 15.3 Differential diagnosis of the vegetative state—cont'd

Condition	Vegetative state	Minimally conscious state (MCS)	Locked-in syndrome	Coma	Death confirmed by brainstem tests
Cerebral metabolism (PET)	Severely reduced	Intermediate reduction	Mildly reduced	Moderately to severely reduced	Severely reduced or absent
Prognosis	Variable: if permanent, continued vegetative state or death	Variable: if permanent, continued MCS or death	Depends on cause but full recovery unlikely	Recovery, vegetative state, or death within weeks	Organ function can be sustained only temporarily with life support

N.B. EEG and measures of cerebral metabolism are *not* required to make these clinical diagnoses. E, eye opening; EEG, electroencephalography; M, motor response; PET, positron emission tomography; V, verbal response. (From Royal College of Physicians. *Prolonged Disorders of Consciousness: National Clinical Guidelines.* London: RCP, 2013; with permission.)

What would you do?

You quickly check the neurological signs and agree this is meningitis. You also note that there is no purpuric rash of meningococcal septicaemia. You try to see the patient's fundi but are unsure whether papilloedema is present. You are worried about doing a lumbar puncture because he is semi-conscious and you are concerned about the possibility of 'coning'. You arrange an immediate CT scan, which is normal. You proceed with a lumbar puncture, and the CSF, which is turbid, is sent urgently to the Microbiologists.

What do you do next?

Investigations

- Blood culture
- CXR

This man has meningitis, presumably bacterial. You recheck for the purpuric spots of meningococcal meningitis.

Information

LUMBAR PUNCTURE

This should be performed with sterile measures. Check there is no papilloedema.

- Obtain patient consent.
- Place patient in lateral decubitus position.
- Identify L4–5 interspace (intersection of imaginary line between iliac crests and spine).
- Clean area with antiseptic, e.g. chlorhexidine.
- Local anaesthetic (2% lidocaine) into skin and subcutaneous tissue.
- Insert lumbar puncture spinal needle (bevel upwards) into skin over L4–5 interspace horizontally and slightly towards the head.
- When needle penetrates the dura mater (a slight decrease in resistance is felt), withdraw stylet and allow a few drops of CSF to escape.
- Measure CSF pressure by connecting manometer to needle (normal CSF pressure is 60–150 mmH$_2$O); it rises and falls with respiration and heart beat.
- Collect CSF in three sterile tubes (2 mL per tube).
- Send to laboratory. Note if clear, cloudy, yellow (xanthochromic) or red.
- Remove needle and apply sterile dressing.
- Patient should lie horizontal for 4 h to avoid headache. Analgesics might be required. Indications and contraindications are shown in Box 15.6.

The CSF results sent through are:
- Protein: 1.5 g/L (normal range 0.2–0.4 g/L)
- Glucose: 1.5 mmol/L
- Leucocytes: 500/mm^3
- Pneumococcus is seen on Gram stain.

Kumar & Clark's Cases in Clinical Medicine

> **Box 15.6** Indications for and contraindications to lumbar puncture
>
> Indications
> - Diagnosis of meningitis, encephalitis and subarachnoid haemorrhage (sometimes)
> - Measurement of CSF pressure, e.g. for idiopathic intracranial hypertension (IIH)
> - Removal of CSF therapeutically (IIH)
> - Diagnosis of conditions, e.g. neoplastic involvement
>
> Contraindications
> - Raised intracranial pressure
> - Local infections at site of puncture area
> - Platelet count $<40 \times 10^9$/L
> - Mass lesion in brain or spinal cord

Table 15.4 Treatment regimens: antibiotics and acute bacterial meningitis

Organism	First choice	Alternative
Unknown	Cefotaxime	Benzylpenicillin + cefotaxime
Meningococcus	Benzylpenicillin	Cefotaxime
Pneumococcus	Cefotaxime	Penicillin if organism sensitive
Haemophilus	Cefotaxime	Chloramphenicol
Listeria	Amoxicillin + gentamicin	

This table demonstrates the value of cefotaxime in clinical practice.

Diagnosis. Pneumococcal meningitis. You immediately start treatment with IV cefotaxime 8 g daily in four divided doses because there is a high incidence of penicillin-resistant pneumococcus (Table 15.4).

Causes of meningitis

These are listed in Box 15.7.

- **Pneumococcal meningitis** most commonly occurs in the debilitated or in those with a chest or sinus infection, valvular disease, splenectomy or a fistula from the paranasal air sinuses to the brain.
- **Meningococcal meningitis** (see also p. 9) occurs in epidemics and is seen in young adults. It is sometimes associated with a petechial and purpuric rash and has a very rapid evolution. Nasopharyngeal swab culture is useful for typing meningococcus and *Haemophilus* (see below).
- ***Staphylococcus aureus* meningitis** generally occurs in the context of systemic infection, abscesses or neurosurgical procedures.
- ***Pseudomonas*** and other Gram-negative enterobacilli are usually a consequence of surgical access to the CSF.

Box 15.7 Causes of meningitis

Bacterial

- *Meningococcus*
- *Pneumococcus*
- *Listeria* spp.
- *Staphylococcus aureus*
- *E. coli*
- *Pseudomonas* spp.

Viral

- Enteroviruses
- Mumps (meningoencephalitides)

Atypical

- Tuberculosis
- *Cryptococcus*
- Leptospirosis

Non-infective

- Subarachnoid haemorrhage
- Chemical meningitis

Recurrent

- Nasal sinus fistula
- Traumatic CSF leak
- Epstein–Barr virus
- Sarcoidosis, Behçet's
- Mollaret's meningitis (herpes simplex virus type 2)

- *Listeria* **meningitis** is quite common. It should be treated with amoxicillin and gentamicin. It is also associated with encephalitis.
- *Haemophilus influenzae* type B used to be extremely common but has been substantially reduced in many countries by immunisation (Hib vaccine) in children.

   Progress. This man made an excellent recovery from his pneumococcal meningitis.

Case history (2)

A 22-year-old Asian man is admitted from A&E with an insidious 2-week history of malaise, headaches and marked confusion. ***On examination**,* he is pyrexial and drowsy, and has neck stiffness and upgoing plantar responses. A presumptive diagnosis of **tuberculous meningitis** is made.

What action would you take?

- Routine blood tests.
- CXR: may show evidence of TB.
- CT scan: an immediate scan is done because, with this man's confusion and possible raised intracranial pressure, coning is a possibility following lumbar puncture. The CT scan is normal.
- Lumbar puncture.

Table 15.5 Typical changes in the CSF in meningitis

	Normal	Viral	Pyogenic	Tuberculosis
Appearance	Crystal clear	Clear/turbid	Turbid/purulent	Turbid/viscous
Mononuclear cells	<5 mm³	10–100 mm³	<50 mm³	100–300 mm
Polymorph cells	Nil	Nil[a]	200–300/mm³	0–200/mm³
Protein	0.2–0.4 g/L	0.4–0.8 g/L	0.5–2.0 g/L	0.5–3.0 g/L
Glucose	2/3 to 1/2 blood glucose	>1/2 blood glucose	<1/2 blood glucose	<1/3 blood glucose

[a]Some polymorph cells may be seen in the early stages of viral meningitis and encephalitis.
(From Feather A, Randall D, Waterhouse M, eds. *Kumar and Clark's Clinical Medicine*, 10th edn. Elsevier, 2021; Box 26.58.)

The CSF results (Table 15.5) sent back to your F1 junior doctor are:
- Glucose 1.8 mmol/L (blood level 6.5, i.e. low glucose)
- Protein 2.3 g/L (very high protein)
- WCC 250 (70% lymphocytes).

Note: the CSF protein can be so high as to cause the formation of a fine clot ('spider web').

Note: tubercle bacilli are seen only occasionally in the CSF, and the CSF must be sent for culture, which takes 6 weeks.

How would you manage this case?

Start anti-tuberculous chemotherapy on the basis of the clinical picture and high protein in the CSF, which strongly suggest tuberculous meningitis. Don't wait for the culture! Give therapy (rifampicin, isoniazid and pyrazinamide) for 6 weeks until the culture and sensitivities come back. Three drugs should be given for 3 months, followed by rifampicin and isoniazid for 9 months, depending on sensitivities. Adjuvant prednisolone 60 mg should be given for 3 weeks. Specialist advice should be sought for treatment, notification and contact tracing.

Progress. This patient made a good recovery. Dexamethasone was also given for the first 3 weeks.

FITS AND FAINTS

Case history (1)

A 16-year-old young woman is referred with a suspected seizure. Earlier that day in her study, she had felt unwell for about an hour. On getting up from her chair she suddenly lost consciousness without warning. She was incontinent of urine. She woke some minutes later, but had nausea and malaise for the rest of the day. Witnesses said that, when unconscious, she was flaccid and pale, and her mouth, hands and feet were twitching.

Table 15.6 Features of fits and faints

	Fit	Faint
Prodrome	None or characteristic brief aura	Short or prolonged. Blood draining, visual darkening, rushing noise. Cardiac syncope may have no prodrome
Posture at onset	Any	Standing unless cardiac
Injury	Common	Rarer. Protective reflexes may act
Incontinence	Sometimes	Sometimes
Skin colour	Normal, flushed or pale	Pale
Recovery	Slow return of consciousness	Rapid, more physical weakness with clear sensorium
Frequency	Rare to many a day	Not repeated attacks each day
EEG	May be abnormal	Normal

Is this a fit or a faint?

The patient has probably suffered a faint. Some factors are good for distinguishing a fit from a faint (Table 15.6), whereas others are unreliable. In this case, it is noted that faints, other than cardiac syncope, occur only on standing; the preceding symptoms are prolonged or ill defined. Twitching is not usually as violent as in a clonic seizure and the underlying muscle tone is not increased.

Investigations

In suspected cardiac syncope include:
- ECG
- 24 h ambulatory monitoring
- Echocardiogram

Vasovagal faints are generally idiopathic but there are often precipitating or predisposing factors.

Associations with faints

- Adolescent, young adult female.
- Low BP.
- Postural hypotension.
- Heavy periods.
- Micturition with prostatic problems.
- Hot, stuffy surroundings.

- Fasting, hypoglycaemia.
- Dehydration.
- Vagal stimuli such as distress or nausea.

Vasovagal attacks must be distinguished from cardiac syncope (see p. 251). In the latter there is often no warning; there may be breathlessness and engorged jugular veins, and the heart rate may be faster than 140 or slower than 40.

Progress. This girl and her parents were reassured that she had had a simple faint.

Case history (2)

A 16-year-old young man presents with repeated brief falls. He does not seem to lose consciousness but has been seen in A&E several times with severe head and facial injuries resulting from these episodes. Recovery, apart from associated injury, is immediate.

What is the diagnosis?

This history is suggestive of **atonic seizures**. This seizure disorder usually presents in childhood, often as one aspect of a complex epileptic syndrome. Not all seizures resulting in falls are generalised tonic—clonic in nature.

The loss of tone is immediate and absolute so that no protective reflexes occur and injury can be severe. Some sufferers need to wear crash helmets.

Progress. The patient was referred to the Neurologists for management of his epilepsy.

Epilepsy

An epileptic seizure is a convulsion or transient abnormal event experienced by the subject as a result of a paroxysmal discharge of cerebral neurones. Epilepsy, by definition, is the continuing tendency to have such seizures. Recurrent seizures can be prevented in most cases by use of anti-convulsant drugs.

Case history (3)

A 28-year-old man is brought to A&E because he was found to be unconscious and shaking in the high street. You are called to see him urgently because he has had a further tonic—clonic generalised seizure.

How would you manage this situation?

Remember

Status epilepticus exists when seizures follow each other without recovery of consciousness.

General measures

- Secure the airway; remove any false teeth and insert oropharyngeal tube.
- Administer 60% oxygen.
- Secure venous access: many anti-convulsants cause phlebitis, so choose large veins and insert two catheters.
- Give glucose, 50 mL of 20% IV, if hypoglycaemia is a possibility (see p. 401).
- Give thiamine, 250 mg by slow IV injection, if patient is a chronic alcohol user.

Control of seizures

- First, intravenous lorazepam 0.1 mg/kg by slow (2 mg/min) IV injection. Give rectal diazepam (10–20 mg) or IM midazolam (0.2 mg/kg) if IV access is difficult.
- If seizures continue, give IV phenytoin/fosphenytoin IV (second catheter):
  - Phenytoin: loading dose of 15 mg/kg at a rate not exceeding 50 mg/min. Give a further bolus up to total loading dose of 30 mg/kg if seizures persist. Continue with a maintenance dose of 100 mg IV at intervals of 6–8 h.
  - Fosphenytoin is pro-drug of phenytoin and can be given faster than phenytoin. Doses are expressed as phenytoin equivalents (1.5 mg of fosphenytoin to 1 mg phenytoin).
- If seizures continue (despite phenytoin), use:
  - Phenobarbital: 15 mg/kg at a rate not exceeding 100 mg/min and repeated at intervals of 6–8 h if necessary; IV clonazepam can also be used.
- If seizures continue despite these measures the patient is given a general anaesthetic, using thiopentone or propofol, and management is continued with full anaesthetic support.

Progress. This patient had no further fits after being given phenytoin. He was known to have epilepsy and was referred back urgently to his normal consultant for management of his drug therapy.

DIFFICULTY WALKING

Case history (1)

A 75-year-old man is referred with a 1-year history of progressive difficulty with his walking. He has hypertension, which is well controlled with ramipril 5 mg daily. His wife says that his memory has been progressively getting worse.

On examination, he has a Mini Mental State score of 22, indicating a cognitive impairment. His grasp and snout (pursing of lips on lightly tapping the closed lips) reflexes are present, indicating frontal lobe disease. His legs are stiff and his walking is disorganised. This is an apraxic gait.

An apraxic gait is typical of frontal lobe pathology and can be regarded as a problem with high-level programming and execution of gait. This man has vascular dementia (multi-infarct dementia). Patients with cerebrovascular disease should always be imaged to exclude a frontal meningioma or other lesion.

Progress. This patient was referred to the Psychogeriatric department for full assessment. He was started on donepezil 5 mg daily (a reversal inhibitor of acetyl cholinesterase).

Case history (2)

A 70-year-old woman has a 3-week history of progressive difficulty in walking and loss of bladder function. For the last 6 months she has had problems with a stiff gait, numbness in the feet and pains down the left arm.

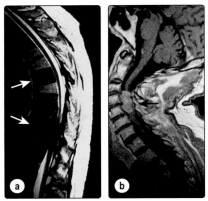

Figure 15.9 MRI showing spinal cord compression. (a) Multiple vertebral metastases (arrows); (b) cervical compression caused by meningioma (arrow).

> ***On examination***, she has wasting and weakness of the hands and brisk triceps reflexes. In the legs there are signs of an upper motor neurone lesion with brisk reflexes and an extensor plantar response. There is also patchy sensory loss in both arms and feet.

What is the diagnosis?

Cervical myelopathy, which at this age is most commonly due to spondylitis. She requires an urgent MRI scan of her cervical spine with a view to early decompression because relatively acute deficits are more potentially reversible. The MRI showed cord compression at the level of C5–6 (Fig. 15.9).

Walking difficulties with upper motor signs in the legs should always be investigated by cervical imaging. Thoracic compression is relatively much less common in the elderly age group.

Other common causes of difficulty in walking are:
- Neurological:
  - Myopathy: proximal, Trendelenburg positive (pelvis drops on the side of the stance leg, suggesting weakness of abductor muscles of the hip), worse on stairs
  - Peripheral neuropathy: foot drop
  - Extra-pyramidal, e.g. shuffling, stooped
  - Spasticity: stiff, circumducting hip
  - Apraxic: upright, high-stepping
  - Ataxic: wide-based.
- Rheumatological/orthopaedic:
  - Polymyalgia
  - Hip joint disease.

Progress. In view of this woman's serious disability and bladder problems, decompressive surgery was performed. This stabilised her condition but without improvement in her bladder function.

HEADACHES

Case history (1)

A 35-year-old woman is admitted to the MAU with a very severe headache of explosive onset. She is slightly drowsy with a GCS of 13, and has photophobia and meningism.

A CT scan shows blood in the subarachnoid space (this has a 95% sensitivity in the first 24 h).

Diagnosis. Subarachnoid haemorrhage.

- Arrange for cerebral MR angiography to identify the source of bleeding.
- If an aneurysm is found, refer to a Neurosurgeon for surgical treatment.
- **Nimodipine** (e.g. 60 mg orally 4-hourly for 2–3 weeks, or 1 mg/h IV) can reduce arterial spasm and reduce further cerebral infarction.
- Avoid hypotension (it may worsen the ischaemic deficit). Treat hypertension if diastolic pressure is persistently >130 mmHg. Aim for a very gradual decrease in BP with careful monitoring and frequent repeat neurological examination.
- Supportive measures include bed rest, analgesia and laxatives (avoid sudden rises in ICP or BP).
- Watch for complications, including hyponatraemia/syndrome of inappropriate antidiuretic hormone secretion (SIADH), hydrocephalus (obstruction of cerebral aqueduct by blood) and vasospasm causing ischaemic deficits.

N.B. If the scan is negative and the history highly suggestive of a sub-arachnoid haemorrhage, a lumbar puncture is necessary.

- A **lumbar puncture** is performed to look for blood-stained CSF and xanthochromia (bilirubin discoloration of CSF due to cell lysis). Xanthochromia may be detected from ~12 h to 3 weeks after subarachnoid haemorrhage. Visible inspection of a centrifuged sample is often sufficient to detect xanthochromia, but laboratory spectrophotometry is more sensitive.

Remember

If a close family member has also had a subarachnoid haemorrhage, the rest of the family should be screened by MR angiography.

Conditions that can mimic subarachnoid haemorrhage include sudden onset of meningitis or viral meningism, migraine, spontaneous subdural haemorrhage and post-coital headache. The last of these is a headache of very sudden onset but is a benign self-limiting condition, perhaps a variant of migraine. With the availability of MR angiography, patients are now often scanned to exclude aneurysms. Finally, low-pressure headache may be of sudden onset. This is a poorly understood condition where headache may occur suddenly on standing and generally settles when lying down. There is meningeal enhancement on MRI and a low CSF pressure. The condition is again self-limiting. At least some cases relate to CSF leaks, sometimes from lumbar puncture (post-lumbar puncture headache) and occasionally from Valsalva manoeuvres.

Progress. In this patient, a posterior communicating aneurysm was found. She was treated with an intravascular coil insertion and made a good recovery.

Case history (2)

A 35-year-old man complains of continuous headache day and night. He used to have a different headache, which was episodic. This previous headache was unilateral and throbbing, and would last a few hours; it was also associated with photophobia, visual scotomata and nausea. The new headache has no such features. He has to take about eight paracetamol tablets a day to control the pain.

What is this new headache due to?

Migraine headache, which was also the cause of this man's original headache. The headache sometimes becomes transformed into a more chronic headache, punctuated by migraine-like exacerbations. Often the patient is given regular analgesia, which has a well-known effect of actually perpetuating headache.

What action should you take?

A brain scan is not often necessary in a clearly chronic headache with no signs, although the patient often expects one. It is more important to take a proper history and institute the correct management.

Management

This is broadly similar for episodic migraine, i.e. sumatriptan prophylaxis is given if the sufferer has more than about two migraines a month or finds them very debilitating. A migraine prophylactic agent should be given (see p. 445).

Progress. This patient was reassured that he did not have malignant or serious disease.

Chronic analgesia abuse should be stopped. This man was advised to reduce this gradually over a month. He was told to expect his headaches to be worse over this period.

Information

Calcitonin-gene related peptide (CGRP) influences neuronal modulation of pain and this may play a role in migraine. Four monoclonal antibodies to the CGRP have been developed and are now being used in chronic migraine, i.e. erenumab, eptinezumab, fremanezumab and galcanezumab.

Case history (3)

A 40-year-old man comes to A&E with severe headache, which then settles on arrival. This has happened before and he has always been discharged immediately. On taking a history, it transpires that an excruciating headache comes on gradually at about the same time every day. The headache is unilateral and pounding, involves the side of the face, and is associated with a watering eye and nose. He jumps up and down in agitation with the pain. The symptoms generally only last about an hour.

What is the cause of this headache?

This description is typical of **cluster headache.** Each cluster may last a few weeks, with several months of relief in between.

Cluster headache

Cluster headache is distinct from migraine and consists of recurrent bouts of excruciating unilateral pain that typically wake the patient. Attacks cluster around one eye. Cluster headache affects adults, mainly males aged 30–40 years. Alcohol and glyceryl trinitrate can provoke attacks. Severe pain can last for several hours and is associated with vomiting. One cheek and nostril become congested. Transient ipsilateral Horner's syndrome is common. One bout of cluster attacks, with pain every few nights, usually lasts 1–2 months. Despite excruciating pain, there are no sequelae. Bouts recur at intervals over several years but tend to disappear after the age of 55.

Progress. In this patient, treatment with analgesics and prophylactic migraine drugs did not help. However, his attacks were attenuated with SC sumatriptan. Oxygen inhalation also helped on occasions. A short course of oral prednisolone reduced the frequency of attacks.

Case history (4)

A 30-year-old woman has a long history of short but severe headaches on one side of the face, lasting only a few minutes but occurring several times a day. There is considerable flushing and rhinorrhoea on the same side during each attack. There is no trigger to the attacks.

What is the cause of this headache?

The patient has **paroxysmal hemicrania**; the attacks are longer in duration than in trigeminal neuralgia but shorter than in cluster headaches or migraine. There is generally some associated autonomic disturbance, as seen here. There is a specific and often extremely rewarding response to indometacin, as occurred in this woman.

Some causes of acute, episodic and chronic headache are given in Box 15.8.

MOVEMENT DISORDERS

- Akinetic–rigid syndromes, i.e. slowed movement with increased tone.
- Dyskinesias – added, uncontrollable movements.
  Both may coexist.

Case history (1)

A 22-year-old woman develops an acute gastrointestinal illness with abdominal pain, vomiting and diarrhoea. After 2 days she becomes generally stiff and has prolonged episodes of painful spasm of the axial muscles with opisthotonic posturing. Her eyes periodically roll upwards involuntarily (oculogyric crises). She had been given metoclopramide for her vomiting.

Diagnosis. Oculogyric crises from metoclopramide.

Acute dystonic reactions can occur in sensitive individuals after relatively modest doses of drugs with central anti-dopaminergic action, such as neuroleptics or certain anti-emetics, e.g. metoclopramide. Neuroleptic malignant syndrome can also occur.

Treatment of oculogyric crisis involves the identification and stoppage of the responsible agent. These acute dystonias respond generally to IV centrally acting anti-muscarinics, e.g. procyclidine 5–10 mg.

Box 15.8 Causes of headache

Very sudden

- Subarachnoid haemorrhage
- First migraine attack
- Subdural haemorrhage
- Meningitis, encephalitis
- Inflammatory meningoencephalitis, e.g. systemic lupus erythematosus (SLE)
- Cerebral abscess
- Raised intracranial pressure
- Low-pressure headache

Episodic

- Tension headache
- Migraine
- Paroxysmal hemicrania
- Cluster headache
- Trigeminal/occipital neuralgia
- Giant cell arteritis (temporal or cranial arteritis)
- Post-coital headache

Chronic

- Tension headache
- Analgesia abuse
- Chronic hemicrania
- Chronic cluster headache
- Cervicogenic headache
- Space-occupying lesions
- Raised intracranial pressure
- Ongoing after many acute headaches
- Associated with depression/anxiety

Anti-emetics, e.g. domperidone, ondansetron or granisetron, do not produce dystonia.

Hypokinetic movement disorders

- Parkinson's disease.
- Multisystem atrophy.
- Progressive supranuclear palsy.
- Dementia with Lewy bodies.
- Corticobasal degeneration.
- Some frontal dementias, mass lesions.
- Tardive dyskinesia (+ hyperkinetic).
- Psychomotor retardation.

Hyperkinetic movement disorder

- Choreo-athetosis.
- Ballismus.
- Dystonia.

- Myoclonus.
- Tics.
- Tremor.
- Psychogenic.

Progress. This woman was given IV procyclidine 5 mg IV. Her dystonia settled within 24 h.

A 40-year-old man has a 1-year history of involuntary facial movements and a shuffling gait. There is a past history of schizophrenia, for which he was given haloperidol. *On examination*, he has intermittent involuntary protrusion of his tongue, grimacing and blepharospasm. He has some writhing movements of his left arm and repetitive rubbing of the soles of his feet on the floor when sitting. Voluntary arm movements are slow. He walks slowly with a shuffling gait and stooped posture.

Diagnosis. Tardive dyskinesia. This develops in patients previously, as well as currently, on anti-psychotic medication. The movement disorder may be a complex mixture of hyperkinetic restlessness (akathisia), dystonia and choreo-athetosis, and hypokinetic bradykinesia. They are late and difficult to reverse. The effects of anti-dopaminergics are thought to be due to long-term dysregulation of dopaminergic pathways. Sometimes, in the short term, increases in anti-psychotic drug doses actually improve the hyperkinetic aspects temporarily (direct anti-dopaminergic action), but this is likely to lead to worsened long-term problems. The drugs that are good for avoiding acute extra-pyramidal side-effects are also good for minimising long-term side-effects.

Progress. In this patient the haloperidol was gradually reduced and stopped. His symptoms improved. He has been told of the risk of recurrence on further anti-psychotic therapy.

GUILLAIN—BARRÉ SYNDROME

This is an acute sensorimotor polyneuropathy that often follows a gastrointestinal infection, e.g. *Campylobacter*, cytomegalovirus or a respiratory infection.

Case history

A 34-year-old woman is brought to A&E by her relatives; she has a 1-week history of difficulty walking. She had had mild gastroenteritis due to *Campylobacter jejuni* about 5 weeks before but had recovered from this. Her relatives thought she was 'putting it on' but became a bit concerned when they found that she was unable to climb the stairs to her flat.

On examination, she looked well and was orientated, but was extremely anxious because she thought she was becoming paralysed. She had a symmetrical weakness in her limbs, which was worse proximally. Reflexes were absent and she had normal plantar responses. There was a mild sensory deficit in a glove and stocking distribution.

What is the diagnosis?

This could be the Guillain—Barré syndrome. *Don't* leave this patient unattended because the progression can be fast and her respiratory muscles can be affected within a few hours.

Kumar & Clark's Cases in Clinical Medicine

Investigations

BLOOD TESTS
- FBC
- U&Es
- CRP
- ABGs

What should you do?

Admit her. Once she is on the ward, perform a lumbar puncture. In this patient the CSF protein is raised. She gets progressively weaker and is having difficulty breathing,

How would you manage this patient?

- Admit her to the HDU.
- Regularly monitor her respiratory function with vital capacity. Intubation and ventilation might be required. Call for expert help.
- Nursing care should take care to avoid pressure ulcers.
- Give orophylaxis to prevent venous thrombosis (low-molecular-weight [LMW] heparin, enoxaparin).
- Steroid therapy is ineffective.
- IV immunoglobulin given in the first 2 weeks reduces duration and severity of weakness. *N.B.* Check IgA levels; severe allergic reactions occur (due to IgG antibodies) with IgA deficiency.

   Progress. This patient was given IV immunoglobulins and gradually improved over the next few months.

Prognosis

Eighty per cent of patients make a full recovery, as occurred in this patient.

SPINAL CORD COMPRESSION

This produces radicular pain at the level of the cord lesion, with a spastic tetraparesis or paraparesis below the level of the lesion; sensory loss below the cord level is also present.

Case history

A 56-year-old man is admitted with a 2-week history of weakness in his legs. He has no other complaints but admits that he is a heavy smoker.

   On examination, there is weakness of both legs, which is more marked distally; the left leg is more severely affected. Knee and ankle jerks are slightly brisk and he has a bilateral extensor plantar response. There are no sensory signs. He has no neurological deficit in his arms.

N.B. This is a medical emergency. This patient has a mild paraparesis and a cord lesion must be excluded.

Investigations

- Routine bloods show an Hb of 100 g/L with an ESR of 100 mm/h.
- CXR was normal, making carcinoma with secondaries unlikely, despite the patient being a heavy smoker.
- Thoracic and lumbar spinal X-rays showed an osteolytic lesion at T10.

The preliminary tests have taken 3 days, and the patient is now incontinent of urine and his leg weakness is worse. Urgent neurological referral is required.

MRI scan shows a lesion at T10. Urgent decompression is performed by a Neurosurgeon but the patient still requires a urinary catheter.

Further blood tests

- Serum protein electrophoresis and immunofixation shows a monoclonal band.
- Bence Jones protein is present in the urine.
- Bone marrow shows infiltration with plasma cells.
  Diagnosis. Multiple myeloma.
  Progress. This patient needed radiotherapy and chemotherapy. He still requires a catheter and is mobilising only slowly with a frame.

Remember

Diagnosis is urgent with cord compression. Prompt diagnosis enables decompression to be performed before severe symptoms develop and potentially before urinary problems; if the latter are present, they are frequently permanent, even with decompression.

Further reading

Diplopia

Gilhus NE. Myasthenia gravis. *New England Journal of Medicine* 2016; **375**: 2570–2581.

Loss of vision

Charles A. Migraine. *New England Journal of Medicine* 2017; **377**: 553–561.

Bell's palsy

De Almeida JR, Al Khabori M, Guyatt GH, et al. Combined corticosteroid and antiviral treatment for Bell palsy: a systematic review and meta-analysis. *Journal of the American Medical Association* 2009; **302**: 985–993.

Stroke/TIA

Albers GW. Thrombosis before thrombectomy. *New England Journal of Medicine* 2020; **382**: 2045–2046.

Brott G, Hobson 2nd RW, Howard G, et al. Stenting versus endarterectomy for treatment of carotid artery stenosis. *New England Journal of Medicine* 2010; **363**: 11–23.

Campbell BCV, Mitchell PJ, Churilov L, et al. Tenecteplase versus alteplase before thrombectomy for ischaemic stroke. *New England Journal of Medicine* 2018; **378**: 1573–1582.

Cramer SC. Brain repair after stroke. *New England Journal of Medicine* 2010; **362**: 1827–1829.

Rothwell PM, Algra A, Amarenco P. Medical treatment in acute and long-term secondary prevention after transient ischaemic attack and ischaemic stroke. *Lancet* 2011; **377**: 1681–1692.

Parkinson's disease

Bressman S, Saunders-Pullman R. When to start levodopa therapy for Parkinson's disease. *New England Journal of Medicine* 2019; **380**: 389–390.

Multiple sclerosis

Frohman EM, Wingerchuk DM. Transverse myelitis. *New England Journal of Medicine* 2010; **363**: 564–572.

Reich DS, Lucchinetti CF, Calabresi PA. Multiple sclerosis. *New England Journal of Medicine* 2018; **378**: 169–180.

Falls

Dykes PC, Carroll DL, Hurley A, et al. Fall prevention in acute care hospitals. *Journal of the American Medical Association* 2010; **304**: 1912–1918.

Meningitis

McGill F, Heyderman RS, Panagiotou S, et al. Acute bacterial meningitis in adults. *Lancet* 2016; **388**: 3036–3047.

Thigpen MC, Whitney CG, Messonnier NE, et al. Bacterial meningitis in the United States, 1998–2007. *New England Journal of Medicine* 2011; **364**: 2016–2025.

Headaches

Lawton MT, Vates GE. Subarachnoid hemorrhage. *New England Journal of Medicine* 2017; **377**: 257–266.

Spinal cord compression

Chari A, Vogl D, Gavriatopoulou M, et al. Oral selinexor-dexamethasone for triple-class refractory multiple myeloma. *New England Journal of Medicine* 2019; **381**: 727–738.

Ropper AE, Ropper AH. Acute spinal cord compression. *New England Journal of Medicine* 2017; **376**: 1358–1369.

DELIRIUM

Delirium (see also p. 140) is the most commonly misdiagnosed psychiatric disorder in the general hospital and many cases go undetected. Yet it is the most common psychosis met in the hospital setting; 10–20% of surgical and medical inpatients have delirium during their admission. It is the best indication that the higher centres of the brain are failing.

Information

DELIRIUM: CENTRAL FEATURES
- Impaired consciousness/attention
- Global disturbance of cognition
- Psychomotor disturbance
- Disturbed sleep/wake cycle
- Emotional disturbance

Case history

You are asked to see a 68-year-old man who had surgery for a fractured hip, sustained after a fall at home 3 days previously. He was awake all night, occasionally shouting out and disturbing the rest of the ward, and he keeps pulling at his intravenous line.

How would you diagnose delirium?

An acute onset and fluctuating course are valuable diagnostically. Delirium represents an acute generalised impairment of cognitive function (see Information box). The primary feature is disorientation in time and place (more rarely, person). A well patient should know the day of the week, the month and the year (people who are well can occasionally get the date and time wrong). They should know that they are in hospital, its name and location, and the name of the ward. Other psychoses do not affect orientation.

- **'Clouding of consciousness':** refers to the variable level of attention seen in delirium, so that the patient cannot learn information and therefore cannot recall it.
- **Visual hallucinations or illusions:** are commonly present, so the patient may mistake a curtain movement in a dimly lit ward as a threatening person, resulting in extreme fear and agitation, especially at night.
- **Persecutory delusions:** are the most common and may make patients refuse food, drink and medicines because they believe that they are being poisoned. Alternatively, these delusions can cause aggression, as patients defend themselves against a perceived threat.

Remember

- Behaviour may be agitated and disturbed or 'quiet', 'hypoactive' and less easily identified.

- Fluctuating presentation and disturbed sleep/wake cycle may conceal abnormalities during the day.
- Emotional disturbance (fear, perplexity, apathy, depression) is common in delirium.

What were the predisposing factors in this patient?

Delirium occurs most commonly in a person with a developing or deteriorating brain, with risk factors such as:

- Extremes of age (the young and old)
- Brain damage or insult:
  - Any dementia (most common)
  - Previous head injury or episode of delirium
  - Previous cerebrovascular accident
  - Alcoholic brain damage
- Newly prescribed or multiple medications
- Prolonged operative procedure and anaesthesia
- Immobilisation and social isolation
- Dislocation to an unfamiliar environment (such as admission to hospital)
- Sleep deprivation
- Sensory deficits (e.g. visual or hearing) and extremes (overload or deprivation).

Specific causes of delirium

These include:

- Brain trauma
- Epilepsy (ictal, inter-ictal, post-ictal)
- Neoplasm (intracranial or extracranial)
- Other brain space-occupying lesions (e.g. abscess)
- Metabolic encephalopathies (e.g. hypoglycaemia, hypoxia, hyponatraemia)
- Infections (intracranial and systemic)
- Drugs and poisons (see p. 489)
- Withdrawal from drugs (e.g. alcohol and sedatives; see p. 491)
- Vascular (cerebral or myocardial)
- Haematological (severe anaemia)
- Extracranial insult (e.g. hypothermia).

How would you investigate this patient?

Corroborative history from family/partner (duration of history, drug history, past medical and psychiatric history, alcohol/drug use).

An EEG shows excess slow waves in 90% (with the exception of drug withdrawal states) and may show sharp waves and spikes in status epilepticus. It is used occasionally as a confirmatory test, if there is doubt about the clinical diagnosis.

Investigations

- Look for infections (MSU, CXR, blood and sputum cultures, lumbar puncture if indicated)
- U&Es (hyponatraemia)
- Calcium
- Blood sugar
- Liver and cardiac enzymes
- ECG (silent myocardial infarct)
- CT brain scan ('silent' parietal infarct; predisposing brain disease/damage)

Nursing care

A carefully controlled, consistent and balanced environment is essential:
- Single room, if available
- Windows that do not allow exits
- Minimal stimulation by noise
- Persistent orientation by nurses and notices (a very disturbed patient may require one-to-one nursing temporarily)
- Minimal visitors: only those the patient knows well
- Some lighting at night
- Reverse dehydration and don't neglect nutrition
- Treat constipation, sleep disturbance
- Perceptive aids, e.g. glasses, hearing aid.

Management

- Delirium requires urgent management because complications (e.g. falls, pressure ulcers and infections) can exacerbate the condition and contribute to significant mortality, particularly in the elderly.
- Find the cause and reverse it.
- A psychiatric opinion can be useful regarding differential diagnosis (see next section) and management.
- Reduce all drug treatments to a minimum (see p. 491). Avoid anti-psychotic drugs unless the patient is a danger to himself/herself (or others) or is distressed, or if the patient's general health is suffering.
- Symptomatic treatments include haloperidol.
- Evaluate progress regularly.

Differential diagnosis

- Other organic brain disorders:
  - Lewy body dementia: fluctuating conscious level and extreme sensitivity to psychotropic drugs
  - Advancing dementia, acute-on-chronic disturbance.
- Functional psychoses/mood disorders:
  - Severe depression (agitation, psychomotor retardation, persecutory ideas)
  - Mania/hypomania (fluctuating mood, nocturnal disturbance, abnormally heightened perceptions).
- Drugs: delirium tremens (see p. 495).

Drug therapy

Doses of tranquillising drugs should start low and be titrated, depending on age (this patient is 68 years old), pre-existing brain damage and response to initial treatment. Patients with delirium are often sensitive to medication and the dose needs to be balanced carefully.
- Haloperidol by mouth: 1.5 mg then 1.5–5 mg up to 3 × daily, depending on level of disturbance, sensitivity to drug and response.

Note: liquid or tablet form; lowest effective dose; beware extra-pyramidal side-effects (EPSEs).

- Phenothiazines are best avoided because of their anti-muscarinic and alpha-blocking actions.

If intramuscular medication is required

- Haloperidol 0.5–1.5 mg IM.
- Repeat 8-hourly as necessary.

Haloperidol should not be given intravenously. If the patient is sensitive to medication and EPSEs are likely or present, use an 'atypical' anti-psychotic drug, e.g. olanzapine or quetiapine. Check doses carefully. Reversal of acute EPSEs can be achieved with a low dose of an anti-muscarinic drug (e.g. procyclidine 5 mg oral/IM).

Progress. Delirium resolved in this patient 48 h following oral haloperidol. This anti-psychotic medication was tailed off gradually over 1 week.

> **Remember**
>
> **EXTRAPYRAMIDAL SIDE-EFFECTS OF ANTI-PSYCHOTIC MEDICATION**
> - Acute dystonic reactions: involuntary muscle contractions involving extra-ocular muscles, face, neck, mouth and tongue.
> - Pseudo-parkinsonism: rigidity and tremor in larger muscles.

What is the prognosis?

There is often a delay of a few days when the underlying condition has improved but the brain is still dysfunctional. Otherwise, the prognosis depends on successful treatment of the main aetiological condition (up to 20% undetermined in the elderly) and the state of the pre-existing brain (25% of the elderly with delirium will have an underlying dementia). Good communication with the patient's primary care doctor is essential because treated, as well as unrecognised, delirium can cause problems after discharge.

DRUGS AND POISONS AS CAUSES OF DELIRIUM

Delirium can occur in response to excessive or normal doses of many drugs, particularly in the elderly. Some drugs are more likely to cause delirium than others.

> **Case history**
>
> An 83-year-old woman is discharged from hospital following an admission for severe breathlessness due to acute-on-chronic heart failure. She was discharged on furosemide, lisinopril, carvedilol and spironolactone.
>
> Three weeks later she is brought to A&E by her carer because she is confused, very aggressive towards her carer and unaware of where she is.
>
> ***On examination,*** she is conscious but completely disorientated in time and place. She is unaware that she is in hospital. Cardiovascular examination shows a pulse of 60 bpm, irregularly irregular, normal venous pressure, and there are no basal crackles or ankle oedema.
>
> You check on her medication with the carer, who confirms that she takes the drugs given to her when she left the hospital on a regular basis. The carer also says she now

takes an additional drug, which has been given to her by her doctor because of an irregular pulse.

Unfortunately, the carer has not brought all the drugs with her. You contact the patient's doctor, who says that she prescribed digoxin because of the irregular pulse, which she thought was atrial fibrillation.

You think this might be the problem, so you check her digoxin levels as well as her urea and electrolytes.

Drugs causing delirium

Cardiac drugs

- Digoxin: check serum level.
- Calcium channel blockers.
- Anti-arrhythmics, e.g. lidocaine.
- Beta-blockers: especially propranolol (lipid-soluble); use a water-soluble beta-blocker, e.g. atenolol.

Therapeutic drugs affecting the brain

- Benzodiazepines: although withdrawal is a more common cause – see later.
- Barbiturates: again, withdrawal is more common.
- Other hypnotics: nitrazepam.
- Lithium: usually a sign of toxicity.
- High-potency anti-psychotics: neuroleptic malignant syndrome (see Information box).
- Anti-convulsants: usually a sign of toxicity.
- Dopamine and its agonists: levodopa and bromocriptine.

Drugs with anti-muscarinic properties (common cause of delirium)

- Atropine: remember eye drops and pre-medication in anaesthesia.
- Other topical cycloplegics and mydriatics.
- Anti-parkinsonian agents: in patients with both Parkinson's disease and pseudo-parkinsonism, caused by dopamine antagonists.
- Anti-depressants: especially tricyclics – amitriptyline most frequently.
- Anti-psychotics: commonly the phenothiazines, especially chlorpromazine.
- Anti-emetics.
- Anti-histamines.
- Anti-spasmodics: uncommon.

What are the physical signs of the anti-muscarinic state?

- Dilated and poorly reactive pupils (blurred vision).
- Flushed face.
- Dry mouth and skin.
- Fever.
- Tachypnoea.
- Tachycardia.
- Hypertension.
- Urinary retention and diminished bowel sounds.

How would you treat anti-muscarinic-induced delirium?

- General supportive nursing measures (see p. 494).
- Management, usually conservative, with observation of vital signs.
- IV line and ECG monitor if symptoms are marked.
- Oral or IM benzodiazepine (e.g. diazepam 10 mg adult dose) for agitation or seizures.
- Cholinergic therapy with an anti-cholinesterase (physostigmine) is potentially hazardous (heart block, bronchospasm, respiratory failure) and is used, if at all, for life-threatening cases (uncontrolled seizures, coma, respiratory depression). Discuss with a senior and/or the Poisons Unit.

Contraindications. Ischaemic heart disease, prolonged PR/QRS intervals, asthma, diabetes, inflammatory bowel disease, bowel or bladder obstruction, glaucoma, pregnancy, hypothyroidism.

Anti-infective agents

- Anti-malarials, e.g. chloroquine and mefloquine.
- Antibiotics: uncommon, but associated diarrhoea may lead to dehydration.

Gastrointestinal drugs

- H_2 antagonists: cimetidine is most commonly reported.
- Bismuth chelate.

Anti-inflammatories

- NSAIDs.
- Corticosteroids: differential diagnosis of affective and paranoid psychoses.
- Interferons.

Chemotherapeutic agents

- Asparaginase.
- Methotrexate.
- Vinca alkaloids.

Anaesthetic agents

- Ketamine.

'Recreational' drugs

- Alcohol (toxic levels).
- Amfetamine.
- Ecstasy (methylene dioxymethamphetamine, MDMA): an amfetamine-like drug.
- Lysergic acid (LSD) and other hallucinogens (magic mushrooms).
- Cannabis (toxic doses).
- Cocaine.
- Phencyclidine ('angel dust'): chemically related to ketamine.
- Gamma-butyric acid.

Poisons

Exposure can be occupational, environmental or by deliberate self-ingestion, e.g.:

- Methanol
- Solvents: adolescents
- Carbon monoxide
- Plant alkaloids
- Many industrial chemicals: always find out the patient's occupation.

How do you treat drug-/poison-induced delirium?

- Stop the delivery of the drug or poison. If in doubt, stop all non-essential medication and/or reduce the dose.
- Treat specific causes (e.g. hyperbaric or mask-delivered oxygen for CO poisoning).
- General measures are covered in the section on delirium (see p. 494).

Drug withdrawal

- Alcohol (see p. 495).
- Sedatives:
  - Benzodiazepines
  - Barbiturates.

Clinical presentation of sedative withdrawal (beyond delirium)

- Mental: anxiety, irritability, agitation, insomnia, nightmares.
- Arousal: tremor, sweating, tachycardia, sensitivity to light, noise and touch, muscle tension, uncommonly convulsions (with the exception of barbiturate withdrawal).
- Physical: nausea, anorexia, 'flu-like' symptoms, metallic taste.

Treatment of sedative withdrawal

- Replace the original class of drug in adequate doses to control the withdrawal symptoms, reducing to the minimum amount to prevent their re-emergence.
- Try to use a long-acting drug (e.g. diazepam), although sometimes the original drug itself is required.
- Therapeutic drug cessation can be achieved gradually later but the patient should be monitored closely and supported. Even patients with long-term dependence can manage some reduction and stabilisation on a reduced dose in the short term.

Remember

Check doses with a senior colleague and with the national formulary.

Progress. This woman's digoxin level was 2 μg/L (toxic range >1.5 μg) and so her digoxin was stopped but her other medication continued. Her serum urea and electrolytes were normal; the serum potassium was 4.3 mmol/L.

Her delirium required a small dose of oral haloperidol 0.5 mg × 2 daily for the first 4 days. She progressively improved and was discharged after

9 days, back to her normal self. In view of her age, she was started on aspirin 150 g daily (not warfarin) and digoxin 62.5 μg daily for her atrial fibrillation.

DEMENTIA

See also page 143.

Dementia is the most common organic brain syndrome seen in elderly inpatients; 7% of people over the age of 65 and up to 33% over the age of 85 have a dementing illness. Treatable causes can be found in 10% of patients with definite dementia, but that figure is considerably higher if the 'pseudo-dementia' of depressive illness is included.

Dementia is a global, acquired, progressive deterioration of intellect, memory and personality. Altered ('clouded') consciousness is not usually involved, in contrast to delirium, although dementia often confers an underlying predisposition for delirium (see p. 490).

Case history

A 74-year-old woman is brought into A&E, having been found wandering in the street at night. She is poorly nourished and dishevelled, and has several bruises on her arms and legs. You find out from her daughter that her husband died 6 months previously.

How does dementia present?

- Loss of memory, especially short-term.
- Episodes of increasing 'confusion'.
- Falls, with or without head injury.
- Wandering and getting lost (getting into the wrong bed), especially at night.
- Insomnia.
- Weight loss.
- Slow recovery and mobilisation after injury (e.g. hip fracture) or illness (e.g. myocardial infarct, pneumonia).
- Incontinence.
- Difficulty dressing: parietal lesion of dressing dyspraxia.
- Behavioural disinhibition: frontal lobe sign.
- Severe extra-pyramidal reaction to dopamine antagonists: Lewy body dementia.

What are the causes?

These are listed in Box 16.1.

Differential diagnosis

- Delirium.
- Amnestic syndrome: relatively specific memory loss, e.g. Wernicke–Korsakoff syndrome (see p. 496).
- Depressive 'pseudo-dementia'.
- Learning disability ('amentia').

Investigations

- A corroborative history: duration, presentation, mood, alcohol, past history

Box 16.1 Causes of dementia

(See Box 7.3 for treatable causes)

Common causes

Over 65
- Alzheimer's disease
- Multi-infarct dementia
- Lewy body disease
- Parkinson's disease

Under 65
- Alzheimer's disease
- AIDS
- Alcoholic dementia
- Head injuries

Less common causes

- Prion disease (Creutzfeldt–Jakob)
- Huntington's
- Fronto-temporal dementia (Pick's)
- Multiple sclerosis
- Wilson's disease

- A Mini-Mental State Examination (MMSE): a brief, structured bedside screening test of memory
- Intelligence quotient (IQ) (performed by a psychologist) to confirm cognitive decline
- Blood tests:
  - Gamma-glutamyl transpeptidase and MCV: raised levels are evidence of excess alcohol consumption
  - Urea, creatinine, eGFR
  - Liver enzymes
  - Free T4 and TSH
  - VDRL
  - Hb
  - ESR or CRP
  - Auto-immune screen to include anti-nuclear antibody (ANA)
  - Serum electrophoresis
  - Glucose levels
  - Vitamin B12 and red cell folate
  - Calcium
- HIV testing after counselling in at-risk group
- MSU
- CXR
- CT/MRI brain scan: tumour, subdural haematoma, normal pressure hydrocephalus and infarcts *might* confirm generalised cerebral atrophy
- ECG: arrhythmias
- EEG: diffuse slow waves are rare before 75 in normal health; a normal EEG would suggest an alternative diagnosis
- Consider lumbar puncture, if diagnosis is unclear

Kumar & Clark's Cases in Clinical Medicine

Examination

- Cardiovascular, neurological and endocrine system: to exclude secondary causes.
- Mental state examination.
- Simple cognitive screening bedside tests: dementia may be suggested by the quality of the responses, e.g. 'perseveration' (repeating a response beyond the relevant question), 'confabulation' (inventing recollections to compensate for memory loss).
- Look for depressed affect.

SIMPLE COGNITIVE SCREENING

- Orientation in time, place and person: ask day, month, year; ward, hospital, town/city, country; identity of relatives or key ward staff
- Attention and concentration: ask patient to recite the days of the week or the months of the year backwards (should be 100% accurate)
- Verbal short-term memory: teach patient to recite immediately a name and address accurately (a test of registration: they should be able to do this in two attempts). Then ask the patient to recall the name and address 5 min later (test of memory recall; should recall 95% of the individual items)
- Long-term memory: tests of general information, e.g. recent news, world events or on a subject of interest to them
- Pre-morbid intelligence (necessary to judge whether there has been a deterioration in intellect): establish level of education achieved and occupation

How would you manage a case of dementia?

- Treat any reversible cause.
- Stop anti-muscarinic drugs, if possible.
- Involve a psychiatrist early regarding diagnosis and management.
- Acetyl cholinesterase inhibitors may be indicated in early Alzheimer's disease (e.g. donepezil, galantamine or rivastigmine), as well as memantine (affects glutamate transmission), in conjunction with specialist advice from the old age Psychiatry team (see p. 143).
- Low-dose haloperidol (e.g. 0.5 mg) can help control agitation and any accompanying delusions.
- Short-acting hypnotics, such as temazepam, can help insomnia.
- While on the ward, ensure adequate fluids, nutrition, and treatment of constipation and any other reversible causes of incontinence.
- If possible, discharge home as soon as possible to avoid disorientating experience of admission.
- Involve the nearest relatives only.
- Refer to old age Psychiatry specialist dementia services.

Progress. This patient improved considerably after a few days in hospital with care from an MDT. Her daughter lived fairly nearby and so was able, with the Occupational Therapist, to arrange for aids at home to allow independent living. This patient was assessed by the Psychogeriatrician, who thought her dementia symptoms might well be related to her depression (pseudo-dementia) following the death of her husband. She was started on citalopram (a selective serotonin re-uptake inhibitor, SSRI) 8 mg daily, with some improvement. She returned home but requires continual supervision.

DELIRIUM TREMENS (DTs)

Delirium tremens is the most severe form of alcohol withdrawal syndrome and is a medical emergency because of the major complications that can arise. It often occurs on the second or third day after admission, due to stopping drinking suddenly, although it can occur after a significant reduction in drinking in those who are highly alcohol-dependent.

Case history

A 49-year-old man was admitted via A&E to the Orthopaedic ward, having had a fall and fracturing his pelvis. On the third day after admission, he became disorientated and restless with visual hallucinations. The Orthopaedic junior doctor wants your advice.

A full history elicits that the patient had been a heavy drinker for 10 or more years and obviously has had no alcohol since the fall. You think he has DTs — particularly as he has had a similar episode in the past.

Remember

Heavy drinkers under-report and conceal alcohol consumption. The problem is suggested by:
- Regular medical presentations
- Injuries/falls
- Anxiety/depression/self-harm
- Marital/family/financial/legal difficulties.

What are the clinical features of DTs?

- Coarse tremor (which may affect the whole body).
- Disorientation in place and time.
- Anxiety (often severe).
- Motor restlessness.
- Nausea and/or diarrhoea.
- Insomnia.
- Nightmares.
- Excessive sympathetic drive:
  - Sweating
  - Tachycardia
  - Hypertension
  - Low-grade fever.
- Reduced attention.
- Illusions: visual.
- Hallucinations: classically visual and frightening, but may be tactile or auditory; small animals (insects, spiders, rats) advance menacingly towards and over the patient.
- Persecutory delusions.
- Convulsions in severe cases.

Remember

COMPLICATIONS OF DTs
- Co-morbid illness or trauma (infection, dehydration, head injury)

- Hypoglycaemia
- Electrolyte disturbances (sodium, potassium, magnesium)
- Convulsions
- Coma
- Death

Investigations

- Serum U&Es (especially hypokalaemia)
- Calcium and magnesium
- Gamma-glutamyl transpeptidase (raised)
- Aspartate transferase
- Bilirubin
- Glucose
- Hb
- MCV (raised)
- MSU
- If necessary, appropriate X-rays to exclude infection (CXR) and trauma (CT brain scan if indicated: ?subdural)

How would you treat DTs?

- Admit the patient to an acute medical bed.
- General measures (see Delirium, p. 487).
- Treat electrolyte and fluid imbalances in particular.
- Treat any co-morbid disorder.
- Oral thiamine 200 mg daily, even in the absence of Wernicke—Korsakoff encephalopathy, the specific signs of which can be missed in the presence of severe withdrawal symptoms. Parenteral thiamine 500 mg daily must be given early if long-term dementia is to be prevented.
- Parenteral high-dose thiamine is necessary in the presence of a thiamine-related encephalopathy.

Information

WERNICKE—KORSAKOFF SYNDROME
Acute confusion, ocular palsies and nystagmus, and ataxic gait, leading to chronic short-term memory loss and confabulation.

Specific drug therapy

- Follow a protocol if your hospital has one.
- Oral treatment is preferred, unless the patient is severely distressed and disturbed. Doses suggested here may not be adequate to control the initial condition, and more may be required:
  - Diazepam 10 mg × 4 daily orally or
  - Chlordiazepoxide 20 mg × 4 daily orally
  - Oxazepam is used in patients with severe liver disease.
- Chlormethiazole capsules should be avoided because of problems with dependence and adverse effects.
- Doses of chlordiazepoxide up to 200 mg spread over the first 24 h may be required initially in uncontrolled, severe, life-endangering withdrawal with fits. The patient must be monitored constantly, with resuscitation facilities available.

- Prophylactic anti-convulsants (e.g. carbamazepine 200 mg × 2 daily) should be given when there is a previous history of withdrawal convulsions or if the current presentation has been complicated by fits.

Progress. This patient improved after 3 days of diazepam treatment and the dose of the medication was tapered to nothing over the next 7 days. More gradual tapering is required in a patient with a history of convulsions, with a longer period (e.g. 3 months) on anti-convulsants. This man was discharged from hospital and provision of long-term care was arranged.

Long-term care

This primarily involves maintaining abstinence from alcohol. Referral to alcohol support agencies requires individual motivation. Acamprosate has been shown to be helpful in reducing craving in conjunction with support from addiction services or group therapy. Those with concurrent psychological problems (e.g. depression, psychosis) need psychiatric referral. This patient remains abstinent and still attends group therapy.

DEPRESSION

See also page 145.

Depressive illness is common but often undetected or inadequately treated (see Information box). The central symptom is usually low mood. Associated symptoms reflecting effects on an individual's behaviour, thoughts, perceptions and cognition become more marked as the severity of the condition increases.

Whereas much depressive illness has an insidious onset and never reaches the attention of acute medical or specialist services, up to one-third of physically ill patients attending hospital have depressive symptoms.

Information

Depressive illness can be missed in medical patients for the following reasons:
- Depression is considered 'understandable' in those physically unwell
- Symptoms of depression are attributed entirely to an underlying medical condition
- Negative attitude to diagnosis of depression and reluctance to report symptoms
- Limited opportunity to discuss emotional issues in a medical setting.

Associations of depression in patients presenting acutely

- Suicide attempt or deliberate self-harm (see p. 502).
- Concurrent physical illness (particularly chronic, painful, life-threatening or disfiguring).
- Unpleasant and demanding treatment for physical illness.
- Destabilisation of a chronic condition, exacerbation of physical symptoms or excessive functional impairment.
- Medical treatment refusal or poor compliance.
- Weight loss, poor nutrition, self-neglect or unusual behaviour (e.g. heavy drinking).
- Increased somatic concern and unexplained physical symptoms.

Case history

A 66-year-old woman is admitted to an MAU for investigation of anaemia, which had made her breathless and tired so that she was unable to cope on her own. Her husband died 6 months previously. The ward nurses have noted that she has been despondent and reluctant to care for herself, and her nutritional intake has been poor. You suspect she may be depressed.

Depression can be broadly categorised as follows:

- Mild: low mood often associated with anxiety symptoms
- Moderate: increasingly low mood, depressive thinking (e.g. suicidal) with biological symptoms (sleep disturbance with early morning waking, mood worse in the morning, reduced appetite, weight and libido)
- Severe: more intense low mood, suicidal thoughts with development of psychotic symptoms, including delusions and hallucinations (most often associated with suicide)

How would you assess this case?

A summary of the key areas of observation and enquiry is provided in Box 16.2.

Box 16.2 Assessment of mental state: key areas

Appearance/behaviour
- General state of health, self-care, facial expression, eye contact, rapport, cooperation, posture and movement

Speech
- Rate, tone, quantity, volume, spontaneity and form

Mood
- Sustained disturbance: depressed, elated, anxious, irritable
- Reactivity: reduced 'blunted', increased 'labile'
- Congruity: appropriateness to circumstances or theme of discussion

Thoughts
- Preoccupations, predominant concerns
- Mood-congruent ideas (e.g. suicidal)
- Delusions: abnormal unshakeable beliefs inconsistent with sociocultural context

Perceptions
- Auditory or visual hallucinations (a perception in the absence of a stimulus), presence of which may be suggested by abnormalities of general behaviour

Cognitive assessment
- See Information box, p. 499

Insight
- Recognition and attribution of illness/awareness of merits of treatment

---

- Full blood screen, including FBC, U&Es, creatinine (eGFR), TFTs, liver biochemistry, serum calcium.
- A CXR may also be helpful.
- Accurate diagnosis requires a detailed history, with a reliable corroborative account if possible, and mental state examination.
- Factors that increase vulnerability to developing depression:
  - Previous history of depression
  - Family history of depression or suicide
  - Stress/life events, particularly with separation or loss
  - Social isolation or adversity
  - Physical illness and its treatment
  - Medication that can cause depression
  - Alcohol/substance misuse.

Differential diagnosis

- Dementia.
- Delirium.
- Alcohol or substance misuse.
- Chronic dysthymia.
- Grief (normal or pathological).

How do you identify a severe case?

In moderate to severe depression, mental state examination may reveal:
- Depressed facial appearance, tearfulness, reduced expression, poor eye contact, retardation of movement or agitation.
- Speech: may be slow and impoverished.
- Persistent, pervasive low mood worse in the morning, anhedonia (loss of interest in pleasure), abulia (inability to make decisions), reduced motivation or energy. *Note:* these complaints are not usually attributable to physical illness alone – psychologically healthy people often cope resiliently with physical illness.
- Suicidal thoughts may be present and should always be enquired about and explored carefully:
  - Have you had any desperate thoughts?
  - Do you feel that life is not worth living?

Biological symptoms are often present. You should ask about feelings of hopelessness (often associated with suicidal contemplation). Other mood-congruent thoughts that might be present include pessimism, feelings of guilt, worthlessness, self-reproach, persecution and impoverishment. In severe depression, thoughts can reach delusional intensity and may be associated with perceptual abnormalities, e.g. condemnatory auditory hallucinations. Tests of cognitive function may be poorly performed due to impaired memory and concentration. In the elderly with fragile but intact cognitive function, severe depression may suggest a dementia ('depressive pseudo-dementia').

Diagnosis. This woman has moderate depression.

How would you manage this case?

- Exclude an organic cause: this patient has anaemia. Investigations show an Hb of 76 g/L, MCV 101, ESR 31 mm/h, WCC 4200.

- *Diagnosis:* A macrocytic anaemia that is probably due to her poor nutritional state and likely to be caused by folate deficiency. You don't want to treat her with folate until you have excluded B_{12} deficiency.
- The laboratory say that the serum levels will be available tomorrow; when they arrive, they show a serum B_{12} of 150 pmol/L, a serum folate of 6 nmol/L and a red cell folate of 70 µg/L, indicating **folate deficiency**. You start her on folic acid 5 mg daily with regular blood monitoring.
- Consider other possible organic causes of depressive symptoms (Box 16.3).
- Specific management depends on the severity:
  - Mild depression may respond to counselling and attempts to resolve problems leading to depression.
  - Mild to moderate depression can respond well to cognitive behavioural therapy, which requires time and available resources.

Box 16.3 Organic causes of depressive symptoms

Endocrine

- Hypothyroidism
- Cushing's syndrome
- Hyperparathyroidism
- Addison's disease
- Hypercalcaemia

Infections

- Viral illness
- Hepatitis
- HIV

Metabolic

- Anaemia (particularly vitamin B_{12} and iron deficiency)
- Renal disease
- Cancer

Neurological

- Multiple sclerosis
- Brain tumour
- Parkinson's disease
- Post-stroke
- Dementias

Drugs

Many drugs have the potential to cause depressive symptoms: check data sheet. Examples include:

- Steroids
- Anti-hypertensives, beta-blockers, digoxin
- Levodopa, methyldopa
- Cimetidine, metoclopramide
- Aminophylline, theophylline
- Regular use of stimulants

- Moderate to severe depression is more likely to present and be detected acutely, and often responds well to medication.
- Establish whether the patient is at risk (see p. 499).
- Refer to the Psychiatric team but explain this to the patient first.
- Assess capacity if the patient is refusing treatment.
- Psychiatric treatment can usually be managed by the liaison team on the medical ward: this is preferable if medical problems require treatment. A Psychiatric Nurse is required to observe the patient.
- The patient will require regular review.
- Psychiatric treatment or admission using the Mental Health Act is considered on the basis of severity and risk.
- Identify aftercare support from family or professionals, having discussed this with the patient.
- Inform her primary care physician.

What medication would you consider and how would you begin treatment?

When prescribing anti-depressants:
- A psychiatric opinion is usually obtained.
- Medication is most effective in moderate and severe depression.
- Compliance is essential and enhanced by good communication. Good prescribing practice includes explanation of:
  - The diagnosis
  - The likelihood of response to treatment (around two-thirds respond well)
  - Common side-effects, which often precede benefits
  - A delay of 2–3 weeks before therapeutic effect
  - The fact that anti-depressants are not addictive (a common misconception).
- Older tricyclic anti-depressants (TCAs) have proven efficacy but significant side-effects (e.g. anti-muscarinic, postural hypotension, cardiotoxic in overdose) and have largely been superseded by newer drugs. TCAs are still useful if newer agents are not tolerated, sedation is desirable, or the patient has had a previous effective response. Avoid prescribing large quantities for outpatients and on discharge.
- The most commonly prescribed newer anti-depressants are selective serotonin reuptake inhibitors (SSRIs), which can cause nausea but in general are better tolerated, cause fewer problematic interactions with other drugs and are less toxic in overdose.
- It is difficult to predict which anti-depressant will be best tolerated in view of the range of side-effects and significant individual variation.
- Elderly patients often require a lower starting dose and more gradual dose increase.
- As a general rule, treatment should continue for at least 6 months after recovery from the acute episode.

Progress. This patient's depression responded to a mixture of bereavement counselling and drug therapy with an SSRI (escitalopram 10 mg daily). Her anaemia was due to dietary folate deficiency and responded well to treatment with oral folic acid, which was continued at home. She is being seen regularly by her GP and her Hb levels are being checked. She is still on escitalopram.

Remember

- Severe depression can be life-endangering (e.g. acutely suicidal, not eating or drinking).
- Refer to the Psychiatric team, who may consider the use of emergency electroconvulsive treatment.

SUICIDE AND DELIBERATE SELF-HARM (DSH)

Presentation to hospital after an attempt to self-harm is a frequent cause of acute medical admissions. The most common method is drug overdose, which is associated with recent alcohol consumption in up to 50% of cases.

The majority of DSH does not represent a serious suicide attempt. Motivations include:

- Escape from overwhelming stress
- Desire to effect a change in personal circumstances ('cry for help')
- Wish to die: serious suicidal intent is evident in up to one-fifth of DSH presentations.

Many of the components of the assessment of DSH can be applied to patients who describe having 'suicidal thoughts'.

Case history

You are called to see a 24-year-old woman, who is accompanied by a friend who called an ambulance to bring the patient to A&E. The woman is tearful, smells of alcohol and says that she took a handful of paracetamol 4 h previously after a violent argument with her boyfriend. She tells you that her mother died 3 months ago and that she wants to join her. She has seen her doctor recently, complaining of poor sleep.

Remember

- Dependants might be at risk (e.g. young children at home): inform a Social Worker if necessary.
- Some hospitals have dedicated staff who assess all patients. In these situations, your task is to identify those who are in need of immediate attention or treatment.

How would you manage this case of DSH?

- Examine the patient and check conscious level (GCS 15), respiratory rate (15/min) and BP (104/72).
- Attend to immediate medical requirements (overdose, see p. 377). Most patients will be admitted to hospital after overdose for specific treatment or observation. They may under-estimate or under-state the number of tablets taken.
- When the medical condition is stable, interview the patient, if possible with a collateral history from reliable informants, and aim to cover the following aspects.

Identify mental illness

- Most completed suicides are associated with a psychiatric diagnosis, most often a depressive illness (see p. 503). Many suicide victims have seen their doctor in the preceding weeks.

- Conversely, clear psychiatric illness is evident in less than one-third of DSH presentations. Most occur after a 'life event', with up to half following a relationship problem.
- The most common diagnoses include depression, alcohol dependence and personality disorders (borderline, anti-social).

Detect patients at risk of completed suicide

- Serious suicide attempts form a minority of DSH presentations but individuals who harm themselves have a greatly increased risk of suicide compared to the general population.
- A high proportion of suicide victims have a previous history of DSH.
- An indication of risk should be documented in the notes with an appropriate plan of action.

FEATURES ASSOCIATED WITH INCREASED SUICIDE RISK

- Demographic: socially isolated (divorced, widowed, never married); male (rates in young men increasing steeply); older age; minority groups (e.g. young Asian women); unemployed; low socioeconomic class; certain professions (doctors, dentists, vets, farmers); individuals with access to means (drug users, gun owners)
- Attempt:
  - Planning: taking care of affairs (cancelled appointments, final acts, e.g. suicide note — the content of which can be helpful)
  - Circumstances: performed in isolation, steps to avoid detection
  - Method: violent, severe overdose or believed likely to be lethal
- History: present or previous psychiatric diagnosis (particularly depression, schizophrenia), recent hospital discharge, previous DSH, recent life event (e.g. bereavement, retirement, divorce), physical illness (chronic painful illness, CNS disorders [multiple sclerosis, epilepsy], cancer, HIV), family history of psychiatric illness/suicide, alcohol/drug misuse, impulsive personality
- Mental state: agitation, depressed mood, suicidal thoughts, hopelessness, delusions, hallucinations, insight in early schizophrenia

Explore suicidal thoughts

- Never avoid detailed but tactful questions concerning suicidal ideas and intentions.
- Responses need to be assessed in the context of the overall presentation, especially if the patient is unforthcoming.
- Establish the patient's thoughts about the episode of self-harm.
- Find out if the patient wishes to die. Ask questions to assess underlying mental state, e.g.:
  - How does the patient see the future?
  - Does the patient see life as completely hopeless?
  - Does the patient feel he/she would be better off dead?
- Assess plans for further attempts: method, circumstances.
- Identify protective factors: reasons for not wishing to die, e.g. change in circumstances, family, dependants.

Identify means of preventing recurrence

The most significant factor predictive of repetition is the number of previous episodes. Assess:

- Current and previous coping resources
- Level of support: identify important relationships
- Possible precipitants (current problems, recent events) and means of addressing them
- Alternative methods of dealing with distress.

Further management: Psychiatric Liaison referral

- Many hospitals have dedicated staff to assess all DSH presentations in liaison with the Psychiatric team. Learn to recognise individuals in need of immediate attention or treatment.
- Most patients do not require further psychiatric intervention.
- If a significant psychiatric disorder is identified, management can be initiated as an inpatient or outpatient in communication with the patient's doctor.
- High-risk cases or those with severe symptoms will require psychiatric admission — if necessary, using compulsory detention. Level of risk and nursing observation required should be communicated and documented.

Difficult management problems

Repeated presenters (e.g. self-laceration, overdose, actual or threatened)

- Behaviour often associated with personality-related vulnerabilities (e.g. borderline personality), dysfunctional coping and intermittent stress in the absence of other clear psychiatric diagnosis.
- A planned, consistent multidisciplinary response coordinated through the Psychiatric team can sometimes help provide containment.
- Reduction in the maladaptive expression of distress may occur with support from a key worker, counselling, psychotherapy or enhanced social support.
- Occasional, psychiatric crisis admissions may be required but these should be kept to a minimum in favour of longer-term strategies.
- Low-dose anti-psychotic medication may help to reduce arousal and subjective distress, avoiding prescriptions for large quantities and identifying a care professional or other reliable, willing carer to help supervise the medication initially if required.

Refusal of medical treatment

- Involve senior colleague and/or Psychiatrist (to determine if mental disorder impairs capacity).
- Explain clearly the risks of not having treatment.
- Assess capacity to make informed decision and record it (see Information box).
- If treatment is considered necessary, attempt persuasion/negotiation, if possible including a friend or relative the patient trusts.
- Continue trying to gain the patient's trust, explaining merits of treatment and risks of refusal. A patient who is frightened, angry or presenting in crisis may choose to cooperate as his/her distress settles.

- If the patient has capacity and refuses treatment, a second opinion from a senior is advisable.
- It is essential for discussions with the patient, management decisions and their reasons to be clearly documented in detail and discussed with a senior colleague.
- The Mental Health Act can be used to detain a patient who is refusing medical treatment in hospital if the patient is exhibiting symptoms of mental disorder that places their health, safety or that of others at risk and provides for the administration of treatment for a mental disorder that might be impairing a patient's capacity to decide on their medical treatment.

ASSESSING CAPACITY TO WITHHOLD CONSENT TO EXAMINATION, INVESTIGATION OR TREATMENT
- Adults are presumed competent to refuse medical advice and treatment.
- Decisions with more serious implications require greater capacity.
- A patient lacks capacity if some impairment or disturbance of mental functioning causes an inability to decide whether to consent to or refuse treatment, which is determined by:
  - Inability to comprehend and retain information on indications and benefits of proposed treatment and in particular the possible risks of refusing it
  - Being incapable of weighing up the information in order to arrive at a decision.
- Temporary incapacity (e.g. due to head injury, altered mood, alcohol) may permit essential life-saving treatment without consent.

Patients unwilling to remain in hospital for further assessment
- The patient's capacity to make this decision should be documented.
- If the patient is considered at risk, appropriate staff should attempt to detain him/her in hospital under common law to permit an urgent mental health assessment by a Psychiatrist and approved Social Worker. Reasons relating to the patient's behaviour, mental state and possible risks should be carefully documented.

Intoxicated or violent patients
- The assistance of hospital security or the police might be necessary.
- Assessment will be more productive if the patient is given time to sober up (in which case, the behaviour may completely settle), as long as the patient or others are not put at risk.
- Consider a psychiatric opinion if an underlying psychiatric disorder is thought likely.

Remember

Enforced physical treatment is given under common law and is not sanctioned by use of the Mental Health Act. The decision to go ahead depends on consideration of:
- The patient's capacity to refuse treatment
- Reasonable professional practice and a doctor's duty of care to the patient
- Necessity of the treatment to save life, or to prevent a serious incident or a deterioration in health
- The decision to treat being in the patient's best interests.

Kumar & Clark's Cases in Clinical Medicine

Progress. This patient had taken approximately 20 tablets of paracetamol (10 g) and was given N-acetylcysteine IV (see p. 383); her liver function remained normal. This was her first episode of DSH and she realised the seriousness of what she had done and the necessity for future counselling.

ACUTE ANXIETY

Case history (1)

You are called to A&E to see a breathless young woman. She is acutely distressed and breathing rapidly. She feels light-headed and has paraesthesiae in her hands and feet.

Differential diagnoses such as a respiratory emergency (e.g. asthma, pulmonary embolus and pneumothorax) must first be excluded (see p. 309). Panic attack (see also p. 316) is suggested by:

- Extreme fear
- Subjective complaint of difficulty breathing in rather than out
- Respiratory alkalosis (causing tetany and relative hypocalcaemia)
- ABGs showing hypocapnia but normal oxygen levels
- Sweating
- Emotional trigger (shock)
- Environmental trigger (crowd phobia).

Management

Hyperventilation is best treated by rebreathing into a paper bag in order to increase pCO_2. However, this did not help this young woman and a minor tranquilliser was given (diazepam 5 mg orally). Lorazepam 1–2 mg, orally or IM, is an alternative; this can be repeated 1 h later if necessary. She was sent home on diazepam with a family member and told to see her own doctor urgently for possible counselling.

Case history (2)

The nursing staff inform you that a 55-year-old man is refusing to have any more haemodialysis, having just started this treatment. A phobic reaction to dialysis is suggested by avoidance, abnormal fear and sympathetic overdrive, during dialysis or talking about it.

Depressive illness is a common association of anxiety and should always be excluded (see p. 497). These phobias are also common in oncology (vomit phobia with chemotherapy).

How would you manage this patient?

- Support and sympathy with explanation of the phobia.
- Minor tranquilliser (see early) for the short term only: up to 2 weeks of diazepam 5 mg × 3 daily (drugs with a long half-life are better).
- Ask a Psychologist to consider graded exposure therapy.
- An SSRI (sertraline, citalopram, paroxetine, fluoxetine) is often required in the presence of co-morbid depressive illness.

Information

Patients can be educated about panic attacks, how to prevent them when they are better (seek behaviour therapy for phobias) and how to use a paper bag during an attack.

What are the physical symptoms and signs of anxiety?

- Dilated pupils.
- Photosensitivity: patient might be wearing dark glasses.
- Phonosensitivity: patient cannot bear any noise.
- Dry mouth.
- Flushed face and neck.
- Sweating.
- Hyperventilation.
- Associated hypocapnia and respiratory alkalosis: cause relative hypocalcaemia (tingling or numbness) in extremities and face, light-headedness and tetany (see p. 317).
- Tachycardia (pulse may be as high as 140 bpm).
- Nausea.
- Diarrhoea.
- Frequency of micturition.
- Increased muscle tension.

What are the psychological symptoms of anxiety?

- Excessive fear.
- Derealisation (patient feels that the environment is less real and solid, with a feeling of detachment).
- Fear of collapse.
- Catastrophic thinking ('I'm about to die from a heart attack').

Always look for the following associations

- Phobias: abnormal fear and avoidance of particular situations or things.
- Depressive illness (see p. 97).
- Obsessive–compulsive disorder: repetitive ruminations that are inconsistent with the personality, along with repeated behaviours; checking excessively or hand-washing because of fear of germs.
  Progress. This man settled quickly with counselling and 5 mg of diazepam. He subsequently continued dialysis without any problems.

OPIATE DEPENDENCE

Drugs in this group include diamorphine (heroin), morphine, pethidine, methadone, dihydrocodeine, buprenorphine, oxycodone and fentanyl.

Effects of opiate use

- Euphoria.
- Analgesia.
- Relaxation.
- Drowsiness.
  Heroin addicts are 16 times more likely to die than individuals of equivalent age, chiefly as a result of overdose. They frequently present in the acute hospital setting.

Case history (1)

You are called to see a 23-year-old man admitted 24 h previously following a road traffic accident. He is verbally abusing nursing staff and wants to leave against medical advice. He is demanding methadone, stating that he is a **heroin addict**.

How would you assess this man?

- Attempt to defuse the situation and prevent an escalation of disturbed behaviour.
- Take a history of drug use, including each drug taken, amount and route.
- Obtain information from other sources:
  - Previously or currently attended drug support agencies if patient admits to having received help. They may be able to tell you if the patient has a regular prescription for methadone.
  - Corroborative history from other reliable informant with patient's consent.
- Examine for evidence of opiate use: withdrawal symptoms begin within 12 h of last use and increase in severity over the first 48 h. With longer-acting opioids such as methadone, onset of withdrawal symptoms can be delayed and their duration increased. Opiate withdrawal that is uncomplicated by other drugs is subjectively unpleasant but not life-threatening, and can present with:
  - Agitation
  - Anxiety
  - Low mood
  - Restlessness
  - Tachycardia
  - Sweating
  - 'Goose flesh'
  - Dilated pupils
  - Yawning
  - Sneezing
  - Vomiting
  - Lacrimation
  - Rhinorrhoea.
- Look for evidence of recent drug use, e.g. needle marks, phlebitis, skin abscesses. Subjective complaints include craving, poor sleep (which can last months), abdominal cramps, nausea, diarrhoea and musculoskeletal pain.

How would you investigate this patient?

- Send urine for drug screen.
- Infection screen (risk of hepatitis B, C, HIV).

How would you manage and treat this patient?

Prescribing methadone

- Oral methadone mixture should be given if you are satisfied a significant habit exists, and this is confirmed by reliable sources or objective evidence of use or withdrawal symptoms.
- If possible, seek advice from a local specialist drug unit.
- There are published guidelines on clinical management of drug use and dependence – a copy should be available in the hospital pharmacy.
- Any registered medical practitioner can prescribe methadone.
- Methadone tablets should not generally be prescribed because of their potential for misuse.
- Dose required to control withdrawal can be carefully titrated in hospital. Start at low dose of methadone, e.g. 10 mL (1 mg per 1 mL mixture).

A further 10 mL at 4-hourly intervals is used until objective signs of withdrawal are controlled. Establish daily requirement.

- Doses >40 mL (40 mg) daily should be taken only if there is reliable information that the patient has been receiving higher regular prescription, but even in this case dose should be gradually titrated upwards.

Remember

Avoid high doses. Methadone overdose causes respiratory arrest — patients can overstate their requirements and physical tolerance of opiates can change quickly.

Symptomatic treatment of withdrawal symptoms

This may be indicated and includes the following:

- Give ibuprofen for pain.
- Give loperamide for diarrhoea.
- Patients may demand more methadone than required to control withdrawal symptoms in order to promote sleep. This should be avoided. Short-term use of hypnotic medication is an alternative. Diazepam also helps muscle spasm and anxiety.
- Observe for evidence of withdrawal from other drugs, e.g.:
  - Alcohol: DTs (see p. 495)
  - Benzodiazepines: risk of convulsions.
- Co-morbid psychiatric disorder can be present:
  - Depressive illness (see p. 497)
  - Psychotic symptoms (if polydrug use includes stimulants or hallucinogenic drugs).

When condition is stable

Gradually reduce methadone by 10% per day if aiming for abstinence. This patient wishes to remain on methadone in the longer term and was already receiving regular prescription prior to admission. He requests referral to the local drug support service. The reduction regimen may require some flexibility to promote cooperation.

Remember

Patients should be warned of the risks even of relatively low doses of methadone and be cautioned about its safe-keeping, particularly if there are children at home (5–10 mL could be lethal for a child).

Progress. On discharge, as drug service support is required, arrange planned transfer of care and be specific about who will prescribe and when. The patient's doctor should be informed and may be willing to prescribe. Avoid giving large prescriptions. Methadone should generally be prescribed for collection on a daily basis but drug services can advise on this. This patient continues on methadone supplied by the local drug support service.

Case history (2)

A young man is rushed to A&E in a comatose state. His girlfriend tells you he used heroin after an abstinence of 4 weeks.

Kumar & Clark's Cases in Clinical Medicine

How do you proceed?

- Careful history: dose, timing and type of heroin used:
  - Two doses of heroin were obtained from an illicit source; dose unknown. The patient's girlfriend says that a number of tablets were obtained and she was fairly certain that they were not only heroin because they were cheap. The patient had been at a drug help clinic while abstinent and was aware of fentanyl being contaminated with illicit supplies of heroin.
- Urgent cardiorespiratory support should be available.
- Assess evidence of opiate toxicity (an acute medical emergency):
  - Conscious level — GCS 13
  - Respiratory depression — 12 bpm
  - Bradycardia — 52/min
  - Miosis — present
  - Hypothermia — 36.4°.
- Examine for other causes of impaired consciousness (e.g. head injury).
- Administer the opiate antagonist naloxone (0.8–2 mg):
  - IV naloxone has a high affinity for opiate receptors and reverses the signs of toxicity by displacing ingested opiates.
  - Life-threatening symptoms may recur in view of the relatively short half-life (minutes) of naloxone, which may need to be re-administered, depending on the half-life of the opiate taken (e.g. half-life of methadone is >24 h).

Information

Naloxone is an opioid antagonist that often requires repeated doses if respiratory depression continues. Naloxone must be readily available for use in the community.

Heroin overdose, causing life-threatening respiratory depression, can occur after a period of abstinence as physical tolerance is reduced. Prior overdose is a strong predictor of further overdoses and of overdose death.

Clinicians are well aware of the potency of fentanyl; it binds the Mu-receptor 50–100 times more strongly than morphine.

Remember

All patients need to be monitored in hospital for at least 24 h, even if they make a brisk recovery.

Progress. This patient made a rapid recovery with the use of repeated naloxone and agreed to be referred back to the Drug Dependency Unit.

THE DISTURBED PATIENT

A behaviourally disturbed patient is often distressed and frightened by their subjective experiences or the circumstances in which they find themselves. The behaviour may place the individual or others at risk.

Typical presentations

- Agitation and restlessness.
- Over-activity.

- Communication of distress, e.g. self-injury or mutilation, threats to harm self.
- Fluctuating and unpredictable behaviour.
- Intimidating, defensive or over-sensitive behaviour.
- Verbally loud, aggressive or violent conduct.

Underlying causes of disturbed behaviour

Organic mental disorders

- Dementia: patients can be restless and aggressive, and may wander because of disorientation. Their dementia may be exaggerated by coexistent physical conditions, e.g. acute infection, constipation.
- Delirium (see p. 485): arising from a number of causes and commonly associated with disturbed behaviour due to misinterpretation of surroundings. Conscious level is impaired, often with fearfulness, perceptual abnormalities (visual or auditory hallucination) and abnormal thinking (e.g. persecutory delusions).
- Epilepsy: ictal (e.g. temporal lobe) or post-ictal.

Other psychiatric disorders

- Major psychoses:
  - Schizophrenia: delusional thinking or abnormal sensory experience (e.g. auditory hallucination) may be driving behaviour
  - Manic psychosis: elevation in mood can be associated with hyperactive and disorganised behaviour.
- Anxiety and depression (see pp. 506 and 497): can be associated with agitation, restlessness and high arousal. Major depression is associated with suicidality and self-harm.

Substance use

This includes alcohol intoxication or withdrawal (see p. 496), and use of other drugs, e.g. stimulants, hallucinogens, solvents.

Physical illness

Individuals may have a physical cause to explain their disturbed behaviour, e.g. chronic pain, side-effects of medication.

Personality factors in the absence of physical or psychiatric disorder

Personality vulnerabilities or 'disorders' can give rise to several distinct patterns of problematic behaviour, which may be associated with circumstances, crises, stress or intoxication. This can include exaggerated propensities to express anger, violent, explosive or anti-social conduct, or self-mutilating and cutting.

Case history

A young man walks into A&E. He is unkempt, preoccupied and suspicious. His behaviour is bizarre, disorganised and unpredictable. He has been argumentative and intimidating, causing distress to staff and other patients.

Management

- Aim to identify the cause and take control of the situation.
- Of paramount concern is the safety of the patient, other patients, yourself and colleagues.
- Disturbed patients should be assessed in a safe area with adequate staff support (medical, nursing, security) and access to a panic alarm.
- Consider the possibility that the patient might be concealing a weapon.
- Specific management depends on the severity of the disturbed behaviour and the cause.
- Clues to the diagnosis can often be found by carefully observing an uncooperative patient, even from a distance while awaiting staff support, e.g. impairment of the conscious level may suggest delirium or drug intoxication; a smell of alcohol may be apparent. A major psychotic mental illness may be suggested from the appearance, behaviour and speech, e.g. preoccupation, suspiciousness, over-activity, thought disorder, delusional ideas.
- Additional background information from reliable informants is invaluable but not always possible.

  After an initial assessment of the situation and with appropriate staff support, a further attempt to calm this patient should be made.

Use interpersonal skills/de-escalation

- Approach the patient in a non-confrontational manner, avoiding invasion of their personal space. Disturbed patients may misinterpret their surroundings and the motives of others, and whereas their behaviour can create fear in those around them, they are often defensive and frightened themselves. The likelihood of cooperation is enhanced if the patient feels safe.
- Clear communication with sensitive statements and questions is often helpful.
- Ask the patient what he/she wants; listen and offer advice and reassurance.
- Attempt to interview the patient in a safe, relaxed setting.
- If initial attempts to engage the patient fail, and providing the situation has not escalated, give the patient some space and time before trying again. Make sure the patient is appropriately observed. The time can be used to consider alternative management.

If the patient remains uncooperative

An uncooperative patient whose behaviour is of concern and suggests a mental health problem will require an urgent mental health assessment. An approved 'clinician' — under the Mental Health Act (often the duty Psychiatrist) — is required to sign a medical recommendation that the patient be detained on mental health grounds. If this is appropriate, the patient will be transferred to the Psychiatric team. Should the patient's behaviour be considered to present a risk to him-/herself or others before this can be completed, the use of restraint and possibly medication under common law should be considered. The reasons for this course of action should be clearly documented and suitable staff should be available.

  Following implementation of the Mental Health Act. As the patient's behaviour remains disturbed and he is a risk to himself and others, safe restraint should be used as a coordinated response by suitably trained nursing staff. This involves sufficient numbers so that at least one can hold each limb, with two nurses taking responsibility for giving the medication.

Medication

- Reduction in arousal can be achieved by a carefully planned regimen of anti-psychotic medication, preferably given orally and in liquid form in the first instance.
- Before IM medication is decided on, all non-invasive measures to calm the patient and secure cooperation should be attempted. Even patients who present as highly disturbed initially may agree to take oral medication when it becomes clear that the situation is under control.
- Giving IM medication to a potentially resistive and aroused patient is not without risk, which must be outweighed by risks of inaction and clearly documented.
- Resuscitation equipment must be available.
- A patient receiving IM medication under restraint should be held in the prone position to protect the airway. The patient is released gently when signs of relaxation and calming become evident, and placed under constant observation.
- The dose of anti-psychotic medication can be reduced by combination with a sedating benzodiazepine in the short term.
- Start at low doses, oral if possible, and increase gradually, depending on response. A suitable regimen is:
  - Haloperidol oral 2.5–5 mg
  - Lorazepam oral 1–2 mg; IM 0.5–1 mg.
- Vital signs (pulse, temperature, BP, conscious level) should be monitored every 15 min.
- While the behaviour continues to present a risk, the dose may be repeated at intervals of 30 min to 1 h until the patient is settled, subject to regular monitoring of vital signs.

Remember

Particular caution should be used in patients who have never received anti-psychotic medication previously ('neuroleptic-naïve') because of the possibility of adverse effects such as a hypersensitivity reaction or acute dystonia.

When the patient is more settled

Further assessment can be carried out to establish an accurate diagnosis prior to starting regular treatment.

Progress. This patient's doctor is eventually contacted and you are told that a diagnosis of schizophrenia was made 5 years ago. The patient had been well but the doctor said he had not attended the clinic (despite reminders) in the last 3 months and suspects he has run out of medication. He has been on olanzapine 10 mg daily. This information is passed on to the Psychiatric team, who continue his management.

Further reading

Delirium
Marcantonio ER. Delirium in hospitalized older adults. *New England Journal of Medicine* 2017; **377**: 1456–1466.

National Institute for Health and Care Excellence (NICE). Delirium: Prevention, diagnosis and management. Clinical guideline CG103. 2019. https://www.nice.org.uk/guidance/cg103.

Drugs and poisons as causes of delirium

Bleck TP. Dopamine antagonists in ICU delirium. *New England Journal of Medicine* 2018; **379**: 2569–2570.

Suicide and deliberate self-harm

Fazel S, Runeson B. Suicide. *New England Journal of Medicine* 2020; **382**: 266–274.

Acute anxiety

Craske MG, Stein MB. Anxiety. *Lancet* 2016; **388**: 3048–3059.

Opiate dependence

Babu KM, Brent J, Juurlink DN. Prevention of opioid overdose. *New England Journal of Medicine* 2019; **380**: 2246–2255.

Bisaga A. What should clinicians do as fentanyl replaces heroin? *Addiction* 2019; **114**(5): 782–783.

Wood E. Strategies for reducing opiate overdose deaths. *New England Journal of Medicine* 2018; **378**: 1565–1567.

A SWOLLEN RED LEG

Case history

The A&E doctor asks you to come and see a 50-year-old man who is unwell and has a red, swollen leg. He thinks he needs anti-coagulation for a possible DVT.

On arrival, you check if this was of sudden onset or a chronically swollen leg. You ask if there is a past history of DVT or whether there are any risk factors, such as a long car journey, air travel, immobility or a family history of clotting disorders. You also ask about any recent illness, e.g. heart failure, blood disorder.

What should you do next?

You do a full medical examination.

On examination, the patient weighs 102 kg and has a temperature of 38°C. The leg is indeed red, swollen, hot and tender below the knee. You note a small ulcer on the medial side of the leg above the ankle. Dorsalis pedis pulse is palpable.

What is your diagnosis?

Cellulitis, probably due to streptococci gaining entry via the venous ulcer.

Differential diagnosis

- DVT.
- Ruptured Baker's cyst.
- Lipodermatosclerosis.
- Acute allergic contact dermatitis: e.g. to dressings.
- Necrotising fasciitis: black necrotic areas within cellulitic area.

Information

LIPODERMATOSCLEROSIS
- Hot, red and woody hard 'atrophic' skin
- Long-standing venous disease
- Can mimic cellulitis but the patient is well, there is no pyrexia, and it may be bilateral

Investigations

- Streptococcal titres: anti-streptolysin O titre (ASOT), ADB (anti-DNase B)
- Swab/blood cultures rarely helpful

How do you treat?

Penicillin V plus flucloxacillin 500 mg × 4 daily, having ascertained that he is not allergic to penicillin. Oral therapy should be for 10–14 days. When the cellulitis is very severe, parenteral benzylpenicillin 1.2 g × 4 daily and flucloxacillin 1 g × 4 daily, i.e. 3 days' IV therapy, should be given initially, followed by 10 days' oral therapy.

Progress. The patient's leg improved with antibiotics and he was discharged after 3 days. He was given compression stockings for his venous hypertension and referred to a Dietitian for advice on weight reduction.

Leg ulceration

Take a full history of associated diseases (diabetes mellitus, rheumatoid arthritis, past history of DVT, varicose veins, heart disease, hypertension, vasculitis, sickle cell, scleroderma).

Causes and signs

- Venous hypertension:
  - Ulcer: chronic and recurrent; site − internal malleolus
  - Oedema
  - Venous eczema
  - Skin discoloration: atrophie blanche (stellate scarring with telangiectasia), erythema, haemosiderin pigmentation
  - Skin texture: lipodermatosclerosis.
- Arterial disease:
  - Ulcer: punched out; site − often lateral or higher up on leg (painful)
  - Pulses: absent dorsalis pedis or posterior tibial
  - Cool leg.
- Vasculitis: non-blanching purpura.
- Neuropathic: sensory signs of decreased sensation present, particularly over pressure areas on feet; common in diabetics.

> **Investigations**
>
> - General: FBC, U&Es, liver biochemistry, auto-antibodies (vasculitis), blood sugar, vitamin B$_{12}$, *Treponema pallidum* enzyme immunoassay (neuropathic ulcer)
> - Venous: Doppler ultrasound − always perform before compression bandaging
> - Arterial: Doppler ultrasound, digital subtraction angiography

Management

- **Venous ulcers:** elevation, exercise, compression dressings. Antibiotics if infected (always check Doppler pressures before considering compression, as many ulcers have mixed venous and arterial aetiology). Adequate analgesia.
- **Arterial ulcers:** investigate arterial supply, dressings with *no* compression. Adequate analgesia.
- **Vasculitic ulcers:** vasculitic screen, e.g. anti-neutrophil cytoplasmic antibody (ANCA), anti-nuclear antibody (ANA), rheumatoid factor.
- **Neuropathic ulcers:** keep ulcer clean and remove pressure or trauma from affected area.

  Note: Operating on varicose veins rarely helps venous insufficiency problems − 'replumbing' of the veins is not possible.

  Contact your hospital's Tissue Viability Nurse for assistance with dressings and compression bandaging, and for arranging longer-term community nursing follow-up.

COMPRESSION BANDAGES

- Four-layer bandaging provides high levels of graduated compression with pressure decreasing up the leg.
- 80% of ulcers can be healed within 6 months.

ERYTHEMA NODOSUM

Erythema nodosum is a hypersensitivity reaction to various antigens (e.g. drugs, infectious agents and unknown antigens), producing an inflammation in the dermis and subcutaneous layer (panniculitis).

It presents with painful, tender, dusky blue—red nodules, usually on the shins and lower limbs (Fig. 17.1).

Case history

An unmarried 16-year-old Asian young woman presents to an inner-city A&E with her mother. She has painful red lumps on her shins and arthralgia. Walking has become pain-ful. She is otherwise well, with no relevant previous medical history.

On examination, she has tender, red/purple lumps on her shins but no other signs. The clinical picture was of erythema nodosum.

Make the diagnosis

- Spontaneous onset over days; evolution over a few days or weeks.
- Single or multiple deep, bruise-like nodules 1—10 cm in diameter (better felt than seen).

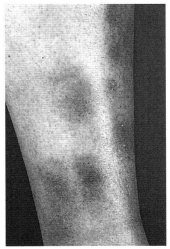

Figure 17.1 Erythema nodosum.

- Tender and warm to touch.
- Predominantly affecting limbs (shins or lower limbs).
- No age or sex limitation (but young females more common).
- Sometimes associated with arthralgia.
- Always do a CXR looking for hilar lymphadenopathy or tuberculosis.

What is the cause?

- Drugs:
    - Oral contraceptives
    - Aspirin and other NSAIDs
    - Sulphonamides.
- Infection:
    - Streptococcal
    - Tuberculosis
    - Leprosy (patient from endemic area)
    - Chlamydia (rare).
- Sarcoidosis.
- Inflammatory bowel disease.
- Idiopathic (common).
- Pregnancy.

Initial treatment

- Aspirin 600 mg as required (unless this is the identified cause of the erythema nodosum).
- Bed rest if severe.
- Tubigrip support bandages.
- If severe symptoms and/or cutaneous ulceration, use dapsone (up to 100 mg daily)/steroids (30 mg daily decreasing course).
  Note: Monitor for haemolytic anaemia and avoid dapsone if there is a glucose-6-phosphate dehydrogenase (G6PD) deficiency.

When should she be referred?

- Recurrent or unresolving symptoms.
- Ulceration.
- Sarcoidosis/tuberculosis/leprosy/inflammatory bowel disease suspected.
- Systemically unwell patient.
  Progress. This young woman went home with her mother, reassured that her illness would settle. After 7 days with occasional aspirin therapy, she was much better and was able to restart school. Her CXR showed hilar lymphadenopathy. With erythema nodosum this is characteristic of **sarcoidosis**.
  She returned to the hospital after 6 months for a follow-up CXR, which was normal.

URTICARIA AND ANGIO-OEDEMA

Urticaria or **hives** is characterised by short-lived dermal swelling (weals) anywhere on the body (Fig. 17.2). These usually itch and, except in some sub-types, resolve without bruising within 24 h (often within 10–20 min). They can form bizarre serpiginous or annular-shaped lesions. The latter show central clearing, not central necrosis as seen in erythema multiforme.

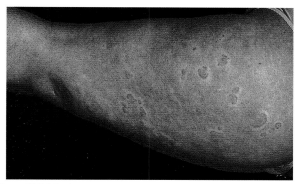

Figure 17.2 Urticaria.

Angio-oedema is a deeper form of swelling affecting the dermis and sub-cutis, usually involving the mucous membranes, e.g. eyes, lips, tongue, genitals, and much less commonly the larynx and gastrointestinal tract. It is generally not itchy but can be painful and disappears within 72 h. It may occur in isolation or with urticaria (45% cases).

The incidence of urticaria/angio-oedema is about 15% in a person's lifetime and both conditions are more common in atopics.

Case history

A 22-year-old woman presents in A&E with a 6 h history of a florid raised red rash all over the body. It is very itchy and distressing, and has caused swelling around her eyes and her right hand. Previous medical history was of atopic eczema as a child and mild hay fever.

On examination, she had red, raised weals all over her body and periorbital swelling.

Diagnosis. Urticaria with angio-oedema.

Classification of urticarias

Acute

By definition, this lasts <6 weeks. Few cases have an identifiable allergen. They are IgE-mediated. In the most severe form there is an anaphylactic reaction but this is fortunately very rare.

- Acute idiopathic urticaria and angio-oedema: accounts for >90% of urticaria. A good history (not type 1 allergy testing) should exclude an allergic cause. Viral infections will sometimes set off an acute urticaria.
- Acute allergic urticaria: drug reactions, insect bites and foods (e.g. peanuts or seafood) can cause this type of reaction, as well as contact urticaria caused by, for example, latex or tomatoes. A history of an almost immediate reaction (seconds to minutes) after contact with an allergen should alert the clinician to this form.

Chronic

By definition, this persists for >6 weeks. Only 2–4% of cases have an identifiable cause and extensive investigation is not indicated. Some cases are autoimmune, and functionally significant IgG (which acts against the high-affinity IgE receptors on mast cells) can be demonstrated in the patient's serum. In a few individuals an acute illness (hepatitis, brucellosis), focal sepsis (e.g. dental abscess), or dermatophyte or parasitic infections can precipitate a reaction but this is very rare.

Physical

Reproducible wealing occurs in response to a specific physical stimulus, e.g. friction, pressure, cold, heat, water, sun. The diagnosis might be suspected from the patient's history or the site of urticaria, i.e. pressure sites in cases of dermographism or delayed pressure urticaria.

General management

- Explanation of condition and likelihood of not identifying specific cause.
- Avoidance of non-specific factors, e.g. aspirin, NSAIDs, opiates.
- H_1 anti-histamines (non-sedating or combination of daytime non-sedating H_1 blockers and sedating H_1 blocker at night); 90% of cases will respond to a non-sedating anti-histamine.
- H_2 anti-histamines, e.g. loratadine 10 mg daily.
- Immunotherapy:
  - Short-term: a short, 7-day course of oral prednisolone 30 mg daily may be given in A&E to settle an attack quickly (especially if angio-oedema is prominent) while waiting for anti-histamines to work.
  - Long-term: dapsone, corticosteroids, IV immunoglobulin, ciclosporin. For very severe cases, refer to the Dermatology department.

Preferred regimens if no contraindications

- Loratadine 10–20 mg daily or cetirizine 10–20 mg daily or fexofenadine 180 mg daily (all non-sedating anti-histamines).
- Sedative anti-histamines, e.g. hydroxyzine 25–50 mg at night.
  Refer: to Dermatology department if no response to anti-histamines.
  Refer: to type 1 Allergy Clinic (usually different to Dermatology) *only* if allergic urticaria is suspected from history.

Management of severe angio-oedema

See page 389.
- Adrenaline (epinephrine): 1 : 1000 (1 mg/mL) IM. Adult dose 0.5–1.0 mL.
- IV chlorphenamine: 10–20 mg (max. 40 mg/24 h).
- IV hydrocortisone succinate: 100–300 mg.

Home (injectable adrenaline) pens

These should never be prescribed lightly and then only after full investigation in an Allergy Clinic, when relevant allergens have been proven and where a genuine anaphylactic reaction has occurred. They are most commonly used in those severely allergic to nuts. Injectable adrenaline pens are *not* appropriate for isolated severe cutaneous urticaria or angio-oedema.

Patients/parents need to attend an Allergy Clinic to be instructed in both when and how to use the pens and, indeed, how frequently, if the first injection gives only temporary relief (two pens should be prescribed).

Adrenaline (epinephrine) 1 : 1000 (1 mg/mL) is available in pre-loaded injections to deliver a dose of 0.3 or 0.5 mg (adult) or 0.15 mg (paediatric), and injections should be carried out by the patient.

Progress. This patient was given prednisolone 30 mg daily for 7 days and started on loratadine 20 mg daily. The nature of the complaint was explained to her; no specific antigen was identified. She was seen by her doctor after 4 days and was completely free of symptoms. She continued with loratadine for 1 month.

Hereditary angio-oedema (HAE)

Skin lesions may develop and laryngeal obstruction can occur. Lesions appear as deep swellings with associated enlarging oedematous borders that last up to 2–4 days. Urticaria does not occur as part of HAE. Patients generally suffer from recurrent attacks of painful angio-oedema, which can be precipitated by minor trauma, emotional upset, infections and temperature change. Involvement of the gastrointestinal tract can cause severe acute pain and simulate a surgical emergency. Recurrent abdominal pain often occurs and starts in childhood. HAE is inherited in an autosomal dominant fashion with either a functional or absolute deficiency of C1 esterase inhibitor (C1-INH). Eighty per cent of cases give a positive family history (e.g. of sudden death). Acquired forms are seen in systemic lupus erythematosus (SLE) or lymphoma.

> **Remember**
>
> **HEREDITARY ANGIO-OEDEMA (HAE)**
> Patients can develop laryngeal obstruction requiring urgent treatment.

> **Investigations**
>
> Two blood samples need to be sent for both absolute levels and functional assay of C1-INH (discuss with laboratory first). Do this test only in patients with recurrent angio-oedema who do not have urticaria. Refer all such patients to a local Immunologist/Dermatologist, depending on local expertise.

Management

Patients are unresponsive to anti-histamines, which can exacerbate the condition, systemic steroids and adrenaline (epinephrine). Refer all patients for management; the acute treatment of choice in A&E is IV (C1-INH) concentrates. If unavailable, fresh frozen plasma can be used. Most cases/families already diagnosed will know where local supplies of C1-INH are to be found. Icatibant (a bradykinin antagonist) and ecallantide (a kallikrein inhibitor) are also of benefit in acute attacks.

In adults, chronic treatment or 'prophylaxis' with lanadelumab, a recombinant fully human monoclonal antibody, produces sustained inhibition of kallikrein and is now the treatment of choice.

SUN-INDUCED RASH

> **Case history**
>
> A 24-year-old arrived in A&E with blisters on her face and arms. She had fallen asleep on the beach in the sun. She had applied factor 4 sunscreen and was surprised that she had

developed an itchy rash. ***On examination,*** she had papules and a few vesicles over the exposed areas.

Remember

- Always take a drug history in somebody who is photosensitive (e.g. doxycycline, amiodarone).
- Always keep SLE and porphyrias in mind for any photosensitivity case where diagnosis is not obvious.

What is the diagnosis?

This is **polymorphic light eruption**, which occurs in 10—20% of the population. The rash appears some hours after the exposure and can last for several hours or a few days following exposure. The rash may be papular or papulovesicular. This patient also had evidence of sunburn — remember, factor 4 does not protect for very long.

Differential diagnosis

Common

- Polymorphic light eruption.
- Sunburn.
- Sunscreen allergy leading to photocontact dermatitis (presents as eczema rather than papules/vesicles).
- Drug-induced photosensitive rash (e.g. doxycycline, amiodarone).

Rare

- Photosensitive eczema.
- Lupus erythematosus (all forms).
- Porphyrias.
- Actinic prurigo.
- Solar urticaria (very rare): gives rise to a rash immediately after sun exposure.

Note: 'prickly heat' or 'heat rash' (miliaria) are incorrect labels often given to polymorphic light eruption. This is an intensely itchy papular eruption in the flexures in hot humid conditions. It is due to blockage of the sweat ducts and does not require sun exposure; neither is it found on sun-exposed skin.

Information

Ultraviolet A and B (UVA/UVB)

- Medium wavelengths 280—310 nm (UVB): cause sunburn and long-term skin changes, e.g. ageing/cancer
- Long wavelengths 310—400 nm (UVA): do not cause sunburn (unless high doses through glass) but do cause photodermatoses. Also contribute to long-term skin damage
- Sunscreen preparations protect against UVB: the sun protection factor (SPF) number gives an indication of the amount of time that a person is protected against burning compared to unprotected skin. Most sunscreens also protect against UVA by utilizing reflectants or chemical absorbers

Most sunscreens are insufficiently applied (and not re-applied after bathing) and so do not give the protection suggested by the SPF factor.

How would you treat this patient?

No treatment was necessary for this young woman because she was virtually asymptomatic. She was given a leaflet on sun exposure and told that her type of rash usually tended to improve over the summer period.

Refer: to the Dermatology department if the condition is not controlled by use of sun block and advice to increase sun exposure slowly in spring/early summer.

If the rash becomes worse each year, consider desensitizing with low-dose PUVA (psoralens + UVA) each spring or short bursts of oral prednisolone 30 mg daily for 1 week for an attack.

GENERALISED RASH OR ERUPTION

Erythroderma means red skin. By definition, it is the term used when >90% of the skin is involved. Erythroderma is not an extensive maculopapular rash.

Case history

A 63-year-old man presents in A&E unwell, shivering and red all over. He has suffered with chronic plaque psoriasis for 40 years and has been managed on topical therapy only. He smells of alcohol and admits to being a heavy drinker.

Examination reveals **erythroderma** and multiple tiny pustules over the trunk. He has a pyrexia of 39.5°C and is clinically dehydrated.

History and clinical examination

Take a comprehensive history of onset, past history, previous skin disease, family history, medication, occupation and other systemic symptoms. These include chills, flu-like symptoms and itching and burning of the skin. A full skin examination, including nails, mouth, genitals, scalp and hair, should be performed, as well as a general examination of lymph nodes and organomegaly.

Differential diagnosis

- Eczema.
- Psoriasis.
- Drug eruption.
- Idiopathic.
- Cutaneous T-cell lymphoma (mycosis fungoides, Sézary syndrome).
- Pemphigus foliaceus.

Are there any complications you should look out for?

- High-output cardiac failure from increased blood flow.
- Hypothermia from heat loss.
- Fluid loss.
- Hypoalbuminaemia.
- Increased basal metabolic rate, i.e. catabolic.
- Capillary leak syndrome in very severe cases of psoriasis: can give rise to ARDS. (*Note:* this can be seen in severe drug rash.)

Management

- Bed rest.
- Rehydrate, plenty of fluids orally or IV.
- Keep warm (space blankets).
- Moisturize the skin.
- Refer all cases to Dermatology urgently.
- Regular (hourly) observations, e.g. BP, pulse, fluid input/output chart, core temperature, weight.

Investigate for cause and treat as appropriate, according to primary skin disease.

Investigations

- FBC
- U&Es
- Liver biochemistry
- CXR
- Culture of blood, skin, urine, sputum if pyrexial
- Skin biopsy (later)

Progress. This man was treated initially with IV glucose/saline with added potassium, then oral fluids. His core temperature fell to 37.2°, so he was kept warm with space blankets in a heated room.

He remained unwell for 2 weeks but then gradually improved.

PRURITUS

Differentiate between a visible rash that is itchy and 'normal-looking' skin (with no rash other than scratch marks) that is itchy.

Case history

A 19-year-old white man presents with a 6-week history of an itchy skin, which has been 'driving him mad', especially at night-time, and he can't sleep. He is fed up with his doctor, who said he had scabies and has treated him four times with malathion without benefit. There is nothing relevant in his past medical history or social history. He had bad asthma as a child.

On examination, he had multiple small red papules on the trunk, around nipples, wrists and axillae, and on the penis. These were accompanied by marked excoriations. No burrows were seen. A few lesions were seen on the soles of the feet.

Diagnosis. Scabies. The diagnosis of scabies was made on clinical grounds. Burrows are not always present but the distribution of non-specific papules (occasionally vesicles) is highly suggestive. Sites commonly involved are axillae, nipples, penis, wrists, palms, soles and web spaces. The face/head is spared in adults. Scabies can be confirmed by skin scraping and microscopy. He lived with his girlfriend (who was unaffected) and had recently visited a prostitute, who may have been the source of infection.

Causes of pruritus

Diseases of the skin associated with pruritus

- Eczema (Fig. 17.3).
- Scabies.

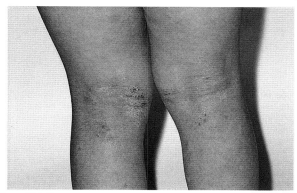

Figure 17.3 Eczema.

- Urticaria.
- Psoriasis.
- Lichen planus.
- Dermatitis herpetiformis.
- Pemphigoid.

Systemic diseases associated with pruritus

- Hypothyroidism.
- Iron deficiency.
- Advanced chronic kidney disease.
- Liver disease (especially primary biliary cholangitis and hepatitis C).
- Lymphoma/myeloproliferative disease.
- Coeliac disease.

General management of urticaria

Treat the primary skin disease and refer to Dermatology.
- Eczema: moisturisers and topical corticosteroids.
- Psoriasis: tar, vitamin D_3 ointments, mild to moderate topical steroids, dithranol (causes staining).
- Urticaria: non-sedating anti-histamines (see p. 553).
- Lichen planus: superpotent topical steroids/oral steroids.
- Systemic diseases: see individual disease for treatment.

Investigations

- Primary skin diseases: most cases can be diagnosed on clinical grounds but scrapings for direct microscopy (scabies), punch biopsy (+ immunofluorescence) and serum IgE for atopic disease are helpful.

- Systemic diseases: FBC, U&Es, liver biochemistry, iron, folate, vitamin B_{12}, TFTs, auto-immune hepatitis screen, including mitochondrial antibodies, endomysial/gliadin antibodies. Consider serum immunoglobulins/protein electrophoresis/CXR in selected cases.

Progress

- Scabies: malathion was given to the patient and his girlfriend. He was told to be careful in applying malathion all over his body, including crevices of his body and webs of his fingers. This should be washed off after 24 h. Sexual contacts (if known), even if asymptomatic and without rash, should be given two treatments 7 days apart.
- Repeated scabies prescription leads to irritant dermatitis. Patients should be warned that the itching can go on for 1 month after successful treatment of scabies. Therefore give some crotamiton or topical steroid rather than further scabies prescription.

This patient's scabies was treated successfully, on this occasion, because he was meticulous in the application of malathion.

CUTANEOUS ADVERSE DRUG REACTION (ADR)

The true incidence is unknown, as many go unreported, but the skin is the most commonly affected organ, involved in 30% of reported ADRs.

Pre-existing disease (SLE, chronic lymphocytic leukaemia, HIV), advancing age (polypharmacy, reduced renal and hepatic clearance) and sensitivity to other drugs (e.g. penicillins: 10% cross-reactivity with cephalosporins) can all increase susceptibility to the development of ADRs.

Case history (1)

A 24-year-old man developed a severe sore throat and a fever. He was seen by his doctor, who diagnosed a streptococcal sore throat and prescribed amoxicillin. Two days later, he presented with a macropapular rash (Fig. 17.4).

On examination, he was noted to have cervical lymphadenopathy and a small palpable spleen. Infectious mononucleosis (glandular fever) was diagnosed with a Monospot test and the amoxicillin was stopped.

Remember

Never use amoxicillin in a patient unless glandular fever has been excluded.

Case history (2)

A 54-year-old doctor presented with a 1-year history of early morning stiffness of her hands and Raynaud's. She had self-medicated with a number of NSAIDs, which had helped to ease the pain and stiffness. She was seen by a Rheumatologist, who found a slight deformity of her fingers but no other signs of rheumatoid arthritis. In view of the long history, she was prescribed sulfasalazine as a disease-modifying drug. A month later, she developed a severe, itchy, morbilliform rash all over her body. This settled on stopping the sulfasalazine, which contains a sulfonamide and 5-ASA (aminosalicylic acid).

Progress. Both cases resolved on stopping the drugs.

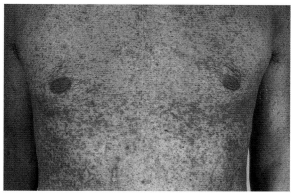

Figure 17.4 Maculopapular rash following amoxicillin therapy in patient with infectious mononucleosis.

> **Remember**
>
> Always discuss the harm/benefit ratio of drugs with your patient. Also, review their current drug therapy and check for interactions.

Classification

- Type A: augmented (~80% of all ADRs) – exaggerated responses to known effects of the drug. Predictable and dose-related, e.g. skin necrosis after extravasation of vincristine, alopecia due to cytotoxic agents, cheilitis due to retinoids, urticaria triggered by opiates causing mast cell degranulation.
- Type B: unpredictable/bizarre – idiosyncratic and therefore more difficult to diagnose (see later).

Physiology

There are a number of mechanisms but the pathogenesis of many cutaneous ADRs remains unknown.

Cutaneous ADRs can also be categorised morphologically into three groups:

1. Skin reactions specific to drugs
2. Rashes potentially caused by drugs
3. Established skin disease exacerbated by drugs.

Skin reactions specific to drugs

Fixed drug eruptions are very rare. They develop within 24 h of drug ingestion and usually affect localised areas showing sharply demarcated, round, red, oedematous (and sometimes bullous) plaques that become violaceous or hyperpigmented with time. Lesions recur at the same site on re-exposure to the drug.

Pigmentation caused by drugs

- Long-term amiodarone or chlorpromazine: purple/slate-grey pigmentation on sun-exposed sites.
- Long-term minocycline: blue/black pigmentation of skin, nails, buccal mucosa, scars (may be irreversible).
- Mepacrine: reversible yellow skin pigmentation.
- Bleomycin: flagellate erythema then hyperpigmentation of trunk.

Rashes potentially caused by drugs

There are many different reaction patterns and only a few common ones will be considered here.

Maculopapular/exanthematic eruptions

This is the most common type of cutaneous ADR. It is thought to be a cell-mediated reaction (may also be immune complex) involving CD8 T cells (Table 17.1). There are widespread, symmetrical, itchy eruptions. Macules and papules may become confluent and develop into a sheet-like erythema, sometimes with fever and eosinophilia. When due to a drug, the rash usually begins on the trunk. Suspect a viral aetiology if it starts on the face and moves down, and if there is associated lymphadenopathy and conjunctivitis. After withdrawal of the drug, the rash usually settles over 2 weeks.

Note: if this eruption has progressed rapidly over 24 h it may herald the onset of the following:

Erythroderma. More than 90% of the skin surface is erythematous and inflamed. Ten per cent of cases are drug-induced (e.g. sulfonamides, sulfonylureas, penicillins, barbiturates, allopurinol, gold, mercury, arsenicals).

Table 17.1 Pathogenesis of some cutaneous ADRs (hypersensitivity reactions)

Type	Examples
Type 1	
Immediate, IgE-mediated hypersensitivity	Urticaria and anaphylaxis due to penicillins
Type II	
Cytotoxic	Allergic thrombocytopenic purpura
Type III	
Immune complex formation	Morbilliform maculopapular rash Serum sickness Vasculitis, e.g. allopurinol and penicillin
Type IV	
Cell-mediated	Allergic contact dermatitis to topical medicaments Erythema multiforme, toxic epidermal necrolysis Lichenoid drug eruption

Toxic epidermal necrolysis (TEN). The development of vesicles and/or bullae and skin tenderness raises this possibility (this might then be followed by 'sheeting off' of the epidermis, see later). Mucosal involvement also suggests TEN.

Anti-convulsant hypersensitivity syndrome. This is not just a severe ADR from an anti-convulsant but a distinct syndrome that, if undiagnosed, can lead to death if patients are changed to a different anti-convulsant that cross-reacts. The rash normally starts 2–4 weeks after starting any of the aromatic anti-convulsants (carbamazepine, phenytoin, phenobarbital, primidone). The rash is a non-specific maculopapular eruption that may involve mucosal surfaces and occasionally pustulates. The distinguishing clinical features from a 'normal' ADR are any of the following:

- Fever
- Hepatosplenomegaly/lymphadenopathy
- Conjunctivitis/peri-orbital oedema
- Arthralgia
- Pharyngitis
- Severe malaise.
  Blood tests may show:
- Eosinophilia
- Lymphocytosis with atypical lymphocytes
- Raised hepatic transferases.

If the drug is not stopped immediately, the patient may progress to multi-organ failure and need ITU care. *All* aromatic anti-convulsant drugs must be avoided in the future because further exposure is likely to lead to an even more severe reaction. Sodium valproate is a reasonable alternative.

Photosensitivity

(See Box 17.1.) Reactions range from erythema to blistering and characteristically spare the sub-mental area, finger webs, under-eyebrow area and triangle of skin behind the ear lobe.

Lichenoid eruption

(See Box 17.1.) This is similar to idiopathic lichen planus but often more widespread and rarely involves mucous membranes.

Spectrum of erythema multiforme, Stevens–Johnson syndrome and toxic epidermal necrolysis

The classification of these diseases is confusing in the literature.

Erythema multiforme. Ten per cent of cases are drug-related (the majority are post-infectious, e.g. herpes simplex virus, mycoplasma). They are mild and self-limiting, and usually resolve within 2–4 weeks. They are characterised by target lesions of a central dusky erythema (sometimes with blistering), a pale oedematous ring and a peripheral erythematous ring. These usually occur acrally (extremities) and symmetrically on extensor surfaces. They involve palms and soles. Mucosal involvement may be present but is mild and limited to one mucosal surface, e.g. the oral cavity.

Stevens–Johnson syndrome (SJS; also called erythema multiforme major). This is a more severe and extensive eruption. Widespread atypical target lesions appear on the trunk, in which epidermal necrosis results in the formation of blisters and epidermal detachment involving <10% of the body surface area. At least two mucosal surfaces are involved (oral, ocular, genital). Mucosal lesions are often more prominent than

> ### Box 17.1 Common drug associations
>
> **Maculopapular eruption**
> - Antibiotics
> - (Penicillins, sulfonamides)
> - Anticonvulsants
> - (Carbamazepine, phenytoin)
> - NSAIDs
>
> **Photosensitivity**
> - Thiazides
> - Sulfonamides
> - Amiodarone
> - Tetracycline
> - Nalidixic acid
>
> **Lichenoid eruption**
> - Gold
> - Beta-blockers
> - Quinine/anti-malarials
> - Thiazides
> - Allopurinol

skin lesions. Systemic toxicity may occur. SJS usually resolves within 6 weeks.

SJS/TEN overlap. When the extent of epidermal detachment is between 10% and 30% of the body surface area, in the presence of other features of SJS, this is considered an SJS/TEN overlap. The skin lesions are often necrotic blisters rather than target lesions, and mucosal lesions are prominent and severe.

TEN. This is of sudden onset (usually evolves over 24–48 h) with widespread morbilliform or confluent dusky erythema and skin tenderness. This is followed by widespread blistering (necrolysis) of the skin with histological evidence of full-thickness epidermal necrosis, sub-epidermal separation and a sparse or absent dermal infiltrate. The Nikolsky sign is positive. Mucous membrane involvement is usually severe, including ocular, genital, oral, nasopharynx and GI tract; mortality is 20–30%.

Adverse prognostic factors include:
- Age >60 years
- Area of involved skin >50%
- Plasma urea >17 mmol/L
- Neutropenia <1.0×10^9/L
- Idiopathic nature of TEN.
  If extensive:
- Ventilation may be required.
- Contact ITU, Dermatology and Ophthalmology urgently.
  Treatment of TEN
- Early high-dose immunosuppression may help but remains controversial (IV immunoglobulin is also commonly used).
- Analgesia (opiate).
- Dressings/human skin bank/autologous skin grafts.

- Eye protection and review for scarring.
- Pressure-relieving bed.
- ITU supportive therapy.

Remember

- All cases of TEN should be considered to be drug-induced and suspected drug(s) should be stopped immediately.
- The most common drugs responsible are sulfonamides, penicillins, anti-convulsants and NSAIDs.

Established skin disease exacerbated by drugs (see Box 17.1)

- Psoriasis: can be destabilised by lithium and possibly beta-blockers and anti-malarials.
- Acne: can be aggravated by progesterone-containing contraceptives, lithium and corticosteroids.
- Rosacea: worse with topical steroids.
- Peri-oral dermatitis: caused and exacerbated by topical steroids.

Diagnosis of ADRs

The key elements to a diagnosis are a meticulous drug history and a high index of suspicion.

- Exclude other causes by history and examination.
- Take a careful drug history: remember to ask about over-the-counter preparations, e.g. laxatives, tonics, cough medicines, vitamins and complementary treatments.
- Establish the start and stop dates of medication and relationship to onset of the rash.
- When the eruption begins 7–21 days after the first administration of a drug or within 48 h if the drug has caused a similar reaction in the past, this is highly suggestive of an ADR.
- The timing is incompatible with an ADR if the drug was started after the onset of cutaneous or mucous membrane signs. If the onset is within 24 h of the first dose, or more than 21 days after stopping the drug, a drug aetiology is doubtful. If there are several drugs, each should be considered as a potential cause.
- Consult drug information for previous reports.

Investigations

These are of little help!

- Blood eosinophilia (may be found in toxic erythema but is non-specific)
- Biopsy 'may suggest but not prove a drug aetiology':
  - Lots of eosinophils: common
  - Lichenoid pattern: rare
  - SLE pattern: rare
  - Vasculitis: sometimes
- Blood level of drug (may be useful to check for overdosage)
- If a fixed drug eruption is suspected, rechallenge may be helpful (in other situations it is rarely justifiable for fear of precipitating a more severe reaction)

- Patch testing is helpful in patients with suspected allergic contact dermatitis (type IV hypersensitivity reactions) but *cannot* be used for systemic ADRs

Treatment

- Withdraw drug(s): symptomatic treatment with oral anti-histamines, topical steroids and moisturisers.
- Severe reactions (SJS and TEN) require supportive therapy and monitoring of infection, fluid balance and temperature. Patients may need ITU. Use of systemic immunosuppression may be considered if patients are seen within the first 24 h of onset.
- Dressings: leave on.
- Support mattress.
- Opiate analgesia.
- Give written information to patient and doctors to ensure no repeat exposure.

  Fig. 17.5 can be used as a guide to referral.

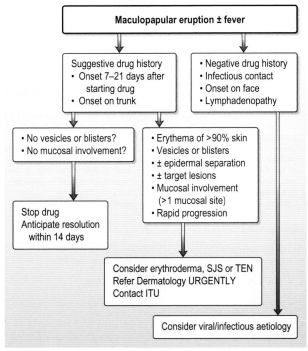

Figure 17.5 When to refer to a Dermatologist in the case of an adverse drug reaction. SJS, Stevens–Johnson syndrome; TEN, toxic epidermal necrolysis.

HIV AND THE SKIN

- Up to 90% of HIV-positive patients will develop a mucocutaneous disease, sometimes related to drug therapy.
- Between 30% and 40% of people with AIDS will suffer from three different dermatoses.
- A rash may be the presenting sign of HIV infection or AIDS (remember that up to 30% receive their diagnosis of AIDS and HIV at the same time, suggesting a large pool of undiagnosed patients).

Case history

Two patients with HIV presented to the clinic with different rashes, both of which are more common in HIV patients. One presented with an eosinophilic folliculitis and the other with Stevens—Johnson/toxic epidermal necrolysis (Fig. 17.6a and b).

Progress. Both patients were referred to the HIV specialist for anti-retroviral therapy (ART).

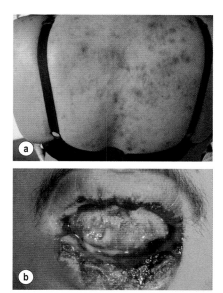

Figure 17.6 Rashes associated with HIV. (a) Eosinophilic folliculitis — a classical HIV dermatosis. (Courtesy of Dr Michael Ardern Jones.) (b) Stevens—Johnson syndrome/toxic epidermal necrolysis is more common in HIV. ((a) Courtesy Dr Michael Arden-Jones. (b) Courtesy of Dr David Paige.)

What dermatoses have commonly been the presenting illness of HIV (or other causes of immunosuppression)?

- Extensive molluscum contagiosum in an adult.
- Kaposi's sarcoma (KS).
- Extensive seborrhoeic dermatitis or eosinophilic folliculitis.
- Pruritic papular eruption (PPE; also called itchy folliculitis) of HIV.
- Extensive oro-pharyngeal candida.
- Hairy leucoplakia.

Why is the skin so frequently affected?

The exact mechanisms are not known but include:
- Immune deficiency: increased infection
- Poor immune surveillance: increased skin tumours
- Post infection: reactive arthritis
- Auto-antibodies: Sjögren's syndrome, polymyositis, idiopathic thrombocytopenic purpura, pemphigoid, vitiligo, alopecia areata
- Aberrant immune function TH1 to TH2 switch: eczema, pruritus, PPE
- Graft-versus-host disease (GVHD): lichen planus, erythroderma.

What types of rash are seen?

There are many different rashes, which can be arbitrarily divided:
- Cutaneous infection
- Opportunistic infection
- Malignancy (basal cell carcinoma [BCC], squamous cell carcinoma [SCC], KS, malignant melanoma)
- Papulo-squamous/inflammatory
- Oral lesions.
  ART has reduced the incidence of all skin lesions.

How would you diagnose the rashes?

The diagnosis can be difficult, as frequently the rash is very extensive or there is an atypical clinical presentation. You should always have a low index for doing:
- Skin biopsies: both for all the routine stains and for culture of bacteria, fungi, viruses and acid-fast bacilli.
- Skin swabs.
- Serology screens.
- Investigation of other 'organs', e.g. blood, stools, sputum, bone marrow. Furthermore, treatment is often problematic, as HIV rashes (even those that are common in immunocompetent people) tend to be resistant to standard therapies and the use of immunosuppressive drugs is usually contraindicated.

Information

CUTANEOUS INFECTIONS IN HIV
Bacterial
- Impetigo (*Staphylococcus aureus*), cellulitis/erysipelas (streptococci): clinically, these infections tend to look much the same as in immunocompetent individuals; deep-seated ecthyma may be seen

Viral

- Herpes: may present with blisters, often extensive and ulcerative, especially peri-anally and orally
- Shingles/varicella zoster virus: often painful, verrucous and extending over more than one dermatome; may be bilateral

Fungal

- Dermatophyte and candidal infections: common in the skin and present typically; often require systemic anti-fungal therapy for eradication (e.g. itraconazole 100 mg × 2 daily for 2—4 weeks)

What opportunistic infections occur in the immunocompromised and how would you distinguish between them?

Information

Failure to diagnose scabies (especially crusted scabies) can lead to a high proportion of medical staff becoming infected.

A variety of normally non-pathogenic organisms have been described in AIDS and other immunosuppressed patients. Clinically they are difficult to distinguish:

- Cutaneous cytomegalovirus may present with blisters, ulcers or a necrotic lesion.
- Fungi are common culprits and may present with nodules (often deep subcutaneous) or scaly papules (*Cryptococcus* is seen in the UK whereas *Histoplasma* is more common in the US).
- Scabies presents typically with itchy papules and burrows in the web spaces, wrists, genitalia and palms/soles. Crusted scabies ('Norwegian scabies') presents atypically with a rather crusted eczematous-looking rash, often centred around the web spaces, and may not be itchy.
- Non-tuberculous or 'atypical' mycobacteria are a particular problem in advanced AIDS and present with papules, nodules, ulcers or sporotrichosis-like lesions.

These infections can be localised to the skin but also present as a systemic infection. Malaise, fever, abdominal pain, headache or diarrhoea may be non-specifically suggestive of systemic infection. Biopsy and culture is the best way to diagnose these rashes.

What causes hairy leucoplakia and what does it look like?

It is due to the Epstein—Barr virus in an immunosuppressed individual and is almost unique to HIV patients. It is a relatively late sign of HIV disease. Clinically, white plaques appear on the sides of the tongue. Vertical ridging or corrugations are seen within the plaques. Unlike candidal infections, there are no small satellite lesions around the edge and the white material cannot be scraped off to leave raw areas underneath.

What types of malignancy occur in immunocompromised patients?

- The two most common types of skin cancer (BCC and SCC) appear to be increased in HIV-positive patients. They look the same as in immunocompetent patients.
- Malignant melanoma may be increased in prevalence. The clinical appearance is typical (Box 17.2).

> **Box 17.2** Clinical criteria for the diagnosis of malignant melanoma
>
> ABCDE criteria (USA)
>
> - **A**symmetry of mole
> - **B**order irregularity
> - **C**olour variegation
> - **D**iameter >6 mm
> - **E**levation
>
> The Glasgow seven-point checklist
>
> *Major criteria*
> - Change in size
> - Change in shape
> - Change in colour
>
> *Minor criteria*
> - Diameter >6 mm
> - Inflammation
> - Oozing or bleeding
> - Mild itch or altered sensation

- Kaposi's sarcoma is more common and more severe in AIDS patients (without available ART therapy) than in classical or African KS. It presents as purplish-brown plaques and nodules. The nose, palate and genitalia seem common sites but remember disease can spread internally. KS is predominantly seen in men who have sex with men with AIDS. There is a strong link between herpes virus type 8 and the development of all types of KS, although other factors might be involved, as not all people with herpes virus type 8 contract KS.
- Lymphomas are more common with HIV and may present with lymphadenopathy, pleural effusions, night sweats and weight loss.

What are the more common 'papulo-squamous' dermatoses encountered in HIV patients?

These are:
- Seborrhoeic dermatitis: 80%
- Unexplained pruritus: 40%
- Xerosis (dry skin), ichthyosis: 30%
- PPE: 20%
- Eczema: 10%
- Psoriasis: 5%
- Drug rashes: 20%.

In general, these rashes become more common (and severe) with progression of the disease.

Seborrhoeic dermatitis

There is an itchy, red and scaly eczematous rash in the seborrhoeic areas (sides of nose, around eyes, forehead, scalp, sternum, glans penis). This looks similar to seborrhoeic dermatitis in immunocompetent patients but is often more extensive. It may appear in early 'asymptomatic' HIV disease.

Therapy. Topical miconazole/hydrocortisone cream, emollients, keto-conazole shampoo. If resistant, consider topical 0.1% tacrolimus ointment, topical lithium and oral itraconazole 100 mg × 2 daily for 2 weeks.

Pruritus and xerosis

These often go together and the aetiology is unclear. Again, they may be early manifestations of advanced HIV disease.

Therapy. Emollients, bath oils, aqueous cream as soap substitute. Sedating anti-histamines (e.g. hydroxyzine or chlorphenamine). Consider 0.5% menthol in aqueous cream or crotamiton. Phototherapy if resistant.

PPE (pruritic papular eruption; also called itchy folliculitis)

This is a unique papular and (at times) pustular eruption centred on hair folli-cles. It is intensely itchy and usually involves the upper trunk, back and proxi-mal arms. Papules tend to arise, grow in size, frequently have the top scratched off and then recede as other new lesions arise. In African—Caribbean patients lesions are often larger and more frequently involve the face. Skin biopsy reveals a lymphohistiocytic infiltrate around blood vessels and hair fol-licles, often accompanied by eosinophils.

The so-called unique HIV rash, 'eosinophilic folliculitis', is probably a variant of PPE.

PPE tends to appear in more advanced HIV disease and becomes worse as CD4 counts fall.

Therapy. Medium-strength topical steroids, oral anti-histamines and low-dose long-term antibiotics (as used in acne) may help. Isotretinoin (20—40 mg daily) or PUVA is effective for resistant cases.

Eczema

The prevalence of eczema is probably increased in HIV patients, reflecting the eosinophilia and high IgE levels that are commonly seen. It looks similar to eczema in immunocompetent patients.

Therapy. As for normal eczema.

Psoriasis

The prevalence of psoriasis is increased in HIV (5% versus 2% in the nor-mal population); 30% may get psoriatic arthropathy (versus 5% of normal psoriatics). The disease can be typical with red, scaly plaques on elbows and knees, and scaling in the scalp. However, psoriasis occasionally becomes severe and widespread in advanced HIV patients. They may become erythrodermic or develop pustular psoriasis, especially on the soles of the feet. When the latter happens, there is clearly an overlap with reactive arthritis.

Therapy. Topical steroids, calcipotriol (a synthetic vitamin D_3 analogue) and tar compounds will help mild cases. UVB or PUVA is useful for more advanced disease. Although there is some in vitro evidence that photother-apy may promote HIV replication, this has not been shown to be a problem in clinical practice.

Oral drugs for severe disease include acitretin or anti-retroviral drugs.

The other drugs used in 'normal' psoriasis include methotrexate, ciclos-porin and hydroxyurea. Biological agents are now being used.

Further reading

A swollen red leg

Thomas KS, Crooke AM, Nunn AJ, et al. Penicillin to prevent recurrent leg ulceration. *New England Journal of Medicine* 2013; **368**: 1695–1703.

Urticaria and angio-oedema

Longhurst HJ. Kallikrein inhibition for hereditary angioedema. *New England Journal of Medicine* 2017; **376**: 788–789.

Sun-induced rash

Lehmann P. Sun exposed skin disease. *Clinics in Dermatology* 2011; **29**: 180–188.

Pruritus

Menter A, Korman NJ, Elmets CA, et al. Guidelines of care for the management of psoriasis and psoriatic arthritis: section 6. *Journal of the American Academy of Dermatology* 2011; **65**: 137–174.

Schneider LC. Ditching the itch with anti-type 2 cytokine therapies for atopic dermatitis. *New England Journal of Medicine* 2017; **376**: 878–879.

Cutaneous adverse drug reaction

Eshki M, Allanore L, Musette P, et al. Twelve-year analysis of severe cases of drug reaction with eosinophilia and systemic symptoms. *Archives of Dermatology* 2009; **145**: 67–72.

Litt JZ. *Drug Eruption and Reaction Manual*. 23rd ed. Boca Raton: CRC Press; 2017.

HIV and the skin

Rodgers S, Leslie KS. Skin infections in HIV-infected individuals in the era of ART. *Current Opinion in Infectious Disease* 2011; **24**: 124–129.

Index

Note: Page numbers followed by "*f*", "*t*" and "*b*" indicate figures, tables and boxes respectively.

A